T0337868

Clinical Guide to Transplantation in Lymphoma

Clinical Guide to Transplantation in Lymphoma

EDITED BY

Bipin N. Savani MD

Professor of Medicine
Director, Long Term Transplant Clinic
Division of Hematology/Oncology
Vanderbilt Ingram Cancer Center
Vanderbilt University Medical Center
Nashville, TN, USA

Mohamad Mohty MD, PhD

Professor
Head, Clinical Hematology and Cellular Therapy Department
Université Pierre et Marie Curie
Hôpital Saint Antoine
INSERM, U938
Paris, France

WILEY Blackwell

This edition first published 2015 © 2015 by John Wiley & Sons, Ltd

Registered Office
John Wiley & Sons, Ltd, The Atrium, Southern Gate, Chichester, West Sussex, PO19 8SQ, UK

Editorial Offices
9600 Garsington Road, Oxford, OX4 2DQ, UK
The Atrium, Southern Gate, Chichester, West Sussex, PO19 8SQ, UK
111 River Street, Hoboken, NJ 07030-5774, USA

For details of our global editorial offices, for customer services and for information about how to apply for permission to reuse the copyright material in this book please see our website at www.wiley.com/wiley-blackwell

The right of the author to be identified as the author of this work has been asserted in accordance with the UK Copyright, Designs and Patents Act 1988.

Library of Congress Cataloging-in-Publication Data
Clinical guide to transplantation in lymphoma / editors, Bipin N. Savani, Mohamad Mohty.
    p. ; cm.
  Includes bibliographical references and index.
  ISBN 978-1-118-86332-9 (cloth)
I. Savani, Bipin N., editor. II. Mohty, Mohamad, editor.
  [DNLM: 1. Lymphoma–surgery. 2. Hematopoietic Stem Cell Transplantation. WH 525]
  RC280.L9
  616.99′446059–dc23

                       2015006391

A catalogue record for this book is available from the British Library.

Wiley also publishes its books in a variety of electronic formats. Some content that appears in print may not be available in electronic books.

Cover image: istockphoto.com/photo/saline-43236562 @donghero

Set in 8.5/12pt Meridien by SPi Global, Pondicherry, India
Printed and bound in Malaysia by Vivar Printing Sdn Bhd

1 2015

Contents

List of contributors, vii

Foreword, xi

Introduction, 1

Section 1: Transplantation in lymphomas

1 Lymphoma and transplantation: historical perspective, 5
Andrew R. Rezvani

2 Lymphoma: working committee and data reporting after transplantation in lymphoma, 13
Wael Saber, Mehdi Hamadani, Shahrukh K. Hashmi and Parameswaran Hari

3 Use of transplantation in lymphoma: adults, 23
Parastoo Bahrami Dahi, Gabriela Soriano Hobbs and Miguel-Angel Perales

4 Hematopoietic stem cell transplantation for lymphoma in children, adolescents, and young adults, 31
Nader Kim El-Mallawany and Mitchell S. Cairo

5 Preparative regimens for lymphoma: autologous hematopoietic stem cell transplantation, 45
Taiga Nishihori, Karma Z. Salem, Ernesto Ayala and Mohamed A. Kharfan-Dabaja

6 Preparative regimens for lymphoma: allogeneic hematopoietic stem cell transplantation, 57
Mohamed A. Kharfan-Dabaja, Najla El-Jurdi, Mehdi Hamadani and Ernesto Ayala

7 Pretransplantation evaluation, comorbidities, and nondisease-related eligibility criteria for transplantation in lymphoma, 69
Melissa Logue

8 Stem cell mobilization in lymphoma patients, 75
Tarah Ballinger, Bipin N. Savani and Mohamad Mohty

9 Allogeneic hematopoietic stem cell transplantation for lymphoma: stem cell source, donor, and HLA matching, 85
Michael Green and Mitchell Horwitz

10 Management of early and late toxicities of autologous hematopoietic stem cell transplantation, 93
Sai Ravi Pingali and Yago Nieto

11 Long-term follow-up of lymphoma patients after allogeneic hematopoietic cell transplantation, 103
Shylaja Mani and Navneet S. Majhail

12 First 100 days of the autologous hematopoietic stem cell transplantation process in lymphoma, 109
Angela Moreschi Woods

13 First 100 days of the allogeneic hematopoietic stem cell transplantation process in lymphoma, 113
Angela Moreschi Woods

Section 2: Management

14 Stem cell transplantation in follicular lymphoma, 119
Satyajit Kosuri and Koen Van Besien

15 Chronic lymphocytic leukemia/small lymphocytic lymphoma, 133
Salyka Sengsayadeth and Wichai Chinratanalab

16 Diffuse large B-cell lymphoma, 145
Lauren Veltri, Bipin N. Savani, Mohamed A. Kharfan-Dabaja, Mehdi Hamadani and Abraham S. Kanate

17 Mantle cell lymphoma, 161
Sascha Dietrich and Peter Dreger

18 Hodgkin lymphoma, 173
Eva Domingo-Domenech and Anna Sureda

19 Peripheral T-cell lymphomas, 187
*Giulia Perrone, Chiara De Philippis, Lucia Farina
and Paolo Corradini*

20 Transplantation in Burkitt and lymphoblastic
lymphoma, 201
Gregory A. Hale

21 Transplantation in adult T-cell
leukemia/lymphoma, 209
Ali Bazarbachi and Olivier Hermine

22 Hematopoietic cell transplantation for
HIV-related lymphomas, 217
Joseph C. Alvarnas

23 Stem cell transplantation for mycosis
fungoides/Sézary syndrome, 233
Eric D. Jacobsen

24 Role of transplantation in lymphoplasmacytic
lymphoma, 241
Silvia Montoto and Charalampia Kyriakou

25 Transplantation outcome in primary mediastinal
large B-cell lymphoma, 247
Amanda F. Cashen

26 Management of post-transplant
lymphoproliferative disorders, 253
Jan Styczynski and Per Ljungman

Appendix I Follow-up calendar after autologous
stem cell transplantation in lymphoma, 261
Angela Moreschi Woods

Appendix II Follow-up calendar after
allogeneic stem cell transplantation
in lymphoma, 263
Angela Moreschi Woods

Index, 265

List of contributors

Joseph C. Alvarnas, MD
Associate Professor
Department of Hematology/Hematopoietic Cell
Transplantation
City of Hope
Duarte, CA, USA

Ernesto Ayala, MD
Department of Blood and Marrow Transplantation
Department of Oncologic Sciences
H. Lee Moffitt Cancer Center
Tampa, FL, USA

Tarah Ballinger, MD
Vanderbilt University Medical Center
Nashville, TN, USA

Ali Bazarbachi, MD, PhD
Department of Internal Medicine
American University of Beirut
Beirut, Lebanon

Mitchell S. Cairo, MD
Departments of Pediatrics, Medicine,
Pathology, Microbiology and Immunology,
and Cell Biology and Anatomy, New York Medical College,
Valhalla, NY, USA

Amanda F. Cashen, MD
Washington University School of Medicine,
St. Louis MO, USA.

Wichai Chinratanalab, MD
Division of Hematology/Oncology
Department of Medicine
Vanderbilt-Ingram Cancer Center
Nashville, TN, USA

Paolo Corradini, MD
Chair of Hematology, University of Milano,
Department of Hematology and Pediatric Onco-Hematology
Division of Hematology and Stem Cell Transplantation
Fondazione IRCCS Istituto Nazionale dei Tumori
Milano, Italy

Parastoo Bahrami Dahi, MD
Adult Bone Marrow Transplantation Service
Memorial Sloan Kettering Cancer Center
Weill Cornell Medical College
NY, USA

Chiara De Philippis
Department of Hematology and Pediatric Onco-Hematology
Division of Hematology and Stem Cell Transplantation
Fondazione IRCCS Istituto Nazionale dei Tumori
Milano, Italy

Sascha Dietrich, MD
Internal Medicine V
University Hospital
Heidelberg, Germany;
Lymphoma Working Party
European Society for Blood and Marrow Transplantation
Paris, France

Eva Domingo-Domenech, MD
Department of Hematology
Institut Català d'Oncologia – Hospital Duran I Reynals
Barcelona, Spain

Peter Dreger, MD
Internal Medicine V
University Hospital
Heidelberg, Germany;
Lymphoma Working Party
European Society for Blood and Marrow Transplantation
Paris, France

Najla El-Jurdi, MD
Department of Internal Medicine
Tufts University School of Medicine
Boston, MA, USA

Nader Kim El-Mallawany, MD
Department of Pediatrics
New York Medical College
Valhalla, NY, USA

Lucia Farina, MD, PhD
Department of Hematology and Pediatric Onco-Hematology,
Division of Hematology and Stem Cell Transplantation,
Fondazione IRCCS Istituto Nazionale dei Tumori
Milano, Italy

Michael Green, MD
Division of Oncology, Hematology,
Hematologic Malignancies and Cellular Therapy.
Duke University Medical Center.
Durham, NC, USA

Gregory A. Hale, MD
Associate Professor of Oncology and Pediatrics,
All Children's Hospital-Johns Hopkins Medicine,
St. Petersburg, FL, USA

Mehdi Hamadani, MD
Division of Hematology-Oncology
Medical College of Wisconsin
Milwaukee, WI, USA

Parameswaran Hari, MD, MRCP, MS
Division of Hematology-Oncology and
Center for International Blood and
Marrow Transplant Research (CIBMTR)
Medical College of Wisconsin
Milwaukee, WI, USA

Shahrukh K. Hashmi, MD, MPH
Assistant Professor of Medicine
Division of Hematology
Department of Internal Medicine
Mayo Clinic
Rochester, MN, USA

Olivier Hermine, MD, PhD
Department of Hematology
Hôpital Necker
Paris, France

Gabriela Soriano Hobbs, MD
Adult Bone Marrow Transplantation Service
Memorial Sloan Kettering Cancer Center
Weill Cornell Medical College
NY, USA

Mitchell Horwitz, MD
Division of Hematologic Malignancies and
Cellular Therapy
Duke University School of Medicine
Durham, NC, USA

Eric D. Jacobsen, MD
Assistant Professor of Medicine
Harvard Medical School;
Clinical Director, Adult Lymphoma Program
Dana-Farber Cancer Institute
Boston, MA, USA

Abraham S. Kanate, MD
Assistant Professor of Medicine
Osborn Hematopoietic Malignancy and Transplantation
Program;
Director of Myeloma/Lymphoma Service
West Virginia University
Morgantown, WV, USA

Mohamed A. Kharfan-Dabaja, MD, FACP
Department of Blood and Marrow Transplantation
Department of Oncologic Sciences
H. Lee Moffitt Cancer Center
Tampa, FL, USA

Satyajit Kosuri, MD
Department of Hematology and Oncology,
Weill Cornell Medical College/New York Presbyterian Hospital
New York, NY, USA

Charalampia Kyriakou, MD, PhD
Department of Haematology
Royal Free Hospital
London, UK
Lymphoma Working Party
European Society for Blood and Marrow Transplantation
Paris, France

Per Ljungman, MD, PhD
Department of Hematology
Karolinska University Hospital and
Division of Hematology
Department of Medicine Huddinge
Karolinska Institutet
Stockholm, Sweden

Melissa Logue, ANP-BC
Adult Nurse Practitioner
The Vanderbilt Clinic
Nashville, TN, USA

Navneet S. Majhail, MD, MS
Blood and Marrow Transplant Program
Cleveland Clinic Taussig Cancer Institute
Cleveland, OH, USA

Shylaja Mani, MD
Blood and Marrow Transplant Program
Cleveland Clinic Taussig Cancer Institute
Cleveland, OH, USA

Mohamad Mohty, MD, PhD
Hôpital Saint Antoine
Université Pierre et Marie Curie
Paris, France

Silvia Montoto, MD
Department of Haemato-oncology
St Bartholomew's Hospital
Barts Health NHS Trust
London, UK
Lymphoma Working Party
European Society for Blood and Marrow Transplantation
Paris, France

Yago Nieto, MD, PhD
Department of Stem Cell Transplantation
and Cellular Therapy
University of Texas M.D. Anderson Cancer Center
Houston, TX, USA

Taiga Nishihori, MD
Department of Blood and Marrow Transplantation
Department of Oncologic Sciences
H. Lee Moffitt Cancer Center
Tampa, FL, USA

Miguel-Angel Perales, MD
Adult Bone Marrow Transplantation Service
Memorial Sloan Kettering Cancer Center
Weill Cornell Medical College
NY, USA

Giulia Perrone
Department of Hematology and Pediatric Onco-Hematology
Division of Hematology and Stem Cell Transplantation
Fondazione IRCCS Istituto Nazionale dei Tumori
Milano, Italy

Sai Ravi Pingali, MD
Department of Stem Cell Transplantation and Cellular Therapy
University of Texas M.D. Anderson Cancer Center
Houston, TX, USA

Andrew R. Rezvani, MD
Division of Blood and Marrow Transplantation
Stanford University
Stanford, CA, USA

Wael Saber, MD, MS
Division of Hematology-Oncology and Center for International
Blood and Marrow Transplant Research (CIBMTR)
Medical College of Wisconsin
Milwaukee, WI, USA

Karma Z. Salem, MD
Faculty of Medicine
American University of Beirut
Beirut, Lebanon

Bipin N. Savani, MD
Professor of Medicine
Director, Long Term Transplant Clinic
Division of Hematology/Oncology
Vanderbilt Ingram Cancer Center
Vanderbilt University Medical Center
Nashville, TN, USA

Salyka Sengsayadeth, MD
Division of Hematology/Oncology
Department of Medicine
Vanderbilt-Ingram Cancer Center
Nashville, TN, USA

Jan Styczynski, MD, PhD
Department of Pediatric Hematology and Oncology
Collegium Medicum
Nicolaus Copernicus University
Bydgoszcz, Poland

Anna Sureda, MD, PhD
Hematology Consultant
Secretary, European Group for Blood and Marrow
Transplantation
Department of Hematology
Institut Català d'Oncologia – Hospital Duran I Reynals
Barcelona, Spain

Koen Van Besien, MD, PhD
Department of Hematology and Oncology,
Weill Cornell Medical College/New York Presbyterian Hospital
New York, NY, USA

Lauren Veltri, MD
Fellow in Hematology/Oncology
Department of Internal Medicine
West Virginia University
Morgantown, WV, USA

Angela Moreschi Woods, MSN, APRN, ACNP-BC
Hematology Nurse Practitioner
Medical Service, Hematology Section
Veterans Affairs Medical Center
Nashville, TN, USA

Foreword

"Doctor, are we then saving the best for last," asked our patient when we mentioned that it was time to discuss stem cell transplantation in relapsed follicular lymphoma as the most favorable option with curative intent. We had not used the word "cure" with the prior therapies that were prescribed. As oncologists, we often use the words "remission" and "cure" and these can be confusing for patients and their caregivers. If an allogeneic stem cell transplant is indeed curative, why did we not proceed with it as initial therapy? A quandary our patients are usually left with.

Oncologists and healthcare providers are faced with challenging malignancies, some curative and others not, due to the nature of the disease driven by its pathology. In the era of newer targeted treatments and exciting novel agents with unique mechanisms of action, oncologists themselves are often perplexed by the timing of stem cell transplant in lymphoma. This book, edited by Professors Savani and Mohty and authored by leaders in the lymphoma field, is indeed an invaluable guide to understanding the current status of stem cell transplantation in lymphoma. Stem cell transplantation should not be considered a treatment of last resort but rather an alternative therapeutic option with curative potential. In that regard, this book discusses the approach to and timing of stem cell transplantation in the various lymphoma subtypes.

Finding a donor at the right time is indeed critical. Matched siblings are preferred donors. However, only one-third of patients will have a healthy matched sibling. There is increasing evidence that unrelated matched donors achieve similar outcomes. Other options, such as cord blood transplant and haploidentical transplant, are gaining popularity and are increasingly safer, mitigating the need to find a sibling match. This book discusses the latest evidence for haploidentical and cord blood transplant procedures pertaining to lymphoma.

Allogeneic stem cell transplantation harnesses antitumor immunity to prevent tumor progression. In the current era, mimicking natural immunity and enhancing host antitumor activity are the characteristics of the immune checkpoint inhibitors, such as program-death (PD-1/PDL-1) inhibitors, with activity in lymphoma. Most of the outcome data in transplantation predates the modern period of small-molecule inhibitors and targeted agents. This book takes a new approach in defining the purpose of transplantation and integrating targeted therapy with the best available evidence. Relapse after allogeneic transplant is still a major issue. The management of post-transplant relapse is a challenge in itself, and exciting avenues of research discussed in this book include the assessment of minimal residual disease at several time points with newer methodologies and increasing the sensitivity of the testing in order to detect early relapse and potentially allow modulation of the immune system with antibodies or adoptive cellular therapies. Another exciting area is the use of chimeric antigen receptor- engineered T cells to provoke an adaptive immune response against hematologic malignancies. There is great potential for this approach to significantly improve patient-specific cancer therapy. The authors highlight the antitumor activity of T cells in various subtypes of lymphoma.

An essential component of stem cell transplant is the conditioning regimen administered prior to the infusion of stem cells. Some of the earlier regimens were dose intense, with or without radiation to eliminate any residual malignancy. Over time, several investigators lowered the dose of radiation and chemotherapeutic agents in the preparative regimen in order to exploit the graft-versus-tumor effect. The authors focus on lymphoablative regimens and regimen-related toxicities. The overall reduction in morbidity and mortality has allowed transplant physicians to offer the option of an allogeneic transplant to the elderly, who were once considered ineligible for transplant. This book offers a very balanced view of the current position of stem cell transplant in patients with Hodgkin and non-Hodgkin lymphoma, and this has never been compiled in such detail.

Most stem cell transplant programs are located at tertiary centers and in some countries access to an academic center is further limited by the added financial constraints. Referral patterns may vary widely throughout the world, but the principles of transplantation and care following transplant are universal and relevant to all physicians and healthcare providers. The topics discussed in this book are pertinent to oncologists, hematologists, transplant physicians and primary care providers.

Chronic graft-versus-host disease and the late complications of chronic immunosuppressive therapy are important challenges with an impact on survival. Transplant centers have therefore established long-term clinics to focus on morbid issues. An orchestrated effort to provide this type of environment for long-term survivors may be feasible at major transplant centers of excellence. In the absence of established clinics, such coordinated follow-up care will need to be managed by the referring oncologist in conjunction with the transplant physician. Referring physicians will also benefit from continued education on the long-term follow-up of survivors.

It is essential to select the optimal time for stem cell transplantation while providing the best long-term care and thus increasing the chances of long-term survival free of this life-threatening malignancy. Therefore referral to a transplant center with expertise in the disease is crucial. This book is also unique in that it serves as a guide to best practice by the oncologist, who is the person resonsible for referral to a transplant center and who is involved with the continued follow-up of the patient. The care delivered by any transplant center is complex and involves coordinated care between specialties.

This book is therefore timely as it provides the most comprehensive method for integrated patient care. The authors and editors deserve to be congratulated on this book and the magnitude of its impact on its readers will be immense.

Finally, this book addresses our patient's question – "Doctor, are we then saving the best for last." To that our answer is, together we are indeed starting a journey to accomplish the best, but certainly not the least, outcome.

Dr Nishitha M. Reddy
Director, Lymphoma Program
Vanderbilt University Medical Center
Nashville, TN, USA

Professor Noel Milpied
CHU de Bordeaux
Bordeaux, France

Professor Christian Gisselbrecht
CHU Saint-Louis, AP-HP
Paris, France

Introduction

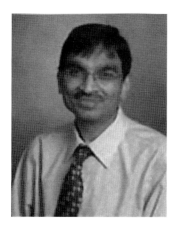

Bipin N. Savani, MD
Professor of Medicine
Director, Long Term Transplant Clinic
Division of Hematology/Oncology
Vanderbilt Ingram Cancer Center
Vanderbilt University Medical Center
Nashville, TN, USA

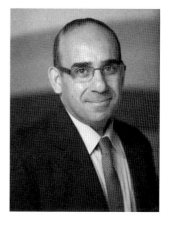

Professor Mohamad Mohty, MD, PhD
Head, Clinical Hematology and Cellular
Therapy Department
Université Pierre et Marie Curie
Hôpital Saint Antoine
INSERM, U938
Paris, France

Lymphoid malignancies are leading causes of cancer with an estimated 100,000 cases projected in the United States in 2014, comprising non-Hodgkin lymphoma (NHL), 70,800; Hodgkin lymphoma (HL), 9190; and chronic lymphocytic leukemia (CLL), 15,720. Although 5-year survival of lymphoid malignancies has improved significantly in the last three decades, it is estimated to account for 25,000 deaths in the United States in 2014 (NHL, 18,990; HL, 1180; CLL, 4600) [1]. This highlights the need for an improvement in upfront and salvage therapy for lymphomas.

Hematopoietic stem cell transplantation (HSCT) provides curative therapy for a variety of diseases. Over the past several decades, significant advances have been made in the field of HSCT and it has now become an integral part of treatment for a variety of lymphoid malignancies. Advances in transplantation technology

Clinical Guide to Transplantation in Lymphoma, First Edition. Edited by Bipin N. Savani and Mohamad Mohty.
© 2015 John Wiley & Sons, Ltd. Published 2015 by John Wiley & Sons, Ltd.

and supportive care have resulted in a significant decrease in transplant-related mortality and relapse rate.

Since the first three cases of successful HSCT in 1968, the number of HSCTs performed annually has increased steadily over the past 30 years [2–6]. It is estimated that by 2015 more than 100,000 patients will receive HSCT (combined allogeneic and autologous) annually worldwide, and numbers are increasing rapidly. We celebrated the one millionth transplant in 2013! With continued improvement in HSCT outcome, the indications for HSCT continue to grow. Furthermore, the sources of stem cells and the number of suitable matches are expanding. At the same time, modified transplantation regimens have facilitated safer procedures despite the increase in patient age and comorbidities. These new findings show that HSCT is more accessible for patients previously not considered good candidates.

Thanks to the advent of reduced-intensity conditioning (RIC) regimens and improvements in supportive care, we now have the ability to safely perform transplantations in older patients and those with comorbid illnesses. In some centers, it is not uncommon to perform autologous or even allogeneic stem cell transplants in patients as old as 75 years. Long-term studies suggest that average health-related quality of life and functional status among survivors, including older patients, recover within a couple of years to pretransplant levels.

In this era, a stem cell source can be found for virtually all patients who have an indication to receive allogeneic HSCT. Since 2006, more allogeneic HSCT procedures have been performed using alternative donor stem cell sources, such as volunteer unrelated donor or cord blood, than related donors [2]. RIC haploidentical related donor or cord blood transplantation has emerged as an alternative for those patients who do not have matched related donor or unrelated donor and the outcome of these types of transplantation are expected to be better than chemotherapy alone or even better than autologous HSCT for selected indications.

Because of the availability of novel substances and treatment strategies, the standard of care in many lymphoid malignancies has changed dramatically. These new approaches include new monoclonal antibodies, immunomodulatory agents, substances interfering with the B-cell receptor signaling pathway, and novel cellular therapies [7]. The choice of HSCT versus a novel agent is one that must be gauged on a patient-by-patient basis.

A very exciting new active immunotherapy strategy is chimeric antigen receptor (CAR) T-cell therapy. CAR technology has recently emerged as a novel and promising approach for specifically targeting malignant cells with precisely engineered T cells. Several clinical trials have reported impressive results with anti-CD19 CAR T cells in both CLL and acute lymphoblastic leukemia and have been investigated in other malignancies [8–10]. Recent data from the National Cancer Institute showed that the infusion of donor-derived allogeneic anti-CD19 CAR T cells caused regression of highly treatment-resistant B-cell malignancies after allogeneic HSCT (anti-CD19 CAR T-cell donor lymphocyte infusion or DLI). Results showed that infusions were not associated with graft-versus-host disease (GVHD) [11]. Relapse of malignancy is a leading cause of death in patients undergoing allogeneic HSCT. B-cell malignancies persisting despite allogeneic HSCT are often treated with unmanipulated DLI. However, DLI has inconsistent efficacy and is associated with significant morbidity and mortality from GVHD. Allogeneic anti-CD19 CAR T cells have significant anti-malignancy activity when administered without prior chemotherapy [11].

As there are no direct comparisons between HSCT and novel agents, general evidence-based recommendations are very difficult to make at this point. Instead, we need to understand the limitations of each approach, and carefully weigh the chances and risks of each procedure on a case-by-case basis. In general, the availability of treatments, their expected benefit and side effects, and individual treatment histories and pretransplant characteristics as determined by the variety of risk score systems need to be taken into consideration.

However, as the success of HSCT is highly dependent on the remission state at the time of HSCT, it seems very desirable to focus on achieving control of the disease first. This can be facilitated by novel substances. As they are well tolerated and show only moderate toxicities, they seem a good option as a bridge until HSCT, and maybe even to postpone HSCT to a later point in the disease. How these substances should be best combined, if there is the option to completely eliminate the chemotherapy backbone from induction or second-line treatment, and whether they will have an effect on graft-versus-lymphoma and immunomodulation is the major focus of ongoing preclinical and clinical studies.

Indeed, the use of HSCT continues to grow each year in the United States, Europe, and around the world. In parallel with advances in other cancer treatments, HSCT has evolved rapidly in the past two decades in ways that may be unfamiliar to those who learned about transplant earlier in their careers. Nevertheless, continued underutilization of transplantation in patients who might otherwise benefit suggests that many of the improvements in the field may not be well known among referring providers.

This book is therefore timely and at the same time unique: the first clinical guide to transplantation in lymphoma in the novel therapeutic era. We have assembled what must be the definitive text on this subject and have called upon more than 50 specialists to contribute to this authoritative volume. This book presents the most current knowledge about how to integrate transplantation and novel therapies in patients with lymphoid malignancies. Section 1 sets the stage, with an overview of transplantation in lymphoma including a historical perspective, role of lymphoma working committees, current use of transplantation in children and adults, the variety of conditioning regimens for autologous and allogeneic HSCT, pretransplant evaluation, stem cell mobilization, donor search for patients needing allogeneic HSCT, and management of long-term complications after HSCT for lymphomas and follow-up. Section 2 is devoted to the management of lymphoid malignancies, focusing on standard of care transplant management, timing and preparation of patients for transplantation, management of posttransplant relapses and, most importantly, discussion of novel therapies and their integration in transplantation for lymphomas. These contributions from acknowledged experts in the field from Europe and the United States cover the organizational aspects of transplant patients. Finally, the appendices are a source of practical information that clinicians will find extremely helpful in the management of lymphoma patients.

Declaration of commercial interest

The authors declare no conflict of interest.

References

1 Siegel R, Ma J, Zou Z, Jemal A. Cancer statistics, 2014. *CA Cancer J Clin* 2014;**64**:9–29.

2 Pasquini MC, *Wang Z*. Current use and outcome of hematopoietic stem cell transplantation: CIBMTR Summary Slides, 2013. Available at http://www.cibmtr.org

3 Passweg JR, Baldomero H, Peters C *et al.* Hematopoietic SCT in Europe: data and trends in 2012 with special consideration of pediatric transplantation. *Bone Marrow Transplant* 2014;**49**: 744–50.

4 Passweg JR, Baldomero H, Bregni M *et al.* Hematopoietic SCT in Europe: data and trends in 2011. *Bone Marrow Transplant* 2013;**48**:1161–7.

5 Passweg JR, Baldomero H, Gratwohl A *et al.* The EBMT activity survey: 1990–2010. *Bone Marrow Transplant* 2012;**47**: 906–23.

6 Thomas ED. A history of bone marrow transplantation. In: Appelbaum FR, Forman SJ, Negrin RS, Blume KG, eds. *Thomas' Hematopoietic Cell Transplantation*. Chichester, UK: Wiley-Blackwell, 2009:3–7.

7 Byrd JC, Jones JJ, Woyach JA, Johnson AJ, Flynn JM. Entering the era of targeted therapy for chronic lymphocytic leukemia: impact on the practicing clinician. *J Clin Oncol* 2014;**32**:3039–47.

8 Porter DL, Levine BL, Kalos M, Bagg A, June CH. Chimeric antigen receptor-modified T cells in chronic lymphoid leukemia. *N Engl J Med* 2011;**365**:725–33.

9 Grupp SA, Kalos M, Barrett D *et al.* Chimeric antigen receptor-modified T cells for acute lymphoid leukemia. *N Engl J Med* 2013;**368**:1509–18.

10 Davila ML, Riviere I, Wang X *et al.* Efficacy and toxicity management of 19-28z CAR T cell therapy in B cell acute lymphoblastic leukemia. *Sci Transl Med* 2014;6:224ra25.

11 Kochenderfer JN, Dudley ME, Carpenter RO *et al.* Donor-derived CD19-targeted T cells cause regression of malignancy persisting after allogeneic hematopoietic stem cell transplantation. *Blood* 2013;**122**:4129–39.

CHAPTER 1

Lymphoma and transplantation: historical perspective

Andrew R. Rezvani

Brief history of hematopoietic cell transplantation

The concept of hematopoietic cell transplantation (HCT) dates back more than 100 years. Writing in the *Journal of the American Medical Association* in 1896, Quine credited Brown-Séquard and d'Arsonval with proposing the therapeutic infusion of bone marrow to treat leukemia, and summarized anecdotal reports of bone marrow infusion as an adjunct to then-standard treatments such as arsenic for pernicious anemia [1]. Quine also described the first case of inadvertently transmitted blood-borne infection (malaria) in a marrow recipient. Anecdotal reports of marrow infusion continued to appear in the literature, but often used only several milliliters of bone marrow and were unsuccessful [2,3]. Classified animal experiments were carried out by the US Atomic Energy Commission during World War II on the use of HCT to treat radiation exposure (later published in 1950), but these were similarly unsuccessful [4]. The era of modern HCT is generally understood to have originated with the 1949 publication by Jacobson *et al.* of the observation that mice could survive otherwise lethal irradiation if splenocytes were protected from the radiation and reinfused afterward [5,6]. Subsequent work by Lorenz *et al.* [7] showed that infusion of bone marrow had similarly protective effects in irradiated mice and guinea pigs. Hematopoietic recovery after marrow infusion was initially hypothesized to derive from a humoral or hormonal factor in the infusate, but in the mid-1950s Main and Prehn and others proved

conclusively that donor hematopoietic cells engrafted and persisted in HCT recipient animals [8–11].

The first successful use of HCT to treat leukemia in murine models was reported by Barnes and Loutit in 1956 [12]. These authors outlined the central premises of modern allogeneic HCT: first, that high-dose myeloablative therapy could eliminate hematologic malignancies and, second, that donor hematopoietic cells could mount an immunologic response which would eradicate residual leukemia in the recipient. In 1957, these authors reported that leukemic mice treated with myeloablative irradiation and syngeneic HCT had hematopoietic recovery but died of recurrent leukemia, while mice receiving allogeneic HCT demonstrated eradication of leukemia but died of so-called "secondary disease," a syndrome of diarrhea and weight loss which would today be recognized as graft-versus-host disease (GVHD) [13,14].

Early efforts at allogeneic HCT in humans were carried out nearly simultaneously by Thomas *et al.* in the 1950s [15]. However, as the immunologic basis of histocompatibility was poorly understood at the time, these patients did not engraft. In fact, a summary of the first approximately 200 human recipients of allogeneic HCT, published in 1970, found no survivors [16]. During this time, however, a number of breakthroughs in animal models of HCT laid the groundwork for the future success of this approach. Billingham *et al.* [17,18] described the biological basis of GVHD and alloimmune tolerance, and Uphoff [19] and Lochte *et al.* [20] described the use of methotrexate to prevent GVHD. Thomas *et al.* [21,22]

Clinical Guide to Transplantation in Lymphoma, First Edition. Edited by Bipin N. Savani and Mohamad Mohty.

pioneered the use of canine models of allogeneic HCT. Perhaps most importantly, advances in the understanding of histocompatibility in both the human and the dog provided a basis for donor–recipient matching, a critical component of successful allogeneic HCT [23–25].

In the setting of these advances, allogeneic HCT in humans was revisited with greater success. By 1975, the Seattle group of investigators summarized the results of 110 patients with acute leukemias or aplastic anemia who had received allogeneic HCT from HLA-identical sibling donors. While deaths from recurrent leukemia, GVHD, and opportunistic infection were common, this report was the first to describe long-term survivors of allogeneic HCT [26,27]. Up to this point, allogeneic HCT had been reserved for patients with refractory leukemia; with the application of this approach to patients in first complete remission, substantial improvements in survival were seen [28]. With the advent of HLA typing, the first unrelated-donor transplant was performed using an HLA-matched volunteer donor in 1979 [29]. From these beginnings, HCT has become a fast-growing and increasingly widely used treatment approach for malignant and non-malignant hematologic disease [30].

Much of the benefit from allogeneic HCT derives from the immune effect of the graft against residual tumor (the graft-versus-tumor, or GVT, effect). In contrast, autologous HCT functions on the principle of dose escalation and relies entirely on high-dose, supralethal chemoradiotherapy to eradicate disease. Autologous hematopoietic cells are infused to rebuild the marrow and circumvent otherwise dose-limiting hematologic toxicity. Autologous HCT developed largely in parallel with allogeneic HCT, although without the barriers of histocompatibility, graft rejection, and GVHD. While a number of anecdotal reports and case series of autologous HCT appeared in the 1950s and 1960s, the first patients reported to be cured of otherwise lethal malignancies by this approach were described by Appelbaum *et al.* in 1978 [31,32]. Subsequent studies established autologous HCT as a potentially curative treatment for many lymphomas, and as an effective but not curative treatment for multiple myeloma.

History of autologous HCT in non-Hodgkin lymphoma

The curative potential of autologous HCT was first demonstrated in patients with non-Hodgkin lymphoma (NHL) [32,33], and this approach continues to form a cornerstone of management of relapsed NHL, as described in subsequent chapters. The central principles of autologous HCT for NHL were established in the 1980s. Specifically, chemosensitivity is a key determinant of benefit from autologous HCT; Philip *et al.* [33] reported as early as 1987 that disease-free survival rates were approximately 40% in patients with chemosensitive relapsed NHL, approximately 20% in those with chemotherapy-refractory disease, and nearly zero for patients with primary refractory NHL who had never achieved complete remission. The benefit of autologous HCT in relapsed aggressive NHL was confirmed in a randomized controlled clinical trial comparing standard-dose chemotherapy to high-dose chemotherapy with autologous HCT. The final results of this trial, reported in 1995, showed that both event-free survival (EFS) and overall survival (OS) were superior in the group undergoing autologous HCT (46% vs. 12% for EFS, and 53% vs. 32% for OS) [34]. On the basis of this convincing finding, autologous HCT has come to be considered the standard of care for eligible patients with chemotherapy-sensitive relapsed aggressive NHL.

Autologous HCT has also been studied in patients with indolent NHL, but the historical evidence for benefit is less definitive in this setting than in aggressive NHL. Several trials in the 1990s demonstrated prolonged disease-free survival and possible cure in a subset of patients with indolent NHL undergoing autologous HCT [35,36]. Likewise, a randomized controlled trial of 89 patients published in 2003 showed improved EFS and OS with autologous HCT as compared to conventional chemotherapy alone in patients with relapsed indolent NHL (58% vs. 26% for 2-year EFS, and 71% vs. 46% for 4-year OS) [37]. Despite the positive results of this randomized trial, autologous HCT remains controversial in indolent NHL. The curative potential of autologous HCT in indolent NHL is not universally accepted (in contrast to aggressive NHL), and so there may be greater reluctance to expose patients to the regimen-related toxicities and long-term risks of this approach, which include secondary myelodysplastic syndromes and acute leukemias, which can occur in up to 5% of patients [38]. Additionally, many of the trials supporting autologous HCT in indolent NHL were performed before the advent of rituximab and modern chemoimmunotherapy. For example, treatment with FCR (fludarabine, cyclophosphamide, and rituximab) chemotherapy can produce median disease-free survivals of more than 4 years in patients with relapsed indolent NHL [39]. In the setting of highly active conventional chemotherapy regimens, the appeal of autologous HCT in indolent NHL is reduced. Nonetheless, historical data do support its efficacy as a treatment option, particularly for patients with short remission durations or suboptimal responses to conventional chemoimmunotherapy.

History of autologous HCT in Hodgkin lymphoma

While Hodgkin lymphoma (HL) is among the most curable forms of cancer with upfront treatment, the minority of patients who relapse or who have primary refractory HL have a grim prognosis with conventional chemotherapy alone. Reports of the successful use of autologous HCT in HL began to appear in the literature in the mid-1980s [40–44]. On the basis of these uncontrolled and generally single-institution studies, relapsed HL quickly became one of the most common indications for autologous HCT. As with NHL, chemosensitivity at relapse was felt to be one of the most important determinants of likelihood of cure after autologous HCT.

Since autologous HCT had already entered widespread use, two randomized controlled trials comparing conventional chemotherapy with autologous HCT were performed in the 1990s. The British National Lymphoma Investigation randomized a total of 40 patients with relapsed or refractory HL to receive either BEAM conditioning (carmustine, etoposide, cytarabine, and melphalan) followed by autologous HCT, or reduced-dose BEAM alone. The trial was initially intended to enroll a larger number of patients, but it proved impossible to accrue patients for randomization due to insistence on the part of both patients and physicians for autologous HCT. The trial was thus closed early and suffered from severely limited statistical power, with only 20 patients in each arm of the randomization. Upon publication in 1993, statistically significant differences were seen in EFS in favor of the transplant arm, although the difference in OS did not reach statistical significance [45].

Separately, the European Society for Blood and Marrow Transplantation (EBMT) conducted a randomized clinical trial comparing chemotherapy alone to autologous HCT in 161 patients with chemosensitive relapsed HL, published in 2002. As with the earlier randomized trial, the EBMT group reported

significantly superior EFS, but not OS, with autologous HCT [46]. While neither study showed a statistically significant OS benefit with autologous HCT, the benefit in EFS was felt to be convincing and the studies were acknowledged to be limited in statistical power to detect differences in OS. Thus, on the basis of the earlier uncontrolled trials and these two randomized trials, autologous HCT has become an accepted standard of care for eligible patients with chemosensitive relapsed HL. Additional aspects of autologous HCT for HL, including more recent developments, are covered in more detail in Chapter 18.

History of allogeneic HCT in lymphoma

Historically, autologous HCT has been far more widely employed than allogeneic HCT in the treatment of lymphomas, in part because the earliest clinical trials were unable to definitively establish the existence of an alloimmune graft-versus-lymphoma effect [47]. Likewise, autologous HCT was viewed as more feasible in lymphomas than in leukemias because of the lower incidence of malignant bone marrow involvement in the former. Subsequent experience, however, indicated that tumor contamination of autografts in lymphoma patients contributed to post-transplant relapse [48], underscoring the potential benefit of tumor-free allogeneic grafts in these diseases. Even more importantly, further clinical trials confirmed the existence of potent graft-versus-lymphoma effects [49], underscoring the potential benefit of allotransplantation in lymphoma.

The initial experience with allogeneic HCT in NHL involved the use of myeloablative conditioning with high-dose total body irradiation (TBI) or the combination of busulfan and cyclophosphamide (BU/CY). As a consequence of the intensity of conditioning, allogeneic HCT was generally restricted to patients who were young and healthy enough to tolerate the regimen-related toxicities. These demographics included some patients with HL and aggressive NHL, but excluded the vast majority of indolent NHL patients, who tended to be older at the time of diagnosis. However, even in this young and relatively healthy population, the regimen-related toxicity and transplant-related mortality of allogeneic HCT was substantial, if not prohibitive, ranging from 25 to 50% [47,49–51]. This degree of transplant-related mortality was out of proportion to that seen in leukemia cohorts. Acute and chronic GVHD incidences were no higher than those seen with other transplant indications; the majority of non-relapse deaths in these early trials stemmed from pneumonitis and pulmonary injury, likely because many patients had previously undergone radiation therapy to the chest and were thus predisposed to further pulmonary compromise.

As noted above, the reliance on intensive myeloablative conditioning precluded the vast majority of patients with indolent NHL, who tended to be older and more heavily pretreated than patients with HL or aggressive NHL. In fact, as of 1990, only a total of seven allogeneic transplants for indolent NHL had been reported in the literature [52–54]. Allogeneic HCT was generally not performed for indolent NHL because of good results with conventional therapies, advanced patient age, and the prohibitively high risk of transplant-related mortality.

The most important development in the use of allogeneic HCT for lymphomas has been the introduction of reduced-intensity and non-myeloablative conditioning regimens. These regimens, pioneered by various groups including McSweeney *et al.* [55] in Seattle, Khouri *et al.* [56] at M.D. Anderson Cancer Center, and Lowsky *et al.* [57] at Stanford (among others), are based on the principle that immunologic graft-versus-lymphoma effects rather than conditioning agents are responsible for the majority of benefit from allogeneic HCT. While the specific agents used in reduced-intensity conditioning regimens vary, they are generally selected to permit donor hematopoietic engraftment with minimal regimen-related toxicity. These regimens have little or no intrinsic antitumor effect and instead serve the role of facilitating donor engraftment.

Lymphomas were a natural target disease for newly developed reduced-intensity conditioning regimens, given the older age of the patient population and the high transplant-related mortality seen with myeloablative approaches. Perhaps most importantly, reduced-intensity conditioning made it possible to perform safe allografting in patients who had previously undergone high-dose chemotherapy and autologous HCT (as is common in the course of lymphoma treatment). The prior experience in attempting myeloablative allogeneic HCT in lymphoma patients after a previous autograft was dismal, with a 2-year disease-free survival after allotransplantation of zero [58]. In contrast, non-myeloablative and reduced-intensity regimens quickly proved capable of producing donor engraftment with acceptable regimen-related toxicity in patients with prior autologous HCT.

Over the past 15 years, an extensive literature has arisen describing the successful use of non-myeloablative or reduced-intensity allogeneic HCT to treat lymphoma. These results are described in detail in later chapters, but the overarching theme is that allogeneic HCT is increasingly part of the treatment algorithm for patients with relapsed and refractory lymphomas. For most types of aggressive NHL and for HL, autologous HCT is still generally a standard of care for patients with a first chemosensitive relapse. However, some groups have incorporated allogeneic HCT into the upfront management of patients with indolent NHL in first chemosensitive relapse, based on the excellent results seen in this patient population with modern reduced-intensity approaches [59]. From a historical perspective, the transformation wrought by reduced-intensity conditioning is particularly striking in lymphoma; from a total of only seven patients with indolent NHL transplanted as of 1990 due to prohibitive toxicity, these patients now experience outcomes among the best reported for any allogeneic HCT indication [59,60].

General historical considerations

No historical perspective on HCT would be complete without discussion of improvements in supportive care. Much of the improvement in outcomes with both allogeneic and autologous HCT over the past decades is due to the advent of more effective antimicrobials, surveillance strategies against opportunistic infection, blood-product support, and management of regimen-related toxicities. Common opportunistic infections in the post-transplant period include cytomegalovirus (CMV) reactivation and invasive fungal infections such as pulmonary aspergillosis. In the early days of HCT, these complications were feared and nearly universally fatal. Substantial progress has been made in monitoring CMV reactivation and in determining appropriate thresholds for preemptive antiviral therapy to prevent the development of CMV disease. Likewise, potent modern antifungals such as the triazoles and echinocandins have improved our ability to treat invasive fungal infections, while imaging and endoscopic diagnosis of these infections has improved our ability to detect them.

Substantial progress has been made in the prevention of acute GVHD, with a number of novel prophylactic regimens supplementing standard and proven approaches such as tacrolimus plus methotrexate. In contrast, chronic GVHD remains a poorly understood entity which has proven challenging to prevent or treat, despite decades of clinical investigation.

A recent analysis of transplant outcomes over time confirmed significant reductions in transplant-related mortality and improvements in overall survival over time [61]. Strikingly, the incidence of hepatic acute GVHD, one of the most lethal complications of allogeneic HCT, has declined dramatically over the past 10–15 years. Various explanations have been proposed for this decline, ranging from the increasing use of reduced-intensity and non-myeloablative conditioning regimens to better donor and patient selection to the now-widespread use of prophylactic ursodiol [62]. Regardless, from a historical perspective, improvements in supportive care have transformed HCT and significantly improved outcomes across the range of transplant indications [61].

References

1 Quine WE. The remedial application of bone marrow. *JAMA* 1896;**26**:1012–16.
2 Osgood EE, Riddle MC, Mathews TJ. Aplastic anemia treated with daily transfusions and intravenous marrow. *Ann Intern Med* 1939;**13**:357–67.
3 Morrisson M, Samwick AA. Intramedullary (sternal) transfusion of human bone marrow. *JAMA* 1940;**115**:1708–11.
4 Rekers PE, Coulter MP, Warren SL. Effect of transplantation of bone marrow into irradiated animals. *Arch Surg* 1950;**60**:635–67.
5 Jacobson LO, Simmons EL, Marks EK, Robson MJ, Bethard WF, Gaston EO. The role of the spleen in radiation injury and recovery. *J Lab Clin Med* 1950;**35**:746–70.
6 Jacobson LO, Marks EK, Gaston EO, Robson M, Zirkle RE. The role of the spleen in radiation injury. *Proc Soc Exp Biol Med* 1949;**70**:740–2.
7 Lorenz E, Uphoff D, Reid TR, Shelton E. Modification of irradiation injury in mice and guinea pigs by bone marrow injections. *J Natl Cancer Inst* 1951;**12**:197–201.
8 Main JM, Prehn RT. Successful skin homografts after the administration of high dosage X radiation and homologous bone marrow. *J Natl Cancer Inst* 1955;**15**:1023–9.
9 Trentin JJ. Mortality and skin transplantability in X-irradiated mice receiving isologous, homologous or heterologous bone marrow. *Proc Soc Exp Biol Med* 1956;**92**:688–93.
10 Nowell PC, Cole LJ, Habermeyer JG, Roan PL. Growth and continued function of rat marrow cells in X-radiated mice. *Cancer Res* 1956;**16**:258–61.
11 Ford CE, Hamerton JL, Barnes DW, Loutit JF. Cytological identification of radiation-chimaeras. *Nature* 1956;**177**:452–4.
12 Barnes DW, Corp MJ, Loutit JF, Neal FE. Treatment of murine leukaemia with X rays and homologous bone marrow: preliminary communication. *Br Med J* 1956;**2**:626–7.
13 Barnes DW, Loutit JF. Treatment of murine leukaemia with X-rays and homologous bone marrow.II. *Br J Haematol* 1957;**3**:241–52.
14 Barnes DW, Ilbery PL, Loutit JF. Avoidance of secondary disease in radiation chimaeras. *Nature* 1958;**181**:488.
15 Thomas ED, Lochte HL Jr, Lu WC, Ferrebee JW. Intravenous infusion of bone marrow in patients receiving radiation and chemotherapy. *N Engl J Med* 1957;**257**:491–6.
16 Bortin MM. A compendium of reported human bone marrow transplants. *Transplantation* 1970;**9**:571–87.
17 Billingham RE, Brent L, Medawar PB. Quantitative studies on tissue transplantation immunity. II. The origin, strength and duration of actively and adoptively acquired immunity. *Proc R Soc Lond B Biol Sci* 1954;**143**:58–80.
18 Billingham RE, Brent L, Brown JB, Medawar PB. Time of onset and duration of transplantation immunity. *Transplant Bull* 1959;**6**:410–14.
19 Uphoff DE. Alteration of homograft reaction by A-methopterin in lethally irradiated mice treated with homologous marrow. *Proc Soc Exp Biol Med* 1958;**99**:651–3.
20 Lochte HL Jr, Levy AS, Guenther DM, Thomas ED, Ferrebee JW. Prevention of delayed foreign marrow reaction in lethally irradiated mice by early administration of methotrexate. *Nature* 1962;**196**:1110–1.
21 Thomas ED, Ashley CA, Lochte HL Jr, Jaretzki A III, Sahler OD, Ferrebee JW. Homografts of bone marrow in dogs after lethal total-body radiation. *Blood* 1959;**14**:720–36.
22 Thomas ED, Collins JA, Herman EC Jr, Ferrebee JW. Marrow transplants in lethally irradiated dogs given methotrexate. *Blood* 1962;**19**:217–28.
23 Van Rood JJ, Eernisse JG, Van Leeuwen A. Leucocyte antibodies in sera from pregnant women. *Nature* 1958;**181**:1735–6.
24 Epstein RB, Storb R, Ragde H, Thomas ED. Cytotoxic typing antisera for marrow grafting in littermate dogs. *Transplantation* 1968;**6**:45–58.
25 Storb R, Epstein RB, Bryant J, Ragde H, Thomas ED. Marrow grafts by combined marrow and leukocyte infusions in unrelated dogs selected by histocompatibility typing. *Transplantation* 1968;**6**:587–93.
26 Thomas E, Storb R, Clift RA *et al*. Bone-marrow transplantation (first of two parts). *N Engl J Med* 1975;**292**:832–43.
27 Thomas ED, Storb R, Clift RA *et al*. Bone-marrow transplantation (second of two parts). *N Engl J Med* 1975; **292**:895–902.
28 Thomas ED, Buckner CD, Clift RA *et al*. Marrow transplantation for acute nonlymphoblastic leukemia in first remission. *N Engl J Med* 1979;**301**:597–9.

29 Hansen JA, Clift RA, Thomas ED, Buckner CD, Storb R, Giblett ER. Transplantation of marrow from an unrelated donor to a patient with acute leukemia. *N Engl J Med* 1980;**303**:565–7.

30 Appelbaum FR. Hematopoietic-cell transplantation at 50. *N Engl J Med* 2007;**357**:1472–5.

31 Appelbaum FR, Herzig GP, Ziegler JL, Graw RG, Levine AS, Deisseroth AB. Successful engraftment of cryopreserved autologous bone marrow in patients with malignant lymphoma. *Blood* 1978;**52**:85–95.

32 Appelbaum FR, Deisseroth AB, Graw RG Jr *et al.* Prolonged complete remission following high dose chemotherapy of Burkitt's lymphoma in relapse. *Cancer* 1978;**41**:1059–63.

33 Philip T, Armitage JO, Spitzer G *et al.* High-dose therapy and autologous bone marrow transplantation after failure of conventional chemotherapy in adults with intermediate-grade or high-grade non-Hodgkin's lymphoma. *N Engl J Med* 1987;**316**:1493–8.

34 Philip T, Guglielmi C, Hagenbeek A *et al.* Autologous bone marrow transplantation as compared with salvage chemotherapy in relapses of chemotherapy-sensitive non-Hodgkin's lymphoma. *N Engl J Med* 1995;**333**:1540–5.

35 Rohatiner AZ, Nadler L, Davies AJ *et al.* Myeloablative therapy with autologous bone marrow transplantation for follicular lymphoma at the time of second or subsequent remission: long-term follow-up. *J Clin Oncol* 2007;**25**:2554–9.

36 Freedman AS, Neuberg D, Mauch P *et al.* Long-term follow-up of autologous bone marrow transplantation in patients with relapsed follicular lymphoma. *Blood* 1999;**94**:3325–33.

37 Schouten HC, Qian W, Kvaloy S *et al.* High-dose therapy improves progression-free survival and survival in relapsed follicular non-Hodgkin's lymphoma: results from the randomized European CUP trial. *J Clin Oncol* 2003;**21**:3918–27.

38 Tarella C, Passera R, Magni M *et al.* Risk factors for the development of secondary malignancy after high-dose chemotherapy and autograft, with or without rituximab: a 20-year retrospective follow-up study in patients with lymphoma. *J Clin Oncol* 2011;**29**:814–24.

39 Sacchi S, Pozzi S, Marcheselli R *et al.* Rituximab in combination with fludarabine and cyclophosphamide in the treatment of patients with recurrent follicular lymphoma. *Cancer* 2007;**110**:121–8.

40 Carella AM, Santini G, Santoro A *et al.* Massive chemotherapy with non-frozen autologous bone marrow transplantation in 13 cases of refractory Hodgkin's disease. *Eur J Cancer Clin Oncol* 1985;**21**:607–13.

41 Carella AM, Congiu AM, Gaozza E *et al.* High-dose chemotherapy with autologous bone marrow transplantation in 50 advanced resistant Hodgkin's disease patients: an Italian study group report. *J Clin Oncol* 1988;**6**:1411–16.

42 Philip T, Dumont J, Teillet F *et al.* High dose chemotherapy and autologous bone marrow transplantation in refractory Hodgkin's disease. *Br J Cancer* 1986;**53**:737–42.

43 Phillips GL, Wolff SN, Herzig RH *et al.* Treatment of progressive Hodgkin's disease with intensive chemoradiotherapy and autologous bone marrow transplantation. *Blood* 1989;**73**:2086–92.

44 Jagannath S, Dicke KA, Armitage JO *et al.* High-dose cyclophosphamide, carmustine, and etoposide and autologous bone marrow transplantation for relapsed Hodgkin's disease. *Ann Intern Med* 1986;**104**:163–8.

45 Linch DC, Winfield D, Goldstone AH *et al.* Dose intensification with autologous bone-marrow transplantation in relapsed and resistant Hodgkin's disease: results of a BNLI randomised trial. *Lancet* 1993;**341**:1051–4.

46 Schmitz N, Pfistner B, Sextro M *et al.* Aggressive conventional chemotherapy compared with high-dose chemotherapy with autologous haemopoietic stem-cell transplantation for relapsed chemosensitive Hodgkin's disease: a randomised trial. *Lancet* 2002;**359**:2065–71.

47 Appelbaum FR, Sullivan KM, Buckner CD *et al.* Treatment of malignant lymphoma in 100 patients with chemotherapy, total body irradiation, and marrow transplantation. *J Clin Oncol* 1987;**5**:1340–7.

48 Gribben JG, Freedman AS, Neuberg D *et al.* Immunologic purging of marrow assessed by PCR before autologous bone marrow transplantation for B-cell lymphoma. *N Engl J Med* 1991;**325**:1525–33.

49 Jones RJ, Ambinder RF, Piantadosi S, Santos GW. Evidence of a graft-versus-lymphoma effect associated with allogeneic bone marrow transplantation. *Blood* 1991;**77**:649–53.

50 Jones RJ, Piantadosi S, Mann RB *et al.* High-dose cytotoxic therapy and bone marrow transplantation for relapsed Hodgkin's disease. *J Clin Oncol* 1990;**8**:527–37.

51 Phillips GL, Reece DE, Barnett MJ *et al.* Allogeneic marrow transplantation for refractory Hodgkin's disease. *J Clin Oncol* 1989;**7**:1039–45.

52 Copelan EA, Kapoor N, Gibbins B, Tutschka PJ. Allogeneic marrow transplantation in non-Hodgkin's lymphoma. *Bone Marrow Transplant* 1990;**5**:47–50.

53 Lundberg JH, Hansen RM, Chitambar CR *et al.* Allogeneic bone marrow transplantation for relapsed and refractory lymphoma using genotypically HLA-identical and alternative donors. *J Clin Oncol* 1991;**9**:1848–59.

54 Appelbaum FR, Thomas ED, Buckner CD *et al.* Treatment of non-Hodgkin's lymphoma with chemoradiotherapy and allogenic marrow transplantation. *Hematol Oncol* 1983;**1**:149–57.

55 McSweeney PA, Niederwieser D, Shizuru JA *et al.* Hematopoietic cell transplantation in older patients with hematologic malignancies: replacing high-dose cytotoxic therapy with graft-versus-tumor effects. *Blood* 2001;**97**:3390–400.

56 Khouri IF, Keating M, Korbling M *et al.* Transplant-lite: induction of graft-versus-malignancy using fludarabine-based nonablative chemotherapy and allogeneic blood progenitor-cell transplantation as treatment for lymphoid malignancies. *J Clin Oncol* 1998;**16**:2817–24.

57 Lowsky R, Takahashi T, Liu YP *et al.* Protective conditioning for acute graft-versus-host disease. *N Engl J Med* 2005;**353**: 1321–31.

58 Radich JP, Gooley T, Sanders JE, Anasetti C, Chauncey T, Appelbaum FR. Second allogeneic transplantation after failure of first autologous transplantation. *Biol Blood Marrow Transplant* 2000;**6**:272–9.

59 Khouri IF, McLaughlin P, Saliba RM *et al.* Eight-year experience with allogeneic stem cell transplantation for relapsed follicular lymphoma after nonmyeloablative conditioning with fludarabine, cyclophosphamide, and rituximab. *Blood* 2008;**111**:5530–6.

60 Rezvani AR, Storer B, Maris M *et al.* Nonmyeloablative allogeneic hematopoietic cell transplantation in relapsed, refractory, and transformed indolent non-Hodgkin's lymphoma. *J Clin Oncol* 2008;**26**:211–17.

61 Gooley TA, Chien JW, Pergam SA *et al.* Reduced mortality after allogeneic hematopoietic-cell transplantation. *N Engl J Med* 2010;**363**:2091–101.

62 Ruutu T, Eriksson B, Remes K *et al.* Ursodeoxycholic acid for the prevention of hepatic complications in allogeneic stem cell transplantation. *Blood* 2002;**100**:1977–83.

CHAPTER 2

Lymphoma: working committee and data reporting after transplantation in lymphoma

Wael Saber, Mehdi Hamadani, Shahrukh K. Hashmi and Parameswaran Hari

Introduction

Most chapters in this book discuss the role of hematopoietic cell transplantation (HCT) as an effective and often life-saving treatment strategy for patients with lymphoma. This chapter discusses the process, infrastructure, and resources that are essential for systematically collecting and analyzing data on HCT recipients, allowing unbiased evaluation of the effectiveness of HCT in various settings.

Quality assurance and improvement programs at the national and local levels are critical in ensuring that high-quality patient care is being provided. Organizations such as the Foundation for the Accreditation of Cellular Therapy (FACT) and the Joint Accreditation Committee of ISCT and EBMT (JACIE) have led the effort in developing standards and a uniform system of accreditation that have been widely adopted. However, advances in the field depend on scientifically rigorous research, allowing better appreciation of the impact of various patient, disease, and HCT-related factors on outcomes.

In 1972 the International Bone Marrow Transplant Registry (IBMTR) was established to collect data on HCT being performed in centers around the world. A similar organization was established around the same time focusing on HCT in Europe, the European Society for Blood and Marrow Transplantation (EBMT) [1]. In 1987 the National Marrow Donor Program (NMDP) was founded to develop a panel of unrelated donors for US patients. An NMDP Scientific Registry of outcomes was also established to evaluate the unrelated donor transplants the organization facilitated [2]. Other

national registries have resulted from similar efforts. The establishment of public cord blood banks for HCT was accompanied by efforts on the part of individual large banks and international organizations, such as the IBMTR and Eurocord [3], to systematically collect and analyze data on cord blood transplant outcomes. Recently, other international HCT outcomes registries, such as the Asia-Pacific BMT Registry (APBMT) [4], have been established, with similar efforts ongoing in other regions such as South America and the Middle East. In 2004, the NMDP Scientific Registry and the IBMTR became affiliated to form the Center for International Blood and Marrow Transplant Research (CIBMTR) [5]. All these initiatives have in common the goal of combining data from many centers to increase the ability to address important issues in HCT.

It is well recognized that prospective randomized clinical trials (RCTs) represent the gold standard scientific method of evaluating therapeutic interventions. However, many factors may limit the utility of RCT in evaluating various transplantation strategies. Observational databases, such as the ones maintained by CIBMTR, EBMT, and APBMT [1,4,5], can enhance understanding of HCT outcomes by addressing questions that are difficult to study within the scope of RCTs [6,7]. Although approximately 20,000 HCTs are performed yearly in the United States, only a minority are performed on clinical trials. Challenges unique to the field of HCT, such as small numbers treated at individual centers, the wide variety of indications and multiple competing risks in the peritransplant period, make it difficult to perform adequately powered

Clinical Guide to Transplantation in Lymphoma, First Edition. Edited by Bipin N. Savani and Mohamad Mohty.
© 2015 John Wiley & Sons, Ltd. Published 2015 by John Wiley & Sons, Ltd.

single-center studies. In the United States, a national multicenter transplant study network, the Blood and Marrow Transplant Clinical Trials Network (BMT CTN), has been established. However, clinical trials focus on short- and intermediate-term outcomes and the important need for long-term follow-up of transplant recipients is better addressed through observational databases. Some important questions such as the results of HCT in specific patient groups and rare diseases, analysis of prognostic factors, evaluation of new transplant regimens, comparison of HCT with nontransplant therapy, and defining inter-center variability in practice and outcome are difficult to address in randomized trials. In addition to these, the observational database also provides a platform for analyzing the availability, access, and economics of HCT. A biospecimen repository associated with the CIBMTR database allows the linkage of clinical and immunologic data and has led to important insights into transplant immunobiology.

In this chapter we will focus mainly on the CIBMTR as an example of an international stem cell transplantation outcomes database. Many of the take-home messages are quite relevant to any international outcomes registry.

Registry structure

International organizations such as the CIBMTR that depend on extensive collaboration require an overarching governing structure. For the CIBMTR, this structure is its Assembly, which includes a single representative from each CIBMTR center. An Advisory Committee is then elected from the Assembly to oversee CIBMTR operations.

Working committees

There are 15 disease-focused working committees (Table 2.1). Membership on CIBMTR working committees is open to any individual willing to play an active role in the development of studies using CIBMTR data. Each working committee is headed by two to four chairs appointed by the Advisory Committee to nonrenewable 5-year terms. Working committees are staffed by one or more MD CIBMTR scientific directors, PhD statisticians, and MS statisticians.

Table 2.1 CIBMTR working committees.

Acute leukemia
Autoimmune diseases and cellular therapies
Chronic leukemia
Donor health and safety
Graft sources and manipulation
Graft-versus-host disease (GVHD)
Health services and international issues
Immunobiology
Infection and immune reconstitution
Late effects and quality of life
Lymphoma
Nonmalignant marrow disorders and inborn errors of metabolism
Pediatric cancer
Plasma cell disorders and adult solid tumors
Regimen-related toxicity and supportive care

Data reporting

Many national governments now require transplant centers to report a set of clinical data to a central agency with variable responsibilities for addressing national health policy issues, for assessing center quality, and for research. The amount of data and analytic work required vary by country. Here we focus on the data reporting requirements of the US Stem Cell Therapeutic Outcomes Database (SCTOD). The data reporting requirements for the SCTOD were developed by an international group of investigators and clinicians that took into account the reporting requirements in other countries in order to maximize opportunities for research collaboration.

In 2005, the US government passed legislation establishing the C.W. Bill Young Cell Transplantation Program, which included five components (Figure 2.1). The SCTOD contract was awarded to the CIBMTR at the Medical College of Wisconsin. The legislation that established the C.W. Bill Young Cell Transplantation Program also made it mandatory to report outcomes data for all allogeneic (related or unrelated donor) HCTs performed in a US transplant center or using a US donor or cord blood unit. Before instituting a data collection system for the SCTOD, the CIBMTR convened a series of meetings with representatives of the American Society for Blood and Marrow Transplantation (ASBMT), EBMT,

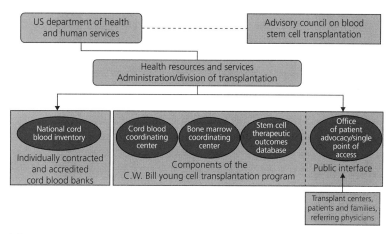

Figure 2.1 Overview of the Stem Cell Therapeutic Research Acts (includes the Stem Cell Therapeutic and Research Act of 2005 and the Stem Cell Therapeutic and Research Reauthorization Act of 2010).

APBMT, US and non-US transplant centers, donor centers, cord blood banks, donor registries, outcomes registries, regulatory agencies, and other organizations involved with HCT to establish consensus on a recommended minimal dataset to be collected for all HCT recipients, whether or not the data were required for the SCTOD. The result of these discussions was agreement on the pre- and post-transplant essential data (TED) forms [8,9]. The APBMT also agreed to utilize the TED form in establishing its own, new registry.

The data collection system for the SCTOD built on not only preexisting forms but also preexisting processes and procedures used by the CIBMTR for many years before the 2005 legislation. An important difference was the implementation of a web-based data collection platform, FormsNet™ 2, in contrast to the paper-based reporting methods used previously. FormsNet™ 2 was launched in December 2007 to be used for both SCTOD reporting and CIBMTR research reporting. FormsNet™ 2 provided bidirectional communication between centers including handling notifications for expected or missing data. It included automated validation checks within and between forms and automatically generated error reports. Some important features were 24/7 accessibility, a flexible system to modify data collection screens to accommodate new data fields, error checks, audit history trail, capability for double data entry and form reconciliation, audit tools for monitoring accuracy, and reporting tools for

continuous process improvement. The CIBMTR developed a newer version of this web-based platform with additional functionality (FormsNet3^SM), which was launched in December 2012. FormsNet3^SM features are aimed at further reducing reporting burden at local centers and enhancing accuracy with new validation tools.

An interface with the NMDP adult donor and cord blood databases allows data on unrelated donor grafts (e.g., HLA, infectious disease markers, donor gender and weight) and cord blood units (e.g., processing procedures, cell counts) to be provided directly from the donor center or cord blood bank to the CIBMTR, also decreasing the reporting burden for HCT centers and the possibility for data entry errors.

Overcoming challenges to data reporting

The major obstacles to establishing outcome registries are the time, effort, and resources required for transplant centers to report data and for registry staff to receive, manage, and analyze data. As mentioned above, the CIBMTR uses a system called FormsNet™ for data collection; the EBMT has a system called ProMISe, and the APBMT uses a system called TRUMP. To minimize data reporting burdens but allow for sophisticated scientific studies, many registries, including the CIBMTR and EBMT, use a two-tier approach for data collection. TED forms are required for all patients. For a subset of these patients a much more comprehensive dataset is obtained on a voluntary basis from centers that have agreed to submit such data (Comprehensive Report Form centers). The CIBMTR uses a weighted randomization scheme to identify patients for comprehensive reporting; the EBMT, in general, collects comprehensive data on a study-by-study basis.

Flow of data

Both the CIBMTR and EBMT try to provide ways in which the data reported to them can be returned to, or accessed by, the centers for their own use. The CIBMTR developed a system whereby transplant centers can provide required data directly to the CIBMTR from their own databases rather than reenter data into FormsNet™. This software, called AGNIS for "A Growable Network Information System," is a point-to-point communications system that "translates" center data into a common standardized language (the National Institutes of Health cancer Data Standards Repository or caDSR) so it can be shared with other centers, registries, and networks that also link to AGNIS (Figure 2.2). Once transferred using the AGNIS communications protocol, the data at the CIBMTR are validated and stored in the CIBMTR research database. AGNIS is an open source mechanism with a long-term goal of enabling an "enter once, use often" capability, reducing centers' submission burden.

Data quality

The CIBMTR ensures procurement of high-quality data by using multiple measures.

1 Consecutive reporting of all HCTs performed by the transplant centers is required to ensure that the data provide unbiased assessment of outcomes and this is verified through on-site audits.

2 Uniform reporting is ensured through several strategies, including FormsNet3SM screen pop-up windows and drop-down lists with an online data manual to supplement these instructions, an assigned clinical research coordinator for each center who is available to resolve data entry questions, posted frequently asked questions on the CIBMTR website, and through multiple web-based and in-person training opportunities.

3 Timely reporting is ensured through applying a continuous process improvement methodology.

4 Accurate reporting is ensured through on-site audits and online validations.

5 Long-term follow-up is ensured through providing "forms-due" reminders to the transplant centers, as well as providing educational tools to the centers to encourage patients to remain in contact with similar on-site audits performed at least once every 4 years [10]. Completeness of follow-up is also ensured during the development stage of studies by estimating a completeness index [11]. Centers with less than 90% completeness are approached to address reasons for incomplete follow-up.

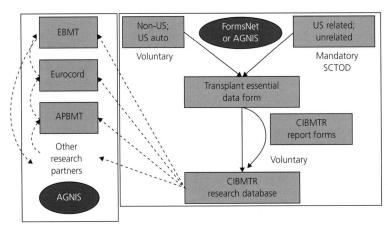

Figure 2.2 Current (solid lines) and future (dashed lines) data flow for CIBMTR and the Stem Cell Therapeutic Outcomes Database (SCTOD). EBMT, European Group for Blood and Marrow Transplantation; APBMT, Asia-Pacific BMT Registry; AGNIS, A Growable Network Information System; CIBMTR, Center for International Blood and Marrow Transplant Research.

The Lymphoma Working Committee

The Lymphoma Working Committee utilizes a two-tier system to capture data used in studies evaluating HCT outcomes among patients with lymphoma (see section Overcoming challenges to data reporting). A limited set of data is collected on the TED forms [8,9], and for a subset of patients a comprehensive set of data is collected on the lymphoma disease specific forms [12,13]. Schedule of forms submission is outlined in Table 2.2. Online manuals have been developed to provide assistance and additional instructions to HCT center data coordinators as they complete these forms [14,15].

These forms capture data on explanatory variables as well as on outcomes post HCT. Recognizing the advances in the field of stem cell transplantation, and balancing the importance of new information and challenges associated with systematic collection of new data, the forms undergo periodic revisions where new variables deemed critical are included and older variables deemed no longer needed are removed. However, inherent limitations of data submitted to a registry (e.g., lack of central pathologic examination) that cannot be resolved through form revisions, and the impact of these limitations on the internal and external validity of studies, must always be considered while drawing inferences.

Statistical methods

It is important to stress that the principles of performing high-quality clinical studies using observational databases are similar to those applied in RCTs. These include clearly stated hypotheses and objectives, inclusion and exclusion criteria that will determine the selection of the population and the external validity of the study, and a study design and an analysis plan that will ensure internal validity.

Type of data

Post-HCT outcomes that are commonly analyzed can represent two different types of data. The first type is survival data, which include incidence of death and treatment failure (combined end points of death or relapse/progression after HCT; in other words, inverse of progression-free survival). Patients either experience the event or are censored at the time of last contact. Kaplan–Meier survival curves are used to summarize these data. The second type of data is the competing risk data, which means that the occurrence of one event precludes the occurrence of another event. Examples of this type include relapse/progression (nonrelapse death being the corresponding competing risk). Similar competing risk events include transplant-related mortality (TRM) or nonrelapse mortality (competing with relapse), neutrophil and platelet recovery (competing with death before engraftment), acute graft-versus-host disease (GVHD), chronic GVHD, infections, and late complications [16] These data are summarized using cumulative incidence function (CIF) to account for the competing risk [16].

Intervals and patient selection

Investigators are frequently interested in summarizing these outcomes or in comparing the incidence between two or more groups of patients. Even though certain outcomes are expected to occur preferentially in a given post-HCT interval (e.g., most TRM occurs early), the occurrence is still random. Therefore, it is critical to handle the "time to event" carefully. To do so, clear definition of the starting point is a must. For example, even though the HCT date is used as the time origin in most studies, if the objective were to compare transplant to nontransplant therapies, the date of diagnosis would represent the most appropriate starting point [16].

It is also critical to define the "at-risk" population. Patients who have no chance of developing the outcome of interest should not be included in the denominator. For example, if an investigator wishes to estimate the incidence of death after GVHD, only patients who developed GVHD should be included in the study population.

Unadjusted comparison

Descriptive studies that only aim to summarize the incidence of post-HCT outcomes can be informative; however, most investigators are interested in comparing groups of patients. Unadjusted comparison is the simplest form of statistical comparative analysis. For this analysis we are only interested in crude comparisons of the groups. It allows us to better understand the distribution of events as they occur in multiple groups. And by comparing the results with subsequent results from adjusted comparisons (see next section), we can have a better understanding of the relationships between

Table 2.2 Form submission schedule.

Form	Baseline	Time post transplant[*]																
		0	7	14	21	28	35	42	49	56	63	70	77	84	91	100	6 months	1 year	2 years
CIBMTR Recipient ID Form	×																		
Transplant Form		×																	
CIBMTR 2400[†]	×																		
CIBMTR 2000, 2004, 2005, 2006, disease specific form[†]		×																	
CIBMTR 2100[‡]																×			
CIBMTR 2200[‡]																×	×	×	×
CIBMTR Disease-Specific Inserts[§]																×	×	×	×
CIBMTR 2900						Event-driven at time of death													

[*]Days, unless stated otherwise.
[†]Used to capture baseline, pretransplant and transplant data, including conditioning regimen and GVHD prophylaxis.
[‡]Used to capture acute and chronic GVHD after day 100, as well as lung injury, VOD/SOS, TMA.
[§]Used to capture relapse/progression after day 100.

multiple variables, and especially if any covariables play a role in actually determining the outcomes (i.e., confounding).

There are three approaches in carrying out this type of analysis [16]. The first involves events that occur early after transplant, such as engraftment. In this situation, we may choose an interval in advance. Patients who experience the event in this interval are considered a "success" while those who were observed for the entire interval but did not develop the event would be considered "failures." The second approach involves comparing survival data or competing risk data at fixed time points, for example an investigator may be interested in comparing survival or TRM at 1 year after HCT. In both of these types of analyses, patients with incomplete follow-up data are excluded from the analysis [16]. The third approach involves comparing the entire survival experience for different groups by comparing their hazard rates. Here we use a weighted log-rank test [16].

Adjusted comparison

As mentioned above, in unadjusted comparisons confounding is a concern. This is especially important given that the assignment in retrospective studies (such as the analyses conducted within a registry) is not random, which means that important risk factors could exhibit serious imbalance between groups of interest. If there is an observed difference in outcomes between the groups, it could be driven by this risk factor imbalance (i.e., confounding is said to be present). Regression models are used to control for this imbalance. The most frequently used regression model is the Cox proportional hazards model. The Cox model uses hazard rate to model timing of events. The hazard rate is the chance of the event of interest occurring in the next instant of time for a patient yet to experience the event. In addition to controlling for confounders, Cox models are often used in studies aiming to identify prognostic factors associated with outcomes of interest. Depending on the sample size available for analysis, these studies often go on to develop risk scores for clinical decision-making [17].

For the results to be valid, the Cox model assumptions must be satisfied. The most important assumption is the proportionality assumption. When there is clear violation of this assumption, ways of addressing this issue include dividing the post-HCT course into distinct time intervals so that within each interval the proportionality assumption holds. Alternatively, when nonproportionality is affecting a specific covariate, we can stratify the Cox model on this covariate [18].

The Cox model can be used to analyze survival data (death and treatment failure) as well as competing risk data. For the latter, it models cause-specific hazard [19], which is defined as the rate at which patients at risk for experiencing the event of interest, as well as the competing event (e.g., if TRM is the event of interest, relapse/progression would be the competing risk), actually experience the event of interest.

Another approach for analyzing competing risk data that is frequently used involves the use of pseudo-value regression [20]. This method allows us to directly model the CIF at a fixed time point as well as compare the entire cumulative incidence curve [20]. Other methods that can directly model the CIF and allow us to compare the entire cumulative incidence curve is the subdistribution hazard model introduced by Fine and Gray [21].

It is important to note that the results of the cause-specific Cox model and pseudo-value regression for competing risk data could be quite different [19]. Therefore, it is critical that the investigator clearly defines the aim of the analysis.

Selected examples from the CIBMTR Lymphoma Committee

Diseases such as lymphoma, for which HCT is indicated, are uncommon. Diffuse large B-cell lymphoma (DLBCL), the most frequent non-Hodgkin lymphoma subtype, occurs with a frequency of 7.14 per 100,000 persons [22]. When we compare the age-adjusted incidence of DLBCL with that of coronary heart disease (17 per 1000 men aged 35–64 and 44 per 1000 men aged ≥65 years [23]), we can appreciate the logistical challenges of launching sufficiently powered RCTs that would accrue in a timely manner for DLBCL relative to coronary heart disease. Indeed, slow accrual was the main barrier that led to the premature termination of a comparative biologic assignment prospective trial comparing autologous HCT to reduced-intensity conditioning (RIC) allogeneic HCT in patients with chemosensitive follicular lymphoma that were beyond their first complete remission

[24]. Whereas such an important question was difficult to tackle in a prospective setting, it was quite feasible in a registry setting [25].

Other examples of studies that can be quite challenging in an RCT setting but which, with careful statistical analyses, could be conducted quite readily within a registry setting include evaluation of allogeneic HCT outcomes among patients with chemorefractory follicular lymphoma/DLBCL and mantle cell lymphoma [26,27], evaluation of the optimal conditioning regimen intensity in allogeneic HCT for follicular lymphoma and DLBCL [28,29], impact of new drugs that have already been widely adopted in routine practice on HCT outcomes [30], and evaluation of optimal type [31,32] and timing of HCT [32].

It is also well known that not all important clinical questions lend themselves to randomization. Studies conducted within the Lymphoma Committee/CIBMTR have successfully addressed a number of these questions. Examples include impact of age [33,34], histology [34], race [35,36], body mass index [37], donor type [31,38–43], and socioeconomic status on HCT outcomes [36].

Other examples where registry-based analysis have already helped to advance the field include identification of risk factors that can independently predict key HCT outcomes for patients with Hodgkin lymphoma [17], and analysis of HCT outcomes among patients with rare types or presenting sites of lymphoma [44–46] or among special populations where the incidence of lymphoma is especially low, as in children [47].

Furthermore, RCTs are best suited to evaluating short- and intermediate-term goals, and since there is a growing population of long-term HCT survivors, there is an urgent need to understand how different HCT strategies can impact long-term outcomes such as second malignancies and additional risk of late mortality [48,49].

Another important role of observational databases is to inform the design of future prospective clinical trials. Analyses of these data can provide average estimates of baseline rates of key clinical outcomes among the population of interest, both overall but also among subgroups of special importance. This information can greatly inform power calculations and sample size estimates. These analyses can also provide estimates of available patients for accrual and this can help in planning of the trial. Furthermore, by providing data on the pattern of occurrence of key events after HCT, the timing of evaluating outcomes post HCT among patients enrolled in an RCT will be better defined. For example, the primary outcome in a Phase III RCT comparing two conditioning regimens among patients with DLBCL undergoing autologous HCT was 2-year progression-free survival [50]. The choice of 2 years was based on data from the CIBMTR that suggested that the hazard for treatment failure (progression/death) was negligible after 2 years. In a recently launched Phase III randomized double-blind clinical trial comparing a novel drug, ibrutinib, to placebo during and after autologous HCT in patients with refractory/relapsed DLBCL of the activated B-cell subtype, based on CIBMTR data the investigators are estimating that nine patients will be accrued per month, and thus with a target accrual goal of 296, the protocol includes a 3-year accrual plan. This affects trial budget and administration plans (BMT CTN 1201; Timothy Fenske, personal communication, April 2014).

Value for young investigators

CIBMTR (and other registries) provide opportunities for members of the transplant community to propose and conduct studies using registry data. By taking an active role in the committees, young investigators can participate in or even lead a study with an international group of senior collaborators. Information about resources available and instructions for proposing a study or requesting data from the CIBMTR can be found at www.cibmtr.org/Studies/Observational.

Value for public and other stakeholders

In addition to systematic enquiries, the large-scale registry data support custom analyses from clinicians, patients, and in fact anyone interested in transplant data. Any interested party can request CIBMTR data using the Custom Information Request Form (inforequest@mcw.edu). Common requests using this mechanism are for descriptive statistics describing populations of interest and univariate analyses of survival. Many requests are related to patient care and clinical decision-making.

Conclusion

Given the rarity of diseases treated by HCT, RCTs aiming to address critical questions are quite challenging to perform, which can be a barrier to advancing the field.

Observational databases, such as the CIBMTR, have helped overcome this barrier by facilitating rigorous scientific evidence-based assessment of HCT outcomes. International collaboration to build and maintain these databases is an integral part of the HCT scientific culture and has served to facilitate progress in the field.

References

1 European Society for Blood and Marrow Transplantation. Available at https://www.ebmt.org/Contents/Pages/Default.aspx (accessed April 10, 2014)

2 National Marrow Donor Program. Available at http://bethematch.org/ (accessed April 16, 2014).

3 EUROCORD. Available at http://www.eurocord.org/index.php?setLang=EN (accessed April 16, 2014).

4 Asia-Pacific Blood and Marrow Transplantation Group. Available at http://www.apbmt.org/ (accessed April 16, 2014).

5 Center for International Blood and Marrow Transplant Research. Available at http://www.cibmtr.org/pages/index.aspx (accessed April 10, 2014).

6 Horowitz M. The role of registries in facilitating clinical research in BMT: examples from the Center for International Blood and Marrow Transplant Research. *Bone Marrow Transplant* 2008;**42**(Suppl 1):S1–S2.

7 Gliklich RE, Dreyer NA. *Registries for Evaluating Patient Outcomes: A User's Guide*, 2nd edn. Rockville, MD: Agency for Healthcare Research and Quality (US), 2010.

8 Center for International Blood and Marrow Transplant Research. Pretransplant essential data. http://www.cibmtr.org/DataManagement/DataCollectionForms/Documents/2400/Rev4.0/Form_2400_R4+.pdf (accessed April 18, 2014).

9 Center for International Blood and Marrow Transplant Research. Post-transplant essential data. http://www.cibmtr.org/DataManagement/DataCollectionForms/Documents/2450/Rev3.0/2450R3.0.pdf (accessed April 18, 2014).

10 Center for International Blood and Marrow Transplant Research. Annual Progress Report. www.cibmtr.org/About/ProceduresProgress/Documents/2012_CIBMTR_Annual_R.pdf (accessed April 18, 2014).

11 Clark TG, Altman DG, De Stavola BL. Quantification of the completeness of follow-up. *Lancet* 2002;**359**:1309–10.

12 Center for International Blood and Marrow Transplant Research. Hodgkin and non-Hodgkin lymphoma pre-HCT data (Form 2018). http://www.cibmtr.org/DataManagement/DataCollectionForms/Documents/2018/Rev3.0/Form_2018_R3+.pdf (accessed April 18, 2014).

13 Center for International Blood and Marrow Transplant Research. Hodgkin and non-Hodgkin lymphoma post-HCT data (Form 2118). http://www.cibmtr.org/DataManagement/DataCollectionForms/Documents/2118/Rev3.0/Form_2118_R3+.pdf (accessed April 18, 2014).

14 Center for International Blood and Marrow Transplant Research. Instructions for Hodgkin and non-Hodgkin lymphoma pre-HCT data (Form 2018). http://www.cibmtr.org/DataManagement/TrainingReference/Manuals/DataManagement/Documents/CIBMTR%202018%20Pre-HCT%20LYM_v2.0.pdf (accessed April 18, 2014).

15 Center for International Blood and Marrow Transplant Research. Instructions for Hodgkin and non-Hodgkin lymphoma post-HCT data (Form 2118). http://www.cibmtr.org/DataManagement/TrainingReference/Manuals/DataManagement/Documents/CIBMTR%202118%20Post-HCT%20LYM_v2.0.pdf (accessed April 18, 2014).

16 Klein JP, Rizzo JD, Zhang MJ, Keiding N. Statistical methods for the analysis and presentation of the results of bone marrow transplants. Part I: unadjusted analysis. *Bone Marrow Transplant* 2001;**28**:909–15.

17 Hahn T, McCarthy PL, Carreras J et al. Simplified validated prognostic model for progression-free survival after autologous transplantation for Hodgkin lymphoma. *Biol Blood Marrow Transplant* 2013;**19**:1740–4.

18 Klein JP, Rizzo JD, Zhang MJ, Keiding N. Statistical methods for the analysis and presentation of the results of bone marrow transplants. Part 2: Regression modeling. *Bone Marrow Transplant* 2001;**28**:1001–11.

19 Logan BR, Zhang MJ, Klein JP. Regression models for hazard rates versus cumulative incidence probabilities in hematopoietic cell transplantation data. *Biol Blood Marrow Transplant* 2006;**12**(1 Suppl 1):107–12.

20 Klein JP, Andersen PK. Regression modeling of competing risks data based on pseudovalues of the cumulative incidence function. *Biometrics* 2005;**61**:223–9.

21 Fine JP, Gray RJ. A proportional hazards model for the subdistribution of a competing risk. *J Am Stat Assoc* 1999;**94**:496–509.

22 Morton LM, Wang SS, Devesa SS, Hartge P, Weisenburger DD, Linet MS. Lymphoma incidence patterns by WHO subtype in the United States, 1992–2001. *Blood* 2006;**107**:265–76.

23 Lerner DJ, Kannel WB. Patterns of coronary heart disease morbidity and mortality in the sexes: a 26-year follow-up of the Framingham population. *Am Heart J* 1986;**111**:383–90.

24 Tomblyn MR, Ewell M, Bredeson C et al. Autologous versus reduced-intensity allogeneic hematopoietic cell transplantation for patients with chemosensitive follicular non-Hodgkin lymphoma beyond first complete response or first partial response. *Biol Blood Marrow Transplant* 2011;**17**:1051–7.

25 van Besien K, Loberiza FR Jr, Bajorunaite R et al. Comparison of autologous and allogeneic hematopoietic stem cell transplantation for follicular lymphoma. *Blood* 2003;**102**:3521–9.

26 Hamadani M, Saber W, Ahn KW et al. Allogeneic hematopoietic cell transplantation for chemotherapy-unresponsive mantle cell lymphoma: a cohort analysis from the Center for International Blood and Marrow Transplant Research. *Biol Blood Marrow Transplant* 2013;**19**:625–31.

27 Hamadani M, Saber W, Ahn KW et al. Impact of pretransplantation conditioning regimens on outcomes of allogeneic transplantation for chemotherapy-unresponsive diffuse large B cell lymphoma and grade III follicular lymphoma. *Biol Blood Marrow Transplant* 2013;**19**:746–53.

28 Hari P, Carreras J, Zhang MJ *et al.* Allogeneic transplants in follicular lymphoma: higher risk of disease progression after reduced-intensity compared to myeloablative conditioning. *Biol Blood Marrow Transplant* 2008;**14**:236–45.

29 Bacher U, Klyuchnikov E, Le-Rademacher J *et al.* Conditioning regimens for allotransplants for diffuse large B-cell lymphoma: myeloablative or reduced intensity? *Blood* 2012;**120**:4256–62.

30 Fenske TS, Hari PN, Carreras J *et al.* Impact of pre-transplant rituximab on survival after autologous hematopoietic stem cell transplantation for diffuse large B cell lymphoma. *Biol Blood Marrow Transplant* 2009;**15**:1455–64.

31 Smith SM, Burns LJ, van Besien K *et al.* Hematopoietic cell transplantation for systemic mature T-cell non-Hodgkin lymphoma. *J Clin Oncol* 2013;**31**:3100–9.

32 Fenske TS, Zhang MJ, Carreras J *et al.* Autologous or reduced-intensity conditioning allogeneic hematopoietic cell transplantation for chemotherapy-sensitive mantle-cell lymphoma: analysis of transplantation timing and modality. *J Clin Oncol* 2014;**32**:273–81.

33 McClune BL, Ahn KW, Wang HL *et al.* Allotransplantation for patients aged ≥40 years with non-Hodgkin lymphoma: encouraging progression-free survival. *Biol Blood Marrow Transplant* 2014;**20**:960–8.

34 Lazarus HM, Carreras J, Boudreau C *et al.* Influence of age and histology on outcome in adult non-Hodgkin lymphoma patients undergoing autologous hematopoietic cell transplantation (HCT): a report from the Center For International Blood and Marrow Transplant Research (CIBMTR). *Biol Blood Marrow Transplant* 2008;**14**:1323–33.

35 Joshua TV, Rizzo JD, Zhang MJ *et al.* Access to hematopoietic stem cell transplantation: effect of race and sex. *Cancer* 2010;**116**:3469–76.

36 Baker KS, Davies SM, Majhail NS *et al.* Race and socioeconomic status influence outcomes of unrelated donor hematopoietic cell transplantation. *Biol Blood Marrow Transplant* 2009;**15**:1543–54.

37 Navarro WH, Loberiza FR Jr, Bajorunaite R *et al.* Effect of body mass index on mortality of patients with lymphoma undergoing autologous hematopoietic cell transplantation. *Biol Blood Marrow Transplant* 2006;**12**:541–51.

38 Hale GA, Shrestha S, Le-Rademacher J *et al.* Alternate donor hematopoietic cell transplantation (HCT) in non-Hodgkin lymphoma using lower intensity conditioning: a report from the CIBMTR. *Biol Blood Marrow Transplant* 2012;**18**:1036–43 e1.

39 Bachanova V, Brunstein C, Burns LJ *et al.* (eds) Alternative donor transplantation for adults with lymphoma: comparison of umbilical cord blood versus 8/8 HLA-matched donor (URD) versus 7/8 URD. *Blood (ASH Annual Meeting Abstracts)* 2013;**122**:161.

40 Lazarus HM, Zhang MJ, Carreras J *et al.* A comparison of HLA-identical sibling allogeneic versus autologous transplantation for diffuse large B cell lymphoma: a report from the CIBMTR. *Biol Blood Marrow Transplant* 2010;**16**:35–45.

41 Freytes CO, Zhang MJ, Carreras J *et al.* Outcome of lower-intensity allogeneic transplantation in non-Hodgkin lymphoma after autologous transplantation failure. *Biol Blood Marrow Transplant* 2012;**18**:1255–64.

42 Bierman PJ, Sweetenham JW, Loberiza FR Jr *et al.* Syngeneic hematopoietic stem-cell transplantation for non-Hodgkin's lymphoma: a comparison with allogeneic and autologous transplantation. The Lymphoma Working Committee of the International Bone Marrow Transplant Registry and the European Group for Blood and Marrow Transplantation. *J Clin Oncol* 2003;**21**:3744–53.

43 Smith SM, van Besien K, Carreras J *et al.* Second autologous stem cell transplantation for relapsed lymphoma after a prior autologous transplant. *Biol Blood Marrow Transplant* 2008;**14**:904–12.

44 Maramattom LV, Hari PN, Burns LJ *et al.* Autologous and allogeneic transplantation for Burkitt lymphoma outcomes and changes in utilization: a report from the Center for International Blood and Marrow Transplant Research. *Biol Blood Marrow Transplant* 2013;**19**:173–9.

45 Maziarz RT, Wang Z, Zhang MJ *et al.* Autologous haematopoietic cell transplantation for non-Hodgkin lymphoma with secondary CNS involvement. *Br J Haematol* 2013;**162**:648–56.

46 Wirk B, Fenske TS, Hamadani M *et al.* Outcomes of hematopoietic cell transplantation for diffuse large B cell lymphoma transformed from follicular lymphoma. *Biol Blood Marrow Transplant* 2014;**20**:951–9.

47 Gross TG, Hale GA, He W *et al.* Hematopoietic stem cell transplantation for refractory or recurrent non-Hodgkin lymphoma in children and adolescents. *Biol Blood Marrow Transplant* 2010;**16**:223–30.

48 Wingard JR, Majhail NS, Brazauskas R *et al.* Long-term survival and late deaths after allogeneic hematopoietic cell transplantation. *J Clin Oncol* 2011;**29**:2230–9.

49 Metayer C, Curtis RE, Vose J *et al.* Myelodysplastic syndrome and acute myeloid leukemia after autotransplantation for lymphoma: a multicenter case-control study. *Blood* 2003;**101**:2015–23.

50 Vose JM, Carter S, Burns LJ *et al.* Phase III randomized study of rituximab/carmustine, etoposide, cytarabine, and melphalan (BEAM) compared with iodine-131 tositumomab/BEAM with autologous hematopoietic cell transplantation for relapsed diffuse large B-cell lymphoma: results from the BMT CTN 0401 trial. *J Clin Oncol* 2013;**31**:1662–8.

CHAPTER 3

Use of transplantation in lymphoma: adults

Parastoo Bahrami Dahi, Gabriela Soriano Hobbs and Miguel-Angel Perales

Introduction

Autologous and allogeneic hematopoietic stem cell transplantation (SCT) are routinely performed in patients with lymphoma. Autologous SCT is the most common transplant for lymphoma, while allogeneic SCT is typically reserved for patients who have failed an autologous SCT or who have particularly high-risk relapsed or refractory disease.

The outcomes of autologous and allogeneic SCT in patients with lymphoma have improved over time, leading to increasing numbers of transplants as well as extension of this procedure to older patients. In particular, the number of transplants facilitated by the National Marrow Donor Program (NMDP) for non-Hodgkin lymphoma (NHL) patients older than 50 years has significantly increased over the last decade [1]. This is attributed to the development of reduced-intensity conditioning (RIC) regimens, improved donor–patient HLA matching, and better post-transplant care.

This chapter provides an overview of indications for transplant in lymphoma based on review of the medical literature, including comprehensive evidence-based reviews and guidelines from the National Comprehensive Cancer Network (NCCN), Center for International Blood and Marrow Transplant Research (CIBMTR), American Society of Bone Marrow Transplant (ASBMT) and NMDP. Because of the heterogeneity of lymphomas, transplant indications are discussed according to histology. Table 3.1 summarizes the transplant indications in lymphomas.

Hodgkin lymphoma

Approximately 9000 individuals are diagnosed with Hodgkin lymphoma (HL) each year in the United States. Most patients are diagnosed between the ages of 15 and 30 years, followed by another peak at age 55 and older [2]. Significant progress has been made in the treatment of patients with HL, with cure rates of 80% or higher using chemotherapeutic approaches [3].

Several studies have shown that high-dose therapy/autologous stem cell transplant (HDT/ASCT) should be the standard treatment for patients with chemosensitive relapsed or refractory HL [4–7]. Using the Deauville criteria for the interpretation of interim or end-of-treatment positron emission tomography (PET) [8], the NCCN recommendation for patients with a Deauville score of 1–3 after second-line chemotherapy is HDT/ASCT [9]. For a Deauville score of 4–5, additional second-line chemotherapy followed by restaging is recommended. Those with a score of 4 can be treated with HDT/ASCT. Patients with disease refractory to second-line chemotherapy who are not chemosensitive should be given a trial of brentuximab vedotin prior to consideration of HDT/ASCT [9].

Different prognostic models have been used to predict outcomes of HDT/ASCT in patients with relapsed or refractory disease. Adverse outcomes have been identified as associated with short remission duration (<12 months), extranodal disease, primary refractory disease, B symptoms, bulky disease at diagnosis, and detectable disease at transplant [10–12]. Pretransplant

Clinical Guide to Transplantation in Lymphoma, First Edition. Edited by Bipin N. Savani and Mohamad Mohty.
© 2015 John Wiley & Sons, Ltd. Published 2015 by John Wiley & Sons, Ltd.

Table 3.1 Transplant indications in lymphomas by histology.

Histology	HL	DLBCL	FL	MCL	PCNSL	PTCL
Autologous SCT	Consolidate in ≥CR2, or relapse/ refractory	Consolidate in ≥CR2, or relapse/ refractory	Consolidate in ≥CR2, or relapse/ refractory	Consolidate in CR1/PR1, or relapse/refractory	Consolidate in ≥CR2, or relapse/ refractory	Consolidate in CR1/PR1, or relapse/refractory
Allogeneic SCT	Relapse/refractory	Relapse/refractory	Relapse/refractory	Relapse/refractory	—	Relapse/refractory

HL, Hodgkin lymphoma; DLBCL, diffuse large B-cell lymphoma; FL, follicular lymphoma; MCL, mantle cell lymphoma; PTCL, peripheral T-cell lymphoma; PCNSL, primary central nervous system lymphoma.

functional imaging status has also been identified as an independent predictor of outcome [13–15].

Allogeneic SCT with myeloablative conditioning (MAC) has been associated with lower relapse rate in patients with relapsed or refractory disease; however, its use has been limited by high transplant-related mortality (TRM) [16]. The advent of RIC transplants has been associated with decreased rates of TRM and has become the standard approach, particularly in patients who have relapsed after autologous SCT [17,18].

Non-Hodgkin lymphoma

NHL represents a highly heterogeneous group of lymphoproliferative disorders originating in B lymphocytes, T lymphocytes, or natural killer (NK) cells. In the United States, B-cell NHL represents 80–85% of cases and T-cell NHL 15–20%; NK cell NHL is rare.

Diffuse large B-cell lymphoma

The addition of rituximab to combination chemotherapy significantly improved outcomes for patients with diffuse large B-cell lymphoma (DLBCL). Despite this, 20–50% of patients either relapse or do not achieve a remission with first-line chemotherapy. This has prompted several studies investigating the role of HDT/ASCT as part of upfront consolidation therapy [19–21]. Most of these studies were done in the pre-rituximab era. More recently, a SWOG study included patients receiving rituximab [22] and demonstrated that upfront autologous SCT prolongs progression-free survival (PFS) but not overall survival (OS). In contrast to upfront therapy, HDT/ASCT is the standard of care in the setting of relapsed disease and is associated with improved OS and PFS [23–25]. Patients with chemosensitive disease

experience response rates of 40–50% and those with refractory disease of 10–20% [25,26].

Early studies using allogeneic SCT for DLBCL utilized MAC and were associated with high TRM [27–29]. Recent studies have reported on both RIC and MAC with encouraging results [30–32]. Additional studies utilizing only RIC show similar outcome, with lower TRM than seen with the use of MAC [33].

Follicular lymphoma

Follicular lymphoma (FL) is the most common subtype of indolent NHL and accounts for about 22% of all newly diagnosed cases of NHL [34]. Although HDT/ASCT improves PFS in FL, it is not recommended as first-line treatment because of no significant improvement in OS, a higher incidence of secondary myelodysplastic syndrome and acute myeloid leukemia, and a lack of comparative data with rituximab-containing regimens [35–38]. Longer follow-up may be needed to identify differences in OS [39]. There are insufficient data to make recommendations on the use of autologous SCT versus nontransplantation therapy as salvage treatment for patients who have had rituximab as part of their salvage therapy [40].

For patients in remission after second-line therapy, maintenance rituximab can be recommended. However, if a patient progressed during or within 6 months of first-line maintenance, the clinical benefit of maintenance in second line is likely minimal. HDT/ASCT is an appropriate consolidative therapy for patients in second or third remission. HDT/ASCT has been shown to prolong OS and PFS in patients with relapsed or refractory disease [38,41–43].

There are insufficient data comparing autologous and allogeneic SCT to recommend one option over the other in relapsed/refractory FL; both appear to have a survival benefit, but have competing risks [44]. Studies have shown RIC allogeneic SCT to be an acceptable alternative approach [38,45–48].

Histologic transformation to DLBCL

Patients with histologic transformation to DLBCL generally have a poor clinical outcome and those responding to initial treatment (complete or partial response) could be considered for consolidation therapy with autologous or allogeneic SCT or a clinical trial [49].

Mantle cell lymphoma

Mantle cell lymphoma (MCL) comprises about 6% of all NHL and usually presents as advanced-stage disease [50]. Although the disease is incurable with chemotherapy alone, several retrospective and prospective studies have shown durable responses with intensive chemotherapies containing rituximab and cytarabine followed by HDT/ASCT [51–57]. Based on these studies, an intensive induction chemotherapy followed by autologous SCT in first remission is recommended for fit patients.

The effect of HDT/ASCT in salvage settings is less clear. Some studies have shown poor outcomes [58,59], while others have shown it to be an acceptable option in salvage setting [60,61].

Despite therapeutic approaches that utilize rituximab-containing intensive chemotherapy followed by autologous SCT, patients experience relapse. Several studies have shown RIC allogeneic SCT to be a feasible and effective treatment for relapsed disease [47,48,60,62–64].

Burkitt lymphoma

Durable remissions following intensive chemotherapy is seen in 60–90% of patients with Burkitt lymphoma [65,66]. Autologous and allogeneic SCT are appropriate options for patients with Burkitt lymphoma beyond first remission and result in comparable outcomes [67,68].

Primary CNS lymphoma

Primary central nervous system (CNS) lymphoma accounts for 3% of primary CNS tumors. HDT/ASCT can be considered for patients with relapsed/refractory disease [69–71].

Peripheral T-cell lymphoma

Peripheral T-cell lymphoma (PTCL) accounts for 10% of NHL [34]. Prognosis is generally poor due to low response rates and less durable responses to conventional chemotherapy. Several retrospective and prospective studies have reported improved outcomes with HDT/ASCT in first remission [72–75]. While HDT/ASCT infrequently results in a durable benefit in patients with relapsed/refractory disease, allogeneic SCT has shown improved outcomes with both MAC and RIC regimens [76–80].

Prognostic tools

Different prognostic tools have been used to predict outcomes of transplant in patients with lymphoma. Hamlin *et al.* [81] have shown second-line age-adjusted international prognostic index (aaIPI) as a tool to predict outcomes of HDT/ASCT in patients with relapsed/refractory DLBCL. Similarly, the second-line aaIPI was also shown to predict outcomes in patients with advanced NHL who underwent allogeneic SCT [82]. Another useful tool is the hematopoietic cell transplantation comorbidity index (HCT-CI), which has been shown to predict risk of TRM and survival after autologous and allogeneic transplantation [83–85].

Maintenance therapies

Maintenance therapy using rituximab at different time points after autologous SCT in MCL has been studied in prospective Phase II studies with improved outcome [86–89]. The timing, dose, and duration of therapy have yet to be determined. Other agents that are currently being investigated for potential maintenance therapy post transplant in MCL include bortezomib, lenalidomide, and ibrutinib. The CORAL study did not show benefit from maintenance rituximab after autologous SCT in DLBCL [90,91]. Romidepsin and vorinostat are being evaluated as maintenance after autologous transplantation in PTCL. The role of maintenance brentuximab vedotin after transplantation in patients with HL is being studied in the AETHERA trial [92].

Novel therapies

In recent years, multiple targeted therapies for patients with lymphoma have been developed. These include, but are not limited to, anti-CD20 monoclonal antibodies (rituximab, obinotuzumab), anti-CD30 monoclonal antibody (brentuximab vedotin), proteasome inhibitors (bortezomib), mTOR inhibitors (temsirolimus, everolimus), immunomodulatory agents (lenalidomide), Bruton's tyrosine kinase (BTK) inhibitors (ibruitinib), and PI3K inhibitors (idelalisib).

Conclusions

Autologous and allogeneic SCT play a significant role in the treatment of patients with lymphoma. With ongoing development and integration of novel agents in the treatment of lymphoma, the applicability and timing of transplantation in these diseases is continuously evolving. At the same time, developments in conditioning regimens and maintenance treatments following autologous and allogeneic SCT should result in improved outcomes of transplantation in lymphoma.

References

1 Pasquini MC, Wang Z. Current use and outcome of hematopoietic stem cell transplantation: CIBMTR Summary Slides, 2013. Available at http://www.cibmtr.org

2 Siegel R, Ma J, Zou Z, Jemal A. Cancer statistics, 2014. *CA: Cancer J Clin* 2014;**64**:9–29.

3 Diehl V, Franklin J, Pfreundschuh M *et al.* Standard and increased-dose BEACOPP chemotherapy compared with COPP-ABVD for advanced Hodgkin's disease. *N Engl J Med* 2003;**348**:2386–95.

4 Linch DC, Winfield D, Goldstone AH *et al.* Dose intensification with autologous bone-marrow transplantation in relapsed and resistant Hodgkin's disease: results of a BNLI randomised trial. *Lancet* 1993;**341**:1051–4.

5 Schmitz N, Pfistner B, Sextro M *et al.* Aggressive conventional chemotherapy compared with high-dose chemotherapy with autologous haemopoietic stem-cell transplantation for relapsed chemosensitive Hodgkin's disease: a randomised trial. *Lancet* 2002;**359**:2065–71.

6 Moskowitz CH, Kewalramani T, Nimer SD, Gonzalez M, Zelenetz AD, Yahalom J. Effectiveness of high dose chemoradiotherapy and autologous stem cell transplantation for patients with biopsy-proven primary refractory Hodgkin's disease. *Br J Haematol* 2004;**124**:645–52.

7 Sirohi B, Cunningham D, Powles R *et al.* Long-term outcome of autologous stem-cell transplantation in relapsed or refractory Hodgkin's lymphoma. *Ann Oncol* 2008;**19**:1312–19.

8 Meignan M, Gallamini A, Itti E, Barrington S, Haioun C, Polliack A. Report on the Third International Workshop on Interim Positron Emission Tomography in Lymphoma held in Menton, France, 26–27 September 2011 and Menton 2011 consensus. *Leukemia Lymphoma* 2012;**53**:1876–81.

9 National Comprehensive Cancer Network Guidelines version 2.2014. Hodgkin lymphoma. http://www.nccn.org/professionals/physician_gls/f_guidelines.asp (accessed April 20, 2014).

10 Brice P, Bouabdallah R, Moreau P *et al.* Prognostic factors for survival after high-dose therapy and autologous stem cell transplantation for patients with relapsing Hodgkin's disease: analysis of 280 patients from the French registry. *Bone Marrow Transplant* 1997;**20**:21–6.

11 Moskowitz CH, Nimer SD, Zelenetz AD *et al.* A two-step comprehensive high-dose chemoradiotherapy second-line program for relapsed and refractory Hodgkin disease: analysis by intent to treat and development of a prognostic model. *Blood* 2001;**97**:616–23.

12 Sureda A, Constans M, Iriondo A *et al.* Prognostic factors affecting long-term outcome after stem cell transplantation in Hodgkin's lymphoma autografted after a first relapse. *Ann Oncol* 2005;**16**:625–33.

13 Jabbour E, Hosing C, Ayers G *et al.* Pretransplant positive positron emission tomography/gallium scans predict poor outcome in patients with recurrent/refractory Hodgkin lymphoma. *Cancer* 2007;**109**:2481–9.

14 Smeltzer JP, Cashen AF, Zhang Q *et al.* Prognostic significance of FDG-PET in relapsed or refractory classical Hodgkin lymphoma treated with standard salvage chemotherapy and autologous stem cell transplantation. *Biol Blood Marrow Transplant* 2011;**17**:1646–52.

15 Moskowitz CH, Matasar MJ, Zelenetz AD *et al.* Normalization of pre-ASCT, FDG-PET imaging with second-line, non-cross-resistant, chemotherapy programs improves event-free survival in patients with Hodgkin lymphoma. *Blood* 2012;**119**:1665–70.

16 Gajewski JL, Phillips GL, Sobocinski KA *et al.* Bone marrow transplants from HLA-identical siblings in advanced Hodgkin's disease. *J Clin Oncol* 1996;**14**:572–8.

17 Alvarez I, Sureda A, Caballero MD *et al.* Nonmyeloablative stem cell transplantation is an effective therapy for refractory or relapsed Hodgkin lymphoma: results of a Spanish prospective cooperative protocol. *Biol Blood Marrow Transplant* 2006;**12**:172–83.

18 Sureda A, Canals C, Arranz R *et al.* Allogeneic stem cell transplantation after reduced intensity conditioning in patients with relapsed or refractory Hodgkin's lymphoma. Results of the HDR-ALLO study: a prospective clinical trial by the Grupo Espanol de Linfomas/Trasplante de Medula Osea (GEL/TAMO) and the Lymphoma Working Party of the European Group for Blood and Marrow Transplantation. *Haematologica* 2012;**97**:310–17.

19 Santini G, Salvagno L, Leoni P *et al.* VACOP-B versus VACOP-B plus autologous bone marrow transplantation for advanced diffuse non-Hodgkin's lymphoma: results of a prospective randomized trial by the non-Hodgkin's Lymphoma Cooperative Study Group. *J Clin Oncol* 1998;**16**:2796–802.

20 Gianni AM, Bregni M, Siena S *et al*. High-dose chemo-therapy and autologous bone marrow transplantation compared with MACOP-B in aggressive B-cell lymphoma. *N Engl J Med* 1997;**336**:1290–7.

21 Martelli M, Gherlinzoni F, De Renzo A *et al*. Early autologous stem-cell transplantation versus conventional chemotherapy as front-line therapy in high-risk, aggressive non-Hodgkin's lymphoma: an Italian multicenter randomized trial. *J Clin Oncol* 2003;**21**:1255–62.

22 Stiff PJ, Unger JM, Cook JR *et al*. Autologous transplantation as consolidation for aggressive non-Hodgkin's lymphoma. *N Engl J Med* 2013;**369**:1681–90.

23 Buadi FK, Micallef IN, Ansell SM *et al*. Autologous hematopoietic stem cell transplantation for older patients with relapsed non-Hodgkin's lymphoma. *Bone Marrow Transplant* 2006;**37**:1017–22.

24 Lazarus HM, Carreras J, Boudreau C *et al*. Influence of age and histology on outcome in adult non-Hodgkin lymphoma patients undergoing autologous hematopoietic cell transplantation (HCT): a report from the Center for International Blood and Marrow Transplant Research (CIBMTR). *Biol Blood Marrow Transplant* 2008;**14**:1323–33.

25 Philip T, Guglielmi C, Hagenbeek A *et al*. Autologous bone marrow transplantation as compared with salvage chemotherapy in relapses of chemotherapy-sensitive non-Hodgkin's lymphoma. *N Engl J Med* 1995;**333**:1540–5.

26 Philip T, Armitage JO, Spitzer G *et al*. High-dose therapy and autologous bone marrow transplantation after failure of conventional chemotherapy in adults with intermediate-grade or high-grade non-Hodgkin's lymphoma. *N Engl J Med* 1987;**316**:1493–8.

27 de Lima M, van Besien KW, Giralt SA *et al*. Bone marrow transplantation after failure of autologous transplant for non-Hodgkin's lymphoma. *Bone Marrow Transplant* 1997;**19**:121–7.

28 Dhedin N, Giraudier S, Gaulard P *et al*. Allogeneic bone marrow transplantation in aggressive non-Hodgkin's lymphoma (excluding Burkitt and lymphoblastic lymphoma): a series of 73 patients from the SFGM database. *Br J Haematol* 1999;**107**:154–61.

29 Peniket AJ, Ruiz de Elvira MC, Taghipour G *et al*. An EBMT registry matched study of allogeneic stem cell transplants for lymphoma: allogeneic transplantation is associated with a lower relapse rate but a higher procedure-related mortality rate than autologous transplantation. *Bone Marrow Transplant* 2003;**31**:667–78.

30 Oliansky DM, Czuczman M, Fisher RI *et al*. The role of cytotoxic therapy with hematopoietic stem cell transplantation in the treatment of diffuse large B cell lymphoma: update of the 2001 evidence-based review. *Biol Blood Marrow Transplant* 2011;**17**:20–47 e30.

31 Bacher U, Klyuchnikov E, Le-Rademacher J *et al*. Conditioning regimens for allotransplants for diffuse large B-cell lymphoma: myeloablative or reduced intensity? *Blood* 2012;**120**:4256–62.

32 van Kampen RJ, Canals C, Schouten HC *et al*. Allogeneic stem-cell transplantation as salvage therapy for patients with diffuse large B-cell non-Hodgkin's lymphoma relapsing after an autologous stem-cell transplantation: an analysis of the European Group for Blood and Marrow Transplantation Registry. *J Clin Oncol* 2011;**29**:1342–8.

33 Rezvani AR, Norasetthada L, Gooley T *et al*. Non-myeloablative allogeneic haematopoietic cell transplantation for relapsed diffuse large B-cell lymphoma: a multicentre experience. *Br J Haematol* 2008;**143**:395–403.

34 The Non-Hodgkin's Lymphoma Classification Project. A clinical evaluation of the International Lymphoma Study Group classification of non-Hodgkin's lymphoma. *Blood* 1997;**89**:3909–18.

35 Ladetto M, De Marco F, Benedetti F *et al*. Prospective, multi-center randomized GITMO/IIL trial comparing intensive (R-HDS) versus conventional (CHOP-R) chemoimmuno-therapy in high-risk follicular lymphoma at diagnosis: the superior disease control of R-HDS does not translate into an overall survival advantage. *Blood* 2008;**111**:4004–13.

36 Lenz G, Dreyling M, Schiegnitz E *et al*. Myeloablative radio-chemotherapy followed by autologous stem cell transplantation in first remission prolongs progression-free survival in follicular lymphoma: results of a prospective, randomized trial of the German Low-Grade Lymphoma Study Group. *Blood* 2004;**104**:2667–74.

37 Gyan E, Foussard C, Bertrand P *et al*. High-dose therapy followed by autologous purged stem cell transplantation and doxorubicin-based chemotherapy in patients with advanced follicular lymphoma: a randomized multicenter study by the GOELAMS with final results after a median follow-up of 9 years. *Blood* 2009;**113**:995–1001.

38 Oliansky DM, Gordon LI, King J *et al*. The role of cytotoxic therapy with hematopoietic stem cell transplantation in the treatment of follicular lymphoma: an evidence-based review. *Biol Blood Marrow Transplant* 2010;**16**:443–68.

39 Brown JR, Feng Y, Gribben JG *et al*. Long-term survival after autologous bone marrow transplantation for follicular lymphoma in first remission. *Biol Blood Marrow Transplant* 2007;**13**:1057–65.

40 Sebban C, Brice P, Delarue R *et al*. Impact of rituximab and/or high-dose therapy with autotransplant at time of relapse in patients with follicular lymphoma: a GELA study. *J Clin Oncol* 2008;**26**:3614–20.

41 Freedman AS, Neuberg D, Mauch P *et al*. Long-term follow-up of autologous bone marrow transplantation in patients with relapsed follicular lymphoma. *Blood* 1999;**94**:3325–33.

42 Rohatiner AZ, Nadler L, Davies AJ *et al*. Myeloablative therapy with autologous bone marrow transplantation for follicular lymphoma at the time of second or subsequent remission: long-term follow-up. *J Clin Oncol* 2007;**25**:2554–9.

43 Schouten HC, Qian W, Kvaloy S *et al*. High-dose therapy improves progression-free survival and survival in relapsed follicular non-Hodgkin's lymphoma: results from the randomized European CUP trial. *J Clin Oncol* 2003;**21**:3918–27.

44 van Besien K, Loberiza FR Jr, Bajorunaite R *et al.* Comparison of autologous and allogeneic hematopoietic stem cell transplantation for follicular lymphoma. *Blood* 2003;**102**:3521–9.

45 Khouri IF, McLaughlin P, Saliba RM *et al.* Eight-year experience with allogeneic stem cell transplantation for relapsed follicular lymphoma after nonmyeloablative conditioning with fludarabine, cyclophosphamide, and rituximab. *Blood* 2008;**111**:5530–6.

46 Khouri IF, Saliba RM, Erwin WD *et al.* Nonmyeloablative allogeneic transplantation with or without 90yttrium ibritumomab tiuxetan is potentially curative for relapsed follicular lymphoma: 12-year results. *Blood* 2012;**119**:6373–8.

47 Freytes CO, Zhang MJ, Carreras J *et al.* Outcome of lower-intensity allogeneic transplantation in non-Hodgkin lymphoma after autologous transplantation failure. *Biol Blood Marrow Transplant* 2012;**18**:1255–64.

48 Sauter CS, Barker JN, Lechner L *et al.* A phase II study of a nonmyeloablative allogeneic stem cell transplant with peritransplant rituximab in patients with B cell lymphoid malignancies: favorably durable event-free survival in chemosensitive patients. *Biol Blood Marrow Transplant* 2014;**20**:354–60.

49 Villa D, Crump M, Panzarella T *et al.* Autologous and allogeneic stem-cell transplantation for transformed follicular lymphoma: a report of the Canadian Blood and Marrow Transplant Group. *J Clin Oncol* 2013;**31**:1164–71.

50 Zhou Y, Wang H, Fang W *et al.* Incidence trends of mantle cell lymphoma in the United States between 1992 and 2004. *Cancer* 2008;**113**:791–8.

51 Khouri IF, Romaguera J, Kantarjian H *et al.* Hyper-CVAD and high-dose methotrexate/cytarabine followed by stem-cell transplantation: an active regimen for aggressive mantle-cell lymphoma. *J Clin Oncol* 1998;**16**:3803–9.

52 Thieblemont C, Antal D, Lacotte-Thierry L *et al.* Chemotherapy with rituximab followed by high-dose therapy and autologous stem cell transplantation in patients with mantle cell lymphoma. *Cancer* 2005;**104**:1434–41.

53 Ritchie DS, Seymour JF, Grigg AP *et al.* The hyper-CVAD-rituximab chemotherapy programme followed by high-dose busulfan, melphalan and autologous stem cell transplantation produces excellent event-free survival in patients with previously untreated mantle cell lymphoma. *Ann Hematol* 2007;**86**:101–5.

54 LaCasce AS, Vandergrift JL, Rodriguez MA *et al.* Comparative outcome of initial therapy for younger patients with mantle cell lymphoma: an analysis from the NCCN NHL Database. *Blood* 2012;**119**:2093–9.

55 Geisler CH, Kolstad A, Laurell A *et al.* Long-term progression-free survival of mantle cell lymphoma after intensive front-line immunochemotherapy with in vivo-purged stem cell rescue: a nonrandomized phase 2 multicenter study by the Nordic Lymphoma Group. *Blood* 2008;**112**:2687–93.

56 Geisler CH, Kolstad A, Laurell A *et al.* Nordic MCL2 trial update: six-year follow-up after intensive immunochemo-therapy for untreated mantle cell lymphoma followed by BEAM or BEAC + autologous stem-cell support: still very long survival but late relapses do occur. *Br J Haematol* 2012;**158**:355–62.

57 Dreyling M, Lenz G, Hoster E *et al.* Early consolidation by myeloablative radiochemotherapy followed by autologous stem cell transplantation in first remission significantly prolongs progression-free survival in mantle-cell lymphoma: results of a prospective randomized trial of the European MCL Network. *Blood* 2005;**105**:2677–84.

58 Freedman AS, Neuberg D, Gribben JG *et al.* High-dose chemoradiotherapy and anti-B-cell monoclonal antibody-purged autologous bone marrow transplantation in mantle-cell lymphoma: no evidence for long-term remission. *J Clin Oncol* 1998;**16**:13–18.

59 Till BG, Gooley TA, Crawford N *et al.* Effect of remission status and induction chemotherapy regimen on outcome of autologous stem cell transplantation for mantle cell lymphoma. *Leukemia Lymphoma* 2008;**49**:1062–73.

60 Fenske TS, Zhang MJ, Carreras J *et al.* Autologous or reduced-intensity conditioning allogeneic hematopoietic cell transplantation for chemotherapy-sensitive mantle-cell lymphoma: analysis of transplantation timing and modality. *J Clin Oncol* 2014;**32**:273–81.

61 Gopal AK, Rajendran JG, Petersdorf SH *et al.* High-dose chemoradioimmunotherapy with autologous stem cell support for relapsed mantle cell lymphoma. *Blood* 2002;**99**:3158–62.

62 Khouri IF, Lee MS, Saliba RM *et al.* Nonablative allogeneic stem-cell transplantation for advanced/recurrent mantle-cell lymphoma. *J Clin Oncol* 2003;**21**:4407–12.

63 Tam CS, Bassett R, Ledesma C *et al.* Mature results of the M. D. Anderson Cancer Center risk-adapted transplantation strategy in mantle cell lymphoma. *Blood* 2009;**113**:4144–52.

64 Cook G, Smith GM, Kirkland K *et al.* Outcome following reduced-intensity allogeneic stem cell transplantation (RIC AlloSCT) for relapsed and refractory mantle cell lymphoma (MCL): a study of the British Society for Blood and Marrow Transplantation. *Biol Blood Marrow Transplant* 2010;**16**:1419–27.

65 Wasterlid T, Brown PN, Hagberg O *et al.* Impact of chemotherapy regimen and rituximab in adult Burkitt lymphoma: a retrospective population-based study from the Nordic Lymphoma Group. *Ann Oncol* 2013;**24**:1879–86.

66 Perkins AS, Friedberg JW. Burkitt lymphoma in adults. *Hematology Am Soc Hematol Educ Program* 2008:**341–8**.

67 Maramattom LV, Hari PN, Burns LJ *et al.* Autologous and allogeneic transplantation for Burkitt lymphoma outcomes and changes in utilization: a report from the Center for International Blood and Marrow Transplant Research. *Biol Blood Marrow Transplant* 2013;**19**:173–9.

68 Gross TG, Hale GA, He W *et al.* Hematopoietic stem cell transplantation for refractory or recurrent non-Hodgkin lymphoma in children and adolescents. *Biol Blood Marrow Transplant* 2010;**16**:223–30.

69 Soussain C, Hoang-Xuan K, Taillandier L *et al*. Intensive chemotherapy followed by hematopoietic stem-cell rescue for refractory and recurrent primary CNS and intraocular lymphoma: Societe Francaise de Greffe de Moelle Osseuse-Therapie Cellulaire. *J Clin Oncol* 2008;**26**:2512–18.

70 Abrey LE, Moskowitz CH, Mason WP *et al*. Intensive methotrexate and cytarabine followed by high-dose chemotherapy with autologous stem-cell rescue in patients with newly diagnosed primary CNS lymphoma: an intent-to-treat analysis. *J Clin Oncol* 2003;**21**:4151–6.

71 Soussain C, Suzan F, Hoang-Xuan K *et al*. Results of intensive chemotherapy followed by hematopoietic stem-cell rescue in 22 patients with refractory or recurrent primary CNS lymphoma or intraocular lymphoma. *J Clin Oncol* 2001;**19**:742–9.

72 d'Amore F, Relander T, Lauritzsen GF *et al*. Up-front autologous stem-cell transplantation in peripheral T-cell lymphoma: NLG-T-01. *J Clin Oncol* 2012;**30**:3093–9.

73 Feyler S, Prince HM, Pearce R *et al*. The role of high-dose therapy and stem cell rescue in the management of T-cell malignant lymphomas: a BSBMT and ABMTRR study. *Bone Marrow Transplant* 2007;**40**:443–50.

74 Jantunen E, Wiklund T, Juvonen E *et al*. Autologous stem cell transplantation in adult patients with peripheral T-cell lymphoma: a nation-wide survey. *Bone Marrow Transplant* 2004;**33**:405–10.

75 Rodriguez J, Conde E, Gutierrez A *et al*. The results of consolidation with autologous stem-cell transplantation in patients with peripheral T-cell lymphoma (PTCL) in first complete remission: the Spanish Lymphoma and Autologous Transplantation Group experience. *Ann Oncol* 2007;**18**:652–7.

76 Le Gouill S, Milpied N, Buzyn A *et al*. Graft-versus-lymphoma effect for aggressive T-cell lymphomas in adults: a study by the Societe Francaise de Greffe de Moelle et de Therapie Cellulaire. *J Clin Oncol* 2008;**26**:2264–71.

77 Beitinjaneh A, Saliba RM, Okoroji G *et al*. Autologous and allogeneic stem cell transplantation for T-cell lymphoma: the M.D. Anderson Cancer Center Experience. *Blood (ASH Annual Meeting Abstracts)* 2011;**118**:Abstract 4118.

78 Corradini P, Dodero A, Zallio F *et al*. Graft-versus-lymphoma effect in relapsed peripheral T-cell non-Hodgkin's lymphomas after reduced-intensity conditioning followed by allogeneic transplantation of hematopoietic cells. *J Clin Oncol* 2004;**22**:2172–6.

79 Kyriakou C, Canals C, Finke J *et al*. Allogeneic stem cell transplantation is able to induce long-term remissions in angioimmunoblastic T-cell lymphoma: a retrospective study from the lymphoma working party of the European Group for Blood and Marrow Transplantation. *J Clin Oncol* 2009;**27**:3951–8.

80 Goldberg JD, Chou JF, Horwitz S *et al*. Long-term survival in patients with peripheral T-cell non-Hodgkin lymphomas after allogeneic hematopoietic stem cell transplant. *Leukemia Lymphoma* 2012;**53**:1124–9.

81 Hamlin PA, Zelenetz AD, Kewalramani T *et al*. Age-adjusted International Prognostic Index predicts autologous stem cell transplantation outcome for patients with relapsed or primary refractory diffuse large B-cell lymphoma. *Blood* 2003;**102**:1989–96.

82 Perales MA, Jenq R, Goldberg JD *et al*. Second-line age-adjusted International Prognostic Index in patients with advanced non-Hodgkin lymphoma after T-cell depleted allogeneic hematopoietic SCT. *Bone Marrow Transplant* 2010;**45**:1408–16.

83 Sorror ML, Maris MB, Storb R *et al*. Hematopoietic cell transplantation (HCT)-specific comorbidity index: a new tool for risk assessment before allogeneic HCT. *Blood* 2005;**106**:2912–19.

84 Plattel WJ, Kluin-Nelemans HC, de Bock GH, van Imhoff GW. Prognostic value of comorbidity for auto-SCT eligibility and outcome in relapsed or refractory aggressive non-Hodgkin's lymphoma. *Bone Marrow Transplant* 2011;**46**:827–34.

85 Pasquini MC, Logan BR, Ho VT *et al*. Comorbidity index (CI) in autologous hematopoietic cell transplantation (HCT) for malignant diseases: validation of the HCT-CI. *Blood (ASH Annual Meeting Abstracts)* 2012;**120**:Abstract 814.

86 Damon LE, Johnson JL, Niedzwiecki D *et al*. Immunochemotherapy and autologous stem-cell transplantation for untreated patients with mantle-cell lymphoma: CALGB 59909. *J Clin Oncol* 2009;**27**:6101–8.

87 Andersen NS, Pedersen LB, Laurell A *et al*. Pre-emptive treatment with rituximab of molecular relapse after autologous stem cell transplantation in mantle cell lymphoma. *J Clin Oncol* 2009;**27**:4365–70.

88 Mangel J, Leitch HA, Connors JM *et al*. Intensive chemotherapy and autologous stem-cell transplantation plus rituximab is superior to conventional chemotherapy for newly diagnosed advanced stage mantle-cell lymphoma: a matched pair analysis. *Ann Oncol* 2004;**15**:283–90.

89 Mangel J, Buckstein R, Imrie K *et al*. Immunotherapy with rituximab following high-dose therapy and autologous stem-cell transplantation for mantle cell lymphoma. *Semin Oncol* 2002;**29**(1 Suppl 2):56–69.

90 Hagberg H, Gisselbrecht C. Randomised phase III study of R-ICE versus R-DHAP in relapsed patients with CD20 diffuse large B-cell lymphoma (DLBCL) followed by high-dose therapy and a second randomisation to maintenance treatment with rituximab or not: an update of the CORAL study. *Ann Oncol* 2006;**17**(Suppl 4):iv31–2.

91 Gisselbrecht C, Schmitz N, Mounier N *et al*. Rituximab maintenance therapy after autologous stem-cell transplantation in patients with relapsed CD20(+) diffuse large B-cell lymphoma: final analysis of the collaborative trial in relapsed aggressive lymphoma. *J Clin Oncol* 2012;**30**:4462–9.

92 A Phase 3 study of brentuximab vedotin (SGN-35) in patients at high risk of residual Hodgkin lymphoma following stem cell transplant (The AETHERA Trial), NCT01100502. Available at http://www.clinicaltrials.gov (accessed April 26, 2014).

CHAPTER 4

Hematopoietic stem cell transplantation for lymphoma in children, adolescents, and young adults

Nader Kim El-Mallawany and Mitchell S. Cairo

Introduction

Upfront chemotherapy protocols for the treatment of lymphomas in children, adolescents, and young adults (CAYA) achieve some of the highest curative rates of any group of malignancies in the field of oncology [1,2]. Depending on the specific type of lymphoma as well as the biological and clinical characteristics of the individual presentation, long-term event-free survival (EFS) rates for CAYA range from 75 to 95%. However, despite these promising statistics, the long-term survival for those patients with refractory or relapsed lymphoma is dismal. For these patients in particular, many of whom are essentially incurable with conventional chemotherapy, it is imperative to define the optimal combination of hematopoietic stem cell transplantation (HSCT) strategies with novel targeted agents.

Lymphomas are the third most common malignancy of childhood (after leukemias and brain tumors) and the most common malignancy of adolescence. While Hodgkin lymphoma (HL) is the most common lymphoma in CAYA, a variety of non-Hodgkin lymphomas (NHL) also occur frequently including Burkitt lymphoma (BL), lymphoblastic lymphoma (LBL), diffuse large B-cell lymphoma (DLBCL), anaplastic large-cell lymphoma (ALCL), and primary mediastinal B-cell lymphoma (PMBL) [3]. While BL and DLBCL have considerable overlap in their clinical presentation and response to treatment, the other lymphomas listed have distinct clinical characteristics, require disease-specific treatment approaches, and are best

discussed as individual entities rather than clumped under one umbrella classification. In general, newly diagnosed lymphomas are highly curable with treatment protocols based on chemotherapy combined with targeted monoclonal antibody-based immunotherapy. Certain subsets of patients with HL will require radiation therapy as well. Ultimately though, excellent outcomes are achieved for CAYA with newly diagnosed lymphoma [1–3].

HSCT in pediatric lymphomas is generally reserved as a strategy for patients with refractory or relapsed disease. The role of HSCT has evolved over the years as the upfront treatment protocols have become progressively more effective. Thirty years ago, when the EFS rates for pediatric lymphomas were below 50%, high-dose chemotherapy with autologous HSCT (auto-HSCT) was effective in salvaging some patients to achieve curative outcomes, most likely due to the fact that patients were, in retrospect, undertreated at the onset of their original diagnosis. However, over the past three decades, as the upfront therapies for pediatric lymphoma have become progressively more intensive and the success rates have effectively doubled, it has become increasingly more difficult to salvage relapsed and refractory disease by simply administering high-dose chemotherapy followed by auto-HSCT (Tables 4.1 and 4.2) [4]. This has led to the utilization of alternative treatment strategies including allogeneic HSCT (allo-HSCT) for certain patients with the goal of achieving a graft-versus-lymphoma (GVL) effect that could potentially maintain a lifelong remission for patients with high-risk disease.

Clinical Guide to Transplantation in Lymphoma, First Edition. Edited by Bipin N. Savani and Mohamad Mohty.
© 2015 John Wiley & Sons, Ltd. Published 2015 by John Wiley & Sons, Ltd.

Table 4.1 Comparison of survival rates for children, adolescents, and young adults with refractory/relapsed Hodgkin lymphoma receiving high-dose chemotherapy and autologous HSCT in multiple cohorts: independent risk factors for relapse determined by individual studies.

	Baker *et al.* [13]	Harris *et al.* [14]	Lieskovsky *et al.* [15]	Williams *et al.* [16]	Claviez *et al.* [17]
Years of cohort	1984–1996	1998–2002	1989–2001	pre-1992	1987–2003
No. of patients	53	39	41	53	74
EFS/FFS/PFS (%)	31	45	53	39	50
Survival (years)	5	3	4	3	5
Risk factors for relapse	Early relapse Chemoresistance	Early relapse Chemoresistance	Refractory disease Advanced stage	Refractory disease Chemoresistance	Early relapse Chemoresistance Multiple relapse

EFS, event-free survival; FFS, failure-free survival; HSCT, hematopoietic stem cell transplantation; PFS, progression-free survival.

Table 4.2 Comparison of survival rates for children, adolescents, and young adults with refractory/relapsed non-Hodgkin lymphoma receiving high-dose chemotherapy and autologous HSCT in multiple cohorts.

Type of NHL	LBL	LBL	ALCL	DLBCL	BL		Mature B-cell NHL	All NHL
Reference	Levine *et al.* [34]	Gross *et al.* [35]	Gross *et al.* [35]	Gross *et al.* [35]	Gross *et al.* [35]	Philip *et al.* [50]	Ladenstein *et al.* [51]	Harris *et al.* [14]
Years of cohort	1989–1998	1990–2005	1990–2005	1990–2005	1990–2005	1984–1987	1979–1991	1998–2002
No. of patients	128	14	24	35	17	14	89	39
EFS/FFS/PFS (%)	39	4	35	52	27	27	39	45
Survival (years)	5	5	5	5	5	4	5	3

ALCL, anaplastic large-cell lymphoma; BL, Burkitt lymphoma; DBLCL, diffuse large B-cell lymphoma; EFS, event-free survival; FFS, failure-free survival; HSCT, hematopoietic stem cell transplantation; LBL, lymphoblastic lymphoma; NHL, non-Hodgkin lymphoma; PFS, progression-free survival.

Principles of autologous and allogeneic HSCT in pediatric lymphomas

High-dose chemotherapy followed by auto-HSCT is a cornerstone for the treatment of pediatric malignancies that are chemosensitive but otherwise incurable with conventional doses of chemotherapy. It is well established that the majority of patients with refractory and/or relapsed lymphomas fail to achieve long-term curative outcomes with conventional chemotherapy. The only exceptions to this general rule are patients with late relapse, and those who initially present with early-stage lymphomas treated with minimally intensive upfront protocols that are designed with the understanding that relapse can still be salvaged with curative intent using conventional-dose chemotherapy.

Starting as early as the late 1970s, high-dose chemotherapy with auto-HSCT has demonstrated the capacity to achieve long-term remission in children with relapsed lymphoma. Building on the foundation of early encouraging results, regimens have utilized chemotherapeutic agents such as carmustine, etoposide, cytarabine, melphalan, cyclophosphamide/ifosfamide, and platinum-based agents. However, while high-dose chemotherapy followed by auto-HSCT has historically been, and still remains, the standard approach for CAYA with chemosensitive refractory and/or relapsed lymphomas, the success rates for auto-HSCT in this group of patients have dwindled over the years. As the upfront regimens have intensified over time, it has become apparent that treating relapse with higher doses of chemotherapy is insufficient to overcome the inherent chemotherapy resistance that develops in refractory and relapsed lymphoma. So although the overall response rates to auto-HSCT are relatively high, maintaining long-term remission in patients is a formidable challenge.

Determining which patients may achieve excellent long-term results with auto-HSCT is critical to defining the optimal treatment strategies for patients with relapsed/refractory disease. While primary refractory lymphoma is nearly a universally poor prognostic factor, various other clinical factors also increase the risk for failure of auto-HSCT including early time to relapse, chemoresistant disease, advanced stage presentation at relapse, multiply relapsed disease, and having received more intensive upfront treatment regimens.

Despite the integration of novel targeted immuno-therapies, most notably the anti-CD20 monoclonal anti-body rituximab in the treatment of mature B-cell lymphomas, significant improvements in the ultimate curative outcomes of relapsed/refractory patients treated with auto-HSCT have not materialized. Therefore, based on the experience in curing otherwise incurable hematologic malignancies such as leukemia with allo-HSCT, as well as the efficacy of allo-HSCT in adult lymphomas [5], treatment paradigms built on the allogeneic GVL effect have been constructed for CAYA as well. As early as the 1990s, a potential GVL effect had been described in lymphoma patients receiving allo-HSCT [6]. Its effect has been deduced primarily from three main principles: the significantly lower relapse rate in lymphoma patients receiving allo-HSCT versus auto-HSCT, the lower relapse rates in those patients who developed graft-versus-host disease (GVHD) post allo-HSCT, and the established efficacy of donor lym-phocyte infusions (DLI) in reinducing remissions in patients who relapse post transplant [7].

The main drawback of utilizing allo-HSCT in patients with relapsed/refractory lymphoma has historically been excessive transplant-related mortality (TRM) and/ or nonrelapse mortality (NRM) rates. Despite the reduced rates of lymphoma relapse post allo-HSCT, the unfavorably high TRM often resulted in equivalent overall survival (OS) rates when comparing autologous versus allogeneic HSCT [8]. However, TRM rates of patients undergoing allo-HSCT continue to decline sig-nificantly in the modern era for the following reasons: significant advances have been achieved in (i) supportive care measures, (ii) the prevention, detection and management of opportunistic infections and GVHD, and (iii) the refining of conditioning regimens and hemato-poietic stem cell processing. In the contemporary era, with success rates of matched unrelated donor allo-HSCT nearing that of matched sibling donors, there is much hope that allo-HSCT will be utilized to reach greater numbers of patients that can benefit from its unique therapeutic potential. Certainly, some of the controversy in analyzing the data on allo-HSCT in pediatric lymphoma arises from

the clouding of historical data, as many of the large-scale analyses of bone marrow transplant registry data have included broad populations of patients usually spanning time periods of more than 10–15 years. While this information is important and useful in directing treatment strategies, results of patients treated more than 15 years ago may not accurately reflect the benefits of contemporary advances in transplant medicine. With all of this in mind, we will examine the data and current HSCT therapeutic strategies for the most common childhood and adolescent lymphomas.

Hodgkin lymphoma

Upfront treatment regimens utilizing chemotherapy with or without radiation therapy for HL achieve long-term EFS rates ranging from 75 to 95% depending on risk stratification [2,3]. However, prognosis for recurrent HL varies widely based on multiple clinical factors. Consequently, the decision to use autologous or even allogeneic HSCT as a therapeutic strategy for refractory and relapsed disease is open for debate. Ultimately, determining prognostic risk factors for those patients with refractory/relapsed disease is the most important step in selecting the optimal treatment approach to improve the long-term curative rates for this very high-risk subset of patients.

While it is widely accepted that primary refractory HL is virtually incurable with conventional doses of chemo-therapy, the treatment approach for CAYA with relapsed HL is not as clear-cut. In theory, late relapse can be salvaged with chemotherapy, while patients with early relapse (defined as <12 months after completion of therapy) fare poorly with nontransplant regimens [9]. Schellong et al. [9] published one of the largest reports on refractory/relapsed pediatric HL, showing that patients who experienced late relapse (defined as >12 months after completion of therapy) achieved a disease-free survival (DFS) of 86%, without requiring an auto-HSCT. However, it is important to point out that patients were enrolled on this study between 1986 and 2003 (17 years). And while the time to relapse was the most important risk factor for failure to achieve DFS and OS, the second most important determinant was the intensity of the initial chemotherapy regimen [9]. Receiving upfront chemotherapy regimens with etopo-side and procarbazine (i.e., more intensive regimens) was a statistically significant risk factor that adversely affected both DFS and OS [9]. Similar to the scenario with childhood NHL, as the primary therapies for HL have become progressively more intensive (and effective), data has surfaced revealing discouraging long-term outcomes for those relapsed patients in the modern era. For adult patients with relapsed HL, the standard approach involves high-dose chemotherapy and auto-HSCT [10,11]. While a definitive randomized controlled trial in CAYA with relapsed HL is lacking, in the contemporary era, for those patients who fail intensive upfront chemotherapy regimens, strong consideration should be given to utilizing an auto-HSCT in the setting of a chemosensitive relapse [12].

The largest reports on auto-HSCT for relapsed and refractory HL in CAYA yield long-term curative rates ranging from 31 to 53% (Table 4.1) [13–17]. Thus although a significant number of patients are long-term survivors with this approach, the majority of patients still remain uncured. Part of the challenge in interpreting this data is the wide heterogeneity of the patient populations. While the actuarial 5-year failure-free survival (FFS) for the 53 patients in the study by Baker *et al.* [13] was only 31%, Lieskovsky *et al.* [15] reported 5-year EFS of 53% for 41 pediatric patients. However, it is important to note that the discouraging results reported by Baker *et al.* included a cohort of patients in which half were characterized by multiply relapsed or refractory disease. Meanwhile, the favorable results for Lieskovsky's group may be reflected in the higher proportion of late relapses in their cohort. The median duration of initial remission among their patients was 23.5 months, indicating that the majority of their cohort experienced a late relapse. Ultimately, each patient with relapsed HL should be evaluated for their individualized clinical scenario, weighing in the presence of the various clinical characteristics known to influence the risk for further treatment failure.

A number of studies have attempted to shed light on the clinical characteristics associated with poor outcomes despite auto-HSCT. The one consistent clinical group experiencing low EFS rates despite auto-HSCT are those patients with primary refractory disease [9,15,16]. However a number of other clinical factors are also associated with poor long-term EFS despite auto-HSCT. These ultra-high-risk patients include those experiencing early relapse within 12 months of completing the original therapy [9,18] – a group of patients characterized by reported risk ratios for treatment failure of 3.1 [13]

and an OS of 34% [14]. Additionally, patients with chemoresistant disease, usually defined as failure to achieve at least partial remission with reinduction chemotherapy, exhibit dismal outcomes with EFS rates below 10% [13,14,17]. Other risk factors that were consistently associated with poor outcomes in the above studies included advanced stage presentation of relapse (including extranodal involvement and the presence of bulky disease) and patients presenting with multiply relapsed disease.

To summarize the role of auto-HSCT for HL in CAYA, it is important to emphasize the need for critical evaluation of each individual clinical scenario. Auto-HSCT has the potential to cure a large percentage of young patients with relapse in the setting of favorable clinical risk factors. On the other hand, based on all the data reviewed above, the ultimate curative outcomes for patients with high-risk clinical characteristics are well below 30% despite the use of high-dose chemotherapy and auto-HSCT. Those high-risk features in the contemporary era of intensive upfront treatment regimens for HL include (i) primary refractory disease, (ii) early relapse within 12 months of completing original therapy, (iii) multiply relapsed disease, (iv) relapse with chemorefractory disease (i.e., failure to achieve at least partial remission with reinduction chemotherapy), and (v) relapse presentation with advanced-stage disease. On critical analysis of the available data in the literature, patients presenting with any of the above five high-risk scenarios have a low likelihood of achieving long-term cure with auto-HSCT, and therefore require novel therapeutic approaches.

Allo-HSCT has traditionally been utilized in the setting of multiply relapsed HL, notably after failure of auto-HSCT. Because of extremely high rates of TRM without any advantage in OS, allo-HSCT was historically reserved as a last-ditch effort [19]. However, with the advent of reduced-intensity conditioning (RIC) regimens and the significant reductions in TRM with modern advances in HSCT, this treatment approach has been revisited in adults with high-risk HL with cautiously optimistic results [20]. RIC regimens have been mostly based on fludarabine–melphalan and fludarabine–busulfan backbones. The largest cohort of adult HL patients treated with RIC allo-HSCT included 285 very heavily pretreated patients with high percentages of multiply relapsed and chemorefractory disease. Despite the overwhelming odds against treatment success, the 2-year progression-free survival (PFS) was 29% [21]. The largest adult HL prospective clinical trial included 78 patients with multiply relapsed disease that received allo-HSCT. The 4-year PFS was 24%, while the NRM was 15% at 12 months [22]. More recently, Thomson et al. [23] reported extremely favorable results utilizing allo-HSCT for a smaller cohort of 25 patients, 20 with refractory disease and four with early relapse. This adult cohort exhibited 80% chemosensitive disease with reinduction chemotherapy, and utilized fludeoxyglucose positron emission tomography (FDG-PET) as the major imaging modality to determine the clinical response. The 3-year PFS was 68% in this high-risk group of patients. Ultimately, these modest PFS rates in patients who had failed multiple prior treatment modalities including auto-HSCT, as well as the more recent data using allo-HSCT as the initial salvage strategy, together offer a glimmer of hope for the potential of allo-HSCT to cure high-risk refractory/relapsed HL.

The modest success of allo-HSCT in refractory/relapsed HL in adults has been conceptually re-enforced by evidence of a GVL effect. The larger cohorts of adult HL allo-HSCT recipients demonstrated a lower risk of relapse in patients who developed GVHD [20–22]. Meanwhile, Peggs et al. demonstrated a significant response rate for patients receiving DLI in two separate studies. In one study, they gave DLI in the setting of post-allo-HSCT progression or mixed chimerism; 56% of 19 patients showed a significant response [24]. In their other study, 46 patients received DLI due to relapse ($N=24$) or mixed chimerism ($N=22$) post allo-HSCT, achieving a significant reduction in relapse rate and durable antitumor response [25].

Building on the experience in treating refractory/relapsed HL in adults with allo-HSCT, Claviez et al. [26] performed a retrospective analysis of the European experience treating refractory/relapsed HL in children and adolescents. In total, 91 patients received allo-HSCT for refractory/relapsed HL; 51 received a RIC allo-HSCT, the other 40 received a myeloablative conditioning (MAC) regimen. NRM was 21% at 1 year; PFS was 30% at 5 years. However, this was a broad cohort of patients receiving allo-HSCT between 1987 and 2005. Notably, patients transplanted in the contemporary era (since 2001) with chemosensitive disease had a 3-year PFS of 60%. While this study did not demonstrate a reduction in risk associated with GVHD, it does shine an encouraging light on the tolerability of allo-HSCT in CAYA and its curative potential for patients with high-risk disease.

More recently, Satwani et al. [27] reported on a multicenter prospective trial for refractory/relapsed lymphoma in CAYA utilizing a tandem approach with MAC chemotherapy (carmustine/etoposide/cyclophosphamide) plus auto-HSCT followed by RIC (busulfan/fludarabine) allo-HSCT. Eligibility for HL required primary refractory disease, early relapse (excluding patients with no prior therapy or radiation only), or late relapse with advanced stage disease. Sixteen patients with HL were enrolled; 13 proceeded to receive the tandem auto/allo-HSCT. Among the 16 enrolled patients, the 10-year EFS was 56.4%. The incidence of TRM for patients receiving the tandem auto/allo-HSCT was 12%, with 22% grade II–IV acute GVHD and 13% chronic GVHD.

Ultimately, although this cohort of patients is small, data from this prospective study, coupled with the encouraging recent results from the European data, offers promising evidence that certain very high-risk patients can achieve formidable curative outcomes with RIC and allo-HSCT despite historically dismal precedents.

Lymphoblastic lymphoma

LBL is the second most common NHL in CAYA. Characterized by overall EFS rates of 75–80%, lymphoblastic lymphoma is derived from T cells in the vast majority of cases [1,28]. While it resides on a spectrum of disease akin to, but biologically different from, acute lymphoblastic leukemia (ALL), patients with both T-cell ALL and T-cell LBL are generally treated on the same upfront treatment protocols. Contemporary regimens are largely based on high-risk ALL chemotherapy backbones, adding in high-dose methotrexate, aggressive intrathecal chemotherapy, as well as usually including cranial radiation therapy to attenuate the increased risk for central nervous system (CNS) relapse as well as the high prevalence of CNS-positive disease [29].

HSCT for patients with LBL is essentially reserved for patients with refractory and relapsed disease. Very little is published about the long-term outcomes of patients with refractory/relapsed disease. The Berlin–Frankfurt–Muenster (BFM) group has published the largest and most relevant contemporary report. Of 324 patients with LBL enrolled in BFM trials between 1990 and

2003, there were 34 patients that experienced relapse, 28 with T-cell LBL and six with B-cell LBL. Of these 34, only 12 were able to achieve a second remission. Ultimately, only five were alive in long-term remission; all five received an allo-HSCT. The overall survival for patients with relapsed LBL was 14%. While the long-term outcomes for patients with refractory/relapsed LBL are dismal in the modern era, it is notable that 5 of 12 patients that received an allo-HSCT were able to achieve long-term remissions (ranging from 48 to 131 months) [30]. Data from Memorial Sloan Kettering Hospital in New York demonstrated similar results for another small cohort of 12 patients with refractory/relapsed LBL, 11 of whom received allo-HSCT, with one patient receiving auto-HSCT. The 10-year OS and DFS were 50%; the single patient that received auto-HSCT died of TRM [31]. Outcomes for patients with relapsed T-cell ALL are very similar [32,33].

The largest study evaluating the use of HSCT in pediatric LBL compared 128 patients receiving auto-HSCT with 76 patients receiving allo-HSCT [34]. It is challenging to apply the results from this retrospective registry data to modern-day clinical practice because this cohort of patients received HSCT between 1989 and 1998 (i.e., 15–25 years ago). Ultimately, the most poignant data reported in this study demonstrated significantly higher relapse rates of 56% in children receiving auto-HSCT versus 34% in allo-HSCT recipients. Nonetheless, the long-term DFS was similar for the two groups (39% auto-HSCT vs. 36% allo-HSCT) because TRM was exceptionally high in those patients receiving allo-HSCT (18% vs. 3%) [34]. However, a retrospective analysis of the Center for International Blood and Marrow Transplant Research (CIBMTR) registry data for CAYA undergoing HSCT for refractory/relapsed lymphoma revealed significantly higher 5-year EFS among 53 patients with LBL receiving allo-HSCT versus auto-HSCT (40% vs. 4%) [35]. Thus while the data for LBL in CAYA is not robust, it is generally accepted that patients with both refractory and relapsed disease are at extremely high risk for recurrence and the standard of care is to attempt reinduction to achieve remission followed by allo-HSCT. Unlike the RIC approach utilized in HL, MAC regimens are still the standard of care for allo-HSCT in LBL, with current debates focusing on whether or not to utilize total body irradiation (TBI)-containing regimens.

Anaplastic large-cell lymphoma

ALCL is the fourth most common NHL in CAYA, accounting for approximately 10% of cases [1]. Typically originating from T lymphocytes, a small portion of ALCL can have a null-cell immunophenotype. ALCL is characterized by a translocation of the *ALK* gene in more than 90% of CAYA. Upfront regimens with alternating combinations of chemotherapy have reported 2- to 5-year EFS rates ranging from 66 to 76% [1,28]. While patients with refractory disease and those who relapse on therapy both have very poor long-term prognoses, many questions still prevail about the patterns of behavior for relapsed ALCL. Widely variable salvage treatment approaches have yielded both favorable and unfavorable results. Ranging from long-term single-agent weekly vinblastine, to combination reinduction chemotherapy, to MAC chemotherapy followed by auto-HSCT or even allo-HSCT, many different approaches have been used in patients with relapsed ALCL [36]. Unfortunately, the data is difficult to interpret because the cohorts of patients reported in the literature are not large and there is considerable variation within each group with regard to the clinical nature of the relapse presentation as well as the initial therapeutic regimens received [36].

The European experience with ALCL in France and Germany has identified specific risk factors that are associated with poor prognosis for relapsed patients. Similar to HL, time to relapse is crucial, with those patients relapsing within 12 months of diagnosis having significantly lower long-term DFS than those with later relapse: 28% versus 68% in the French cohort, and 25% versus 66% in the German study [37,38]. For those patients who relapse while on therapy, there are very few reported survivors in the literature, all of them ultimately having received allo-HSCT. Other poor risk factors associated with relapse include multiply relapsed disease and advanced stage presentation (with CNS or bone marrow involvement) [36]. On the other hand, patients with CD3-negative ALCL seem to have a favorable prognosis [38].

The treatment dilemma for refractory/relapsed ALCL is similar to that for HL. Those patients with favorable-risk relapse have a formidable chance to be cured utilizing auto-HSCT. For patients with refractory disease or high-risk relapse (i.e., early relapse and recurrence with stage IV disease), chances for long-term curative outcomes with auto-HSCT are slim.

Therefore, alternative approaches must be considered for this high-risk subset of patients. The BFM group recently reported encouraging results from a trial utilizing allo-HSCT for refractory or early relapsed ALCL in children and adolescents. Twenty patients received TBI-based MAC regimens; there were eight matched sibling donors, eight unrelated donors, and four haploidentical family donors. EFS at 3 years was 75% in this group of patients with extremely high-risk disease. Notably, all five patients who had relapsed after auto-HSCT survived disease-free [39]. Their experience has been corroborated by smaller case series of patients treated with allo-HSCT in the United States, Italy, and Japan [27,40,41]. Additionally, CIBMTR registry data also demonstrated that CAYA with refractory/relapsed ALCL had a lower rate of relapse after allo-HSCT (20%, $N = 12$) versus auto-HSCT (48%, $N = 24$), although this finding did not reach statistical significance [35].

Based on the available data, the European Inter-Group for Childhood NHL (EICNHL) created a prospective clinical trial for relapsed ALCL risk-stratified into three groups. The highest risk patients include those with refractory disease or CD3-positive ALCL in first relapse and they are recommended to undergo allo-HSCT. Auto-HSCT is recommended for CD3-negative ALCL in early relapse, while those with CD3-negative disease experiencing late relapse are to receive 2 years of monotherapy with vinblastine [36]. Results from this prospective trial will be invaluable to help design the ideal treatment approach for CAYA with refractory and relapsed ALCL.

Mature B-cell lymphomas: Burkitt lymphoma, diffuse large B-cell lymphoma, and primary mediastinal B-cell lymphoma

Mature B-cell lymphomas account for nearly two-thirds of NHL in CAYA [1]. BL is the most common, representing nearly 40% of NHL in CAYA throughout the world. In sub-Saharan Africa, BL is the most common childhood cancer overall and represents up to one-third to half of pediatric oncology diagnoses. DLBCL accounts for approximately 20% of NHL in CAYA. The two diseases have considerable clinical and biological overlap; both are considered aggressive B-cell NHL and respond similarly to treatment. CD20 antigen expression is characteristic of these mature B-cell lymphomas and targeted immunotherapy with the monoclonal antibody rituximab has become an important part of modern day chemoimmunotherapy protocols.

The most recent Children's Oncology Group (COG) protocol for BL and DLBCL integrated rituximab into the standard French–American–British/Lymphomes Malins B (FAB/LMB) backbone chemotherapy with outstanding results. Probability of EFS at 3 years for patients with group B intermediate risk disease was 93% [42]. Even patients with group C high-risk disease, defined as having CNS involvement and/or more than 25% bone marrow involvement, achieve long-term EFS rates of 79% with the FAB/LMB backbone bolstered by the addition of high-dose methotrexate and cytarabine to the regimen [43]. PMBL was once thought of as an uncommon variant of DLBCL, but has recently been characterized by genomic profiling as a biologically distinct disease [44]. While patients with PMBL did not fare as well as those with BL or DLBCL in the aforementioned FAB/LMB chemotherapy protocols, recent data has shown that EFS rates of 93% can be achieved in CAYA using a dose-adjusted EPOCH (etoposide, prednisone, vincristine, cyclophosphamide, doxorubicin)–rituximab protocol without radiotherapy [45,46]. Undoubtedly, these mature B-cell lymphomas carry some of the best prognoses in all of oncology.

The biggest challenge in the management of CAYA with mature B-cell NHL is the treatment approach to patients with refractory and relapsed disease. As the upfront protocols have improved over the past few decades to achieve greater than 90% curative rates, salvaging patients with refractory/relapsed disease has become inordinately difficult. Long-term data for patients who relapsed after treatment on the US collaborative group CCG protocols revealed OS rates of only 12% [47]. Shorter 1-year probability of OS for all patients with relapsed/refractory mature B-cell NHL treated on the recent FAB/LMB 96 protocol was 28% [48]. Data from the FAB/LMB 96 high-risk study revealed probability of 4-year OS of 16% for those with progressive or recurrent disease [43]. In a smaller cohort from Austria/Germany, of nine children with refractory/relapsed mature B-cell NHL, all but one died from progressive disease [49]. These extremely low rates of survival reflect the enormity of the challenge in curing patients with refractory/relapsed disease.

Reports on outcomes for patients with refractory/relapsed B-cell NHL who undergo HSCT are extremely difficult to interpret. While contemporary reports reveal dismal outcomes despite autologous and allogeneic HSCT, large registry data analyses that include patients dating back 20 years sometimes project optimism that may not be relevant in the modern era. Philip *et al.* [50] reported on the French experience with 27 cases of relapsed mature B-cell NHL during the period 1984–1987. Twelve patients received conventional chemotherapy without HSCT; all of them died. Fifteen patients received HSCT (14 auto, 1 allo) and their probability of OS was 27%. Of the four survivors, two had isolated CNS relapse, one had a localized relapse, and the fourth had systemic relapse. All the survivors relapsed within the first year after diagnosis. Ladenstein *et al.* [51] reported on European transplant registry data utilizing auto-HSCT for refractory/relapsed B-cell NHL spanning the years 1979–1991. These data are extremely difficult to apply to the modern era because of the outdated time period in which the study took place. They reported continuous complete remission (CR) in 39% of patients, but the authors emphasized in the discussion that among patients originally treated with the more intensive LMB 86/89 protocols (in which high-dose methotrexate and cytarabine were given), there were no long-term survivors despite auto-HSCT. Additionally, the data from Memorial Sloan Kettering recapitulates these poor outcomes. In their cohort there were nine patients with refractory/relapsed B-cell NHL, five with BL and four with DLBCL. Five patients received auto-HSCT, and four received allo-HSCT (two with BL and DLBCL each). None of the BL patients survived, and two of four with DLBCL were long-term survivors. The paper does not indicate which type of HSCT the survivors received, although the numbers are too small to make any definitive conclusions [31].

There is one single prospective trial evaluating the use of auto-HSCT in CAYA with lymphoma; however, the data for patients with NHL includes BL, DLBCL, LBL and ALCL, and unfortunately the report does not discuss details about which types of NHL ultimately survived. The 3-year EFS for patients with NHL was below 30%. Of the 30 children enrolled with NHL, only 10 proceeded to receive the high-dose chemotherapy plus auto-HSCT, and ultimately only seven survived. The NHL patients enrolled in the study included five with ALCL which, as discussed earlier, especially if presenting with a late relapse, can have very promising outcomes with auto-HSCT [14]. Nonetheless, one finding that was consistently reported by all the above studies was the importance of performing HSCT in patients with chemosensitive disease. Throughout all the reports, patients receiving HSCT in either CR or partial remission had statistically superior outcomes compared to patients with stable, progressive, or refractory disease.

The retrospective CIBMTR registry data analysis examined outcomes for CAYA receiving either autologous or allogeneic HSCT for refractory and relapsed NHL between 1990 and 2005. For 35 patients with DLBCL treated with auto-HSCT, the probability of 5-year EFS was 52%, while for 17 patients with BL receiving auto-HSCT the EFS was only 27%. Interestingly, there was no statistically significant difference in EFS for patients receiving allo-HSCT, despite the TRM rates between auto-HSCT and allo-HSCT being comparable [35]. The authors discussed some of the challenges in interpreting retrospective registry data, stating that although they deliberately started the cohort analysis in 1990 with the goal of capturing mostly those patients treated with contemporary high-intensity chemotherapy regimens upfront, the lack of detail in registry data regarding frontline regimens does present a limitation. Furthermore, patients were more likely to receive auto-HSCT in the earlier years of the cohort, a time period more likely to coincide with less intensive upfront chemotherapy regimens, and perhaps a higher likelihood of being salvaged with HSCT. Nonetheless, as the largest analysis of HSCT in childhood and adolescent NHL, the information is valuable.

Retrospective data from Spain for patients treated in the 1980s revealed very similar outcomes, comparing autologous and allogeneic HSCT for children with refractory/relapsed B-cell NHL. However, the vast majority of their cohort received older less intensive frontline chemotherapy regimens and therefore the data are really not applicable to patients being treated nowadays [52]. This ultimately raises an important question: in light of the dismal outcomes for patients with refractory/relapsed disease despite auto-HSCT, is there a GVL effect that can be optimized in mature B-cell lymphomas via alloHSCT? Although the retrospective CIBMTR data would argue against it, extrapolation from the adult experience with DLBCL [53,54], as well as the evident GVL benefit in LBL and ALCL, serves as motivation to continue to pursue definitive answers. In the cohort of patients reported by Satwani *et al*. [27] utilizing tandem autologous then allogeneic HSCT, there were eight patients with refractory/relapsed mature B-cell NHL. Although the numbers are low, five of eight achieved long-term CR (1.9–8.8 years), with all three of the patients who relapsed doing so after auto-HSCT.

Ultimately, clinicians must make a critical assessment of the individual patient's risk profile, prior therapies received, and the lymphoma's sensitivity to chemotherapy. As indicated by the various aforementioned studies, long-term survival in mature B-cell NHL patients with refractory or relapsed disease in the modern era is meager. In the absence of novel therapies with curative potential at present, novel approaches to therapy are desperately needed. In this setting, nonstandard approaches including the use of allo-HSCT in hopes of driving a GVL effect may be indicated.

Future directions

As detailed in this review of the literature on refractory and relapsed lymphomas in CAYA, curative outcomes are uncommon for the vast majority of patients receiving standard treatment strategies. Undoubtedly, novel directions are desperately needed. Targeted immunotherapies based on monoclonal antibodies directed at CD20 (rituximab and obinituzumab) for mature B-cell NHL, as well as CD30 (brentuximab) for ALCL and HL, have been successfully combined with chemotherapy to improve overall responses. Meanwhile, cellular immunotherapies also offer great promise.

T-cell-based therapies have become an important focal point in the development of novel strategies against hematologic malignancies. Taking advantage of the ability to generate Epstein–Barr virus (EBV)-specific cytotoxic T lymphocytes (CTL), investigators have developed CTL therapy derived from both autologous and allogeneic cell sources to treat refractory/relapsed EBV-positive lymphomas. Targeting the EBV latent membrane proteins (LMP) 1 and 2 that are expressed in types II and III EBV latency programming, these CTL-based therapies have demonstrated enormous potential [55]. Bollard *et al*. [56] recently reported on the use of LMP-CTL therapy derived from autologous dendritic cells in patients with EBV-positive HL or NHL. Of 29 patients with either high-risk or multiply relapsed disease receiving the LMP-CTL therapy while in remission,

28 maintained long-term CR. However, there were eight deaths in CR from late complications including three secondary malignancies. An additional 21 patients received the autologous CTL infusion with refractory/relapsed disease; 11 achieved CR, with nine patients alive in durable remission ranging 2–9 years. Of note, there were 18 patients aged under 29 years included in the trial (14 with HL). Nine received LMP-CTL while in remission and all were alive in CR (range 1–8 years), including two adolescents who received auto-HSCT plus autologous LMP-CTL for primary refractory HL. An additional nine CAYA received autologous LMP-CTL with active disease, among whom two achieved durable CR (4 and 7 years respectively), six had no response, and one relapsed at 4 years. The fact that four patients with multiply relapsed and/or primary refractory disease were able to achieve long-term CR establishes the promising potential of this therapy.

Building on the concept of developing EBV-specific CTL therapy for EBV-positive lymphomas, Bollard and Cairo *et al*. have developed a lymphoma cell therapy consortium for CAYA. Attempting to capitalize on up to 40% of HL being EBV-positive, they have developed a new protocol of RIC followed by EBV-positive matched related or unrelated donor allo-HSCT in children with high-risk refractory/relapsed HL. The allo-HSCT would then be followed by an infusion of donor-derived LMP-CTL to target the EBV-positive lymphoma cells. This therapeutic strategy of utilizing donor-derived EBV-specific CTL has been established in EBV-associated lymphoproliferative disease, chronic active EBV, and the rare EBV-positive hydroavacciniforme-like T-cell lymphoma [55,57,58].

For lymphomas not associated with EBV, T-cell and more recently NK-cell therapies using chimeric antigen receptors (CAR) have been under development. CAR-based therapies combine an extracellular antigen-binding transmembrane domain with intracellular signal transduction domains to direct immune effector cell cytotoxicity. Utilizing antigenic targets such as CD20 and C19, CAR T-cell clinical trials are well underway, albeit with much more momentum for the treatment of leukemia at the moment. In the preclinical domain, antitumor effects of NK cell-based anti-CD20 CAR has been demonstrated for the treatment of BL in mouse models [59,60].

The efficacy of cellular immunotherapies to treat refractory/relapsed lymphomas serves as additional affirmation of the immunogenic nature of hematologic malignancies. Rooted in the concept that MAC chemotherapy followed by auto-HSCT can establish a strong response even in refractory/relapsed disease, the strategy of combining auto-HSCT with a tandem allo-HSCT was pioneered by Carella *et al.* [61] in adult patients. They used an MAC auto-HSCT regimen with carmustine, etoposide, cytarabine and melphalan followed by a nonmyeloablative fludarabine/cyclophosphamide "mini-allograft"; 11 of 15 patients with multiply relapsed and/or refractory lymphomas achieved CR after the tandem transplants, with five patients maintaining long-term CR. The most promising data for the efficacy of tandem auto-HSCT followed by RIC allo-HSCT was reported by Crocchiolo *et al.* [62] in 34 adults with high-risk relapsed NHL, with a 5-year PFS of 68%. The only pediatric data for this tandem approach was discussed earlier in the chapter; in an intent-to-treat analysis of all 30 patients enrolled, 10-year EFS was 56.4% for high-risk relapsed/refractory HL, and 50% for NHL. Among the 23 patients that underwent the tandem auto-HSCT/RIC allo-HSCT, the 10-year EFS was 59.8% for HL and 70% for NHL [27]. Ultimately, while more robust prospective trials are needed to confirm the potential advantage to utilizing MAC auto-HSCT followed by RIC allo-HSCT in CAYA, the promising results lend credence to the concept of a GVL effect to sustain a long-term remission. Furthermore, the relative risk of developing secondary malignancies as a late complication of auto-HSCT may be mitigated by the allo-HSCT.

Ultimately, though, while auto-HSCT and allo-HSCT offer the potential for long-term curative options, the risk for relapse after either treatment strategy is still unfortunately high. Optimizing pre-HSCT treatment regimens to reduce the risk of relapse is essential. The concept of using radioimmunotherapy as a novel therapeutic approach in lymphomas in CAYA is very attractive. Although it has been limited by excessive toxicities in early clinical trials, novel approaches have attempted to incorporate radionuclide-conjugated monoclonal antibodies in the conditioning regimens before HSCT. Radioimmunotherapy in lymphoma has great developmental potential for the following reasons: antigenic targets for the monoclonal antibodies are well established and available, the most success in using radiolabeled antibodies has been established in hematologic malignancies, and lymphomas are very sensitive to radiation therapy. Data for using radiolabeled humoral immunotherapy in combination with chemotherapy in conditioning regimens for auto-HSCT has demonstrated

improved response rates for adult patients with relapsed NHL treated with ^{90}Y-ibritumomab tiuxetan combined with BEAM chemotherapy [63]. While there is need to develop data in CAYA, the potential for benefit using this novel methodology may offer a fresh therapeutic approach in an attempt to bolster the options available to this very high-risk subset of patients.

Conclusions

There is a vitally important role for HSCT in lymphomas in CAYA; it offers a potentially curative therapeutic option for patients with refractory/relapsed disease, a subset of patients that is otherwise essentially incurable.

Table 4.3 Proposed treatment paradigm for children, adolescents, and young adults with refractory and relapsed lymphomas with chemosensitive disease on relapse.

Hodgkin lymphoma

Auto-HSCT
Late relapse
Allo-HSCT
Primary refractory
Early relapse
Multiple relapse

Mature B-cell non-Hodgkin lymphoma

Auto-HSCT
Late relapse
Allo-HSCT
Primary refractory
Early relapse
Multiple relapse

Lymphoblastic lymphoma

Auto-HSCT
Not indicated
Allo-HSCT
Any refractory/relapse

Anaplastic large-cell lymphoma

Auto-HSCT
Late relapse (excluding those with CD3-negative disease with late relapse)
Allo-HSCT
Primary refractory
CD3-positive disease in any relapse

There is a notable exclusion for those patients originally presenting with early-stage disease treated with minimally intensive upfront protocols. Allo-HSCT is suggested in those patients with less than 30% chance for EFS despite the use of auto-HSCT. Use of allo-HSCT can be considered with a tandem auto-HSCT preceding it. Special consideration should be given for EBV-specific CTL immunotherapy in EBV-positive lymphomas.

However, because the characteristics of lymphoma at the time of relapse can be widely heterogeneous, the HSCT-based treatment strategy can vary markedly. Delineating a risk stratification for each individual patient for each specific lymphoma is critical. A proposed treatment algorithm based on disease type and clinical characteristics is summarized in Table 4.3. The emphasis in treatment of CAYA with lymphomas is to achieve cure. Therefore, the most important factor to consider is which patients have a formidable chance for a curative outcome utilizing auto-HSCT. Those with an unacceptably high risk of failing auto-HSCT should be considered for alternative therapeutic strategies in hopes of establishing the optimal treatment that can safely and effectively offer the chance for cure to the greatest number of patients. Ultimately, a well-designed risk stratification-based international multicenter prospective clinical trial offers the best opportunity to answer the many questions regarding the optimal treatment approach in this challenging subset of patients.

References

1 Pinkerton CR, Cairo MS. Childhood non-Hodgkin lymphoma. In: Cairo MS, Perkins SL, eds. *Hematological Malignancies in Children, Adolescents and Young Adults*. Singapore: World Scientific Publishing Co., 2012:299–328.

2 Friedman DL, Younes A. Hodgkin lymphoma in children, adolescents and young adults. In: Cairo MS, Perkins SL, eds. *Hematological Malignancies in Children, Adolescents and Young Adults*. Singapore: World Scientific Publishing Co., 2012:349–61.

3 Hochberg J, Waxman IM, Kelly KM *et al.* Adolescent non-Hodgkin lymphoma and Hodgkin lymphoma: state of the science. *Br J Haematol* 2009;**144**:24–40.

4 Josting A, Muller H, Borchmann P *et al.* Dose intensity of chemotherapy in patients with relapsed Hodgkin's lymphoma. *J Clin Oncol* 2010;**28**:5074–80.

5 Sauter CS, Barker JN, Lechner L *et al.* A phase II study of a nonmyeloablative allogeneic stem cell transplant with peritransplant rituximab in patients with B cell lymphoid malignancies: favorably durable event-free survival in chemosensitive patients. *Biol Blood Marrow Transplant* 2014;**20**:354–60.

6 Jones RJ, Ambinder RF, Piantadosi S *et al.* Evidence of a graft-versus-lymphoma effect associated with allogeneic bone marrow transplantation. *Blood* 1991;**77**:649–53.

7 Bradley MB, Cairo MS. Stem cell transplantation for pediatric lymphoma: past, present and future. *Bone Marrow Transplant* 2008;**41**:149–58.

8 Anderson JE, Litzow MR, Appelbaum FR *et al.* Allogeneic, syngeneic, and autologous marrow transplantation for Hodgkin's disease: the 21-year Seattle experience. *J Clin Oncol* 1993;**11**:2342–50.

9 Schellong G, Dorffel W, Claviez A *et al.* Salvage therapy of progressive and recurrent Hodgkin's disease: results from a multicenter study of the pediatric DAL/GPOH-HD study group. *J Clin Oncol* 2005;**23**:6181–9.

10 Schmitz N, Pfistner B, Sextro M *et al.* Aggressive conventional chemotherapy compared with high-dose chemotherapy with autologous haemopoietic stem-cell transplantation for relapsed chemosensitive Hodgkin's disease: a randomised trial. *Lancet* 2002;**359**:2065–71.

11 Sureda A, Pereira MI, Dreger P. The role of hematopoietic stem cell transplantation in the treatment of relapsed/refractory Hodgkin's lymphoma. *Curr Opin Oncol* 2012;**24**:727–32.

12 Claviez A, Sureda A, Schmitz N. Haematopoietic SCT for children and adolescents with relapsed and refractory Hodgkin's lymphoma. *Bone Marrow Transplant* 2008;**42**(Suppl 2):S16–24.

13 Baker KS, Gordon BG, Gross TG *et al.* Autologous hematopoietic stem-cell transplantation for relapsed or refractory Hodgkin's disease in children and adolescents. *J Clin Oncol* 1999;**17**:825–31.

14 Harris RE, Termuhlen AM, Smith LM *et al.* Autologous peripheral blood stem cell transplantation in children with refractory or relapsed lymphoma: results of Children's Oncology Group study A5962. *Biol Blood Marrow Transplant* 2011;**17**:249–58.

15 Lieskovsky YE, Donaldson SS, Torres MA *et al.* High-dose therapy and autologous hematopoietic stem-cell transplantation for recurrent or refractory pediatric Hodgkin's disease: results and prognostic indices. *J Clin Oncol* 2004;**22**:4532–40.

16 Williams CD, Goldstone AH, Pearce R *et al.* Autologous bone marrow transplantation for pediatric Hodgkin's disease: a case-matched comparison with adult patients by the European Bone Marrow Transplant Group Lymphoma Registry. *J Clin Oncol* 1993;**11**:2243–9.

17 Claviez A, Kabisch H, Suttorp M *et al.* The impact of disease status at transplant and time to first relapse on outcome in children and adolescents with relapsed Hodgkin's lymphoma undergoing autologous stem cell transplantation. *Bone Marrow Transplant* 2005;**35**:S85.

18 Claviez A, Kabisch H, Suttorp M *et al.* The impact of disease status at transplant and time to first relapse on outcome in children and adolescents with Hodgkin's lymphoma undergoing autologous stem cell transplantation. *Blood (ASH Annual Meeting Abstracts)* 2004;**104**:Abstract 1878.

19 Milpied N, Fielding AK, Pearce RM *et al.* Allogeneic bone marrow transplant is not better than autologous transplant for patients with relapsed Hodgkin's disease. European Group for Blood and Bone Marrow Transplantation. *J Clin Oncol* 1996;**14**:1291–6.

20 Sureda A, Robinson S, Canals C *et al.* Reduced-intensity conditioning compared with conventional allogeneic stem-cell transplantation in relapsed or refractory Hodgkin's lymphoma: an

analysis from the Lymphoma Working Party of the European Group for Blood and Marrow Transplantation. *J Clin Oncol* 2008;**26**:455–62.

21 Robinson SP, Sureda A, Canals C *et al*. Reduced intensity conditioning allogeneic stem cell transplantation for Hodgkin's lymphoma: identification of prognostic factors predicting outcome. *Haematologica* 2009;**94**:230–8.

22 Sureda A, Canals C, Arranz R *et al*. Allogeneic stem cell transplantation after reduced intensity conditioning in patients with relapsed or refractory Hodgkin's lymphoma. Results of the HDR-ALLO study: a prospective clinical trial by the Grupo Espanol de Linfomas/Trasplante de Medula Osea (GEL/TAMO) and the Lymphoma Working Party of the European Group for Blood and Marrow Transplantation. *Haematologica* 2012;**97**:310–17.

23 Thomson KJ, Kayani I, Ardeshna K *et al*. A response-adjusted PET-based transplantation strategy in primary resistant and relapsed Hodgkin lymphoma. *Leukemia* 2013;**27**:1419–22.

24 Peggs KS, Hunter A, Chopra R *et al*. Clinical evidence of a graft-versus-Hodgkin's-lymphoma effect after reduced-intensity allogeneic transplantation. *Lancet* 2005;**365**:1934–41.

25 Peggs KS, Kayani I, Edwards N *et al*. Donor lymphocyte infusions modulate relapse risk in mixed chimeras and induce durable salvage in relapsed patients after T-cell-depleted allogeneic transplantation for Hodgkin's lymphoma. *J Clin Oncol* 2011;**29**:971–8.

26 Claviez A, Canals C, Dierickx D *et al*. Allogeneic hematopoietic stem cell transplantation in children and adolescents with recurrent and refractory Hodgkin lymphoma: an analysis of the European Group for Blood and Marrow Transplantation. *Blood* 2009;**114**:2060–7.

27 Satwani P, Jin Z, Bradley MB *et al*. Sequential myeloablative autologous stem cell transplantation and reduced intensity allogeneic hematopoietic cell transplantation is safe and feasible in children, adolescents and young adults with poor-risk refractory or recurrent Hodgkin and non-Hodgkin lymphoma. *Leukemia* 2014. doi: 10.1038/leu.2014.194.

28 El-Mallawany NK, Frazer JK, Van Vlierberghe P *et al*. Pediatric T- and NK-cell lymphomas: new biologic insights and treatment strategies. *Blood Cancer J* 2012;**2**:e65.

29 El-Mallawany NK, Van Vlierberghe P, Ferrando AA *et al*. T-cell malignancies in children and adolescents: state of the clinical and biological science. In: Foss F, ed. *T-Cell Lymphoproliferative Disorders*. New York: Humana Press/Springer Science and Business Media, 2013:179–216.

30 Burkhardt B, Reiter A, Landmann E *et al*. Poor outcome for children and adolescents with progressive disease or relapse of lymphoblastic lymphoma: a report from the Berlin–Frankfurt–Muenster group. *J Clin Oncol* 2009;**27**:3363–9.

31 Giulino-Roth L, Ricafort R, Kernan NA *et al*. Ten-year follow-up of pediatric patients with non-Hodgkin lymphoma treated with allogeneic or autologous stem cell transplantation. *Pediatr Blood Cancer* 2013;**60**:2018–24.

32 Gaynon PS, Harris RE, Altman AJ *et al*. Bone marrow transplantation versus prolonged intensive chemotherapy for children with acute lymphoblastic leukemia and an initial bone marrow relapse within 12 months of the completion of primary therapy: Children's Oncology Group study CCG-1941. *J Clin Oncol* 2006;**24**:3150–6.

33 Raetz EA, Borowitz MJ, Devidas M *et al*. Reinduction platform for children with first marrow relapse of acute lymphoblastic Leukemia: A Children's Oncology Group Study [corrected]. *J Clin Oncol* 2008;**26**:3971–8.

34 Levine JE, Harris RE, Loberiza FR Jr *et al*. A comparison of allogeneic and autologous bone marrow transplantation for lymphoblastic lymphoma. *Blood* 2003;**101**:2476–82.

35 Gross TG, Hale GA, He W *et al*. Hematopoietic stem cell transplantation for refractory or recurrent non-Hodgkin lymphoma in children and adolescents. *Biol Blood Marrow Transplant* 2010;**16**:223–30.

36 Cairo MS, Woessmann W, Pagel J. Advances in hematopoietic stem cell transplantation in childhood and adolescent lymphomas. *Biol Blood Marrow Transplant* 2013;**19**:S38–43.

37 Brugieres L, Quartier P, Le Deley MC *et al*. Relapses of childhood anaplastic large-cell lymphoma: treatment results in a series of 41 children. A report from the French Society of Pediatric Oncology. *Ann Oncol* 2000;**11**:53–8.

38 Woessmann W, Zimmermann M, Lenhard M *et al*. Relapsed or refractory anaplastic large-cell lymphoma in children and adolescents after Berlin–Frankfurt–Muenster (BFM)-type first-line therapy: a BFM-group study. *J Clin Oncol* 2011;**29**:3065–71.

39 Woessmann W, Peters C, Lenhard M *et al*. Allogeneic haematopoietic stem cell transplantation in relapsed or refractory anaplastic large cell lymphoma of children and adolescents: a Berlin–Frankfurt–Munster group report. *Br J Haematol* 2006;**133**:176–82.

40 Cesaro S, Pillon M, Visintin G *et al*. Unrelated bone marrow transplantation for high-risk anaplastic large cell lymphoma in pediatric patients: a single center case series. *Eur J Haematol* 2005;**75**:22–6.

41 Mori T, Takimoto T, Katano N *et al*. Recurrent childhood anaplastic large cell lymphoma: a retrospective analysis of registered cases in Japan. *Br J Haematol* 2006;**132**:594–7.

42 Goldman S, Smith L, Anderson JR *et al*. Rituximab and FAB/LMB 96 chemotherapy in children with Stage III/IV B-cell non-Hodgkin lymphoma: a Children's Oncology Group report. *Leukemia* 2013;**27**:1174–7.

43 Cairo MS, Gerrard M, Sposto R *et al*. Results of a randomized international study of high-risk central nervous system B non-Hodgkin lymphoma and B acute lymphoblastic leukemia in children and adolescents. *Blood* 2007;**109**:2736–43.

44 Rosenwald A, Wright G, Leroy K *et al*. Molecular diagnosis of primary mediastinal B cell lymphoma identifies a clinically favorable subgroup of diffuse large B cell lymphoma related to Hodgkin lymphoma. *J Exp Med* 2003;**198**:851–62.

45 Dunleavy K, Pittaluga S, Maeda LS *et al.* Dose-adjusted EPOCH–rituximab therapy in primary mediastinal B-cell lymphoma. *N Engl J Med* 2013;**368**:1408–16.

46 Gerrard M, Waxman IM, Sposto R *et al.* Outcome and pathologic classification of children and adolescents with mediastinal large B-cell lymphoma treated with FAB/LMB96 mature B-NHL therapy. *Blood* 2013;**121**:278–85.

47 Cairo MS, Sposto R, Perkins SL *et al.* Burkitt's and Burkitt-like lymphoma in children and adolescents: a review of the Children's Cancer Group experience. *Br J Haematol* 2003;**120**:660–70.

48 Cairo MS, Sposto R, Fan J *et al.* Survival in children and adolescents (C+A) with mature B-NHL progressing or relapsing from treatment on FAB/LMB 96: tumor burden and time to relapse are poor prognostic factors [Abstract]. *Pediatr Blood Cancer* 2009;**53**:855.

49 Attarbaschi A, Dworzak M, Steiner M *et al.* Outcome of children with primary resistant or relapsed non-Hodgkin lymphoma and mature B-cell leukemia after intensive first-line treatment: a population-based analysis of the Austrian Cooperative Study Group. *Pediatr Blood Cancer* 2005;**44**:70–6.

50 Philip T, Hartmann O, Pinkerton R *et al.* Curability of relapsed childhood B-cell non-Hodgkin's lymphoma after intensive first line therapy: a report from the Societe Francaise d'Oncologie Pediatrique. *Blood* 1993;**81**:2003–6.

51 Ladenstein R, Pearce R, Hartmann O *et al.* High-dose chemotherapy with autologous bone marrow rescue in children with poor-risk Burkitt's lymphoma: a report from the European Lymphoma Bone Marrow Transplantation Registry. *Blood* 1997;**90**:2921–30.

52 Bureo E, Ortega JJ, Munoz A *et al.* Bone marrow transplantation in 46 pediatric patients with non-Hodgkin's lymphoma. Spanish Working Party for Bone Marrow Transplantation in Children. *Bone Marrow Transplant* 1995;**15**:353–9.

53 Chakraverty R, Mackinnon S. Allogeneic transplantation for lymphoma. *J Clin Oncol* 2011;**29**:1855–63.

54 Klyuchnikov E, Bacher U, Kroll T *et al.* Allogeneic hematopoietic cell transplantation for diffuse large B cell lymphoma: who, when and how? *Bone Marrow Transplant* 2014;**49**:1–7.

55 Heslop HE, Slobod KS, Pule MA *et al.* Long-term outcome of EBV-specific T-cell infusions to prevent or treat EBV-related lymphoproliferative disease in transplant recipients. *Blood* 2010;**115**:925–35.

56 Bollard CM, Gottschalk S, Torrano V *et al.* Sustained complete responses in patients with lymphoma receiving autologous cytotoxic T lymphocytes targeting Epstein–Barr virus latent membrane proteins. *J Clin Oncol* 2014;**32**:798–808.

57 Cohen JI, Jaffe ES, Dale JK *et al.* Characterization and treatment of chronic active Epstein–Barr virus disease: a 28-year experience in the United States. *Blood* 2011;**117**:5835–49.

58 El-Mallawany NK, Geller L, Bollard CM *et al.* Long-term remission in a child with refractory EBV(+) hydroa vacciniforme-like T-cell lymphoma through sequential matched EBV(+)-related allogeneic hematopoietic SCT followed by donor-derived EBV-specific cytotoxic T-lymphocyte immunotherapy. *Bone Marrow Transplant* 2011;**46**:759–61.

59 Chu Y, Ayello J, Lo L *et al.* Expanded natural killer (NK) cells transfected with anti-CD20 chimeric antigen receptor (CAR) mRNA have significant cytotoxicity against poor risk B-cell (CD20+) leukemia/lymphoma (B-L/L). *Blood (ASH Annual Meeting Abstracts)* 2012;**120**:Abstract 3007.

60 Chu Y, Yahr A, Ayello J *et al.* Anti-CD20 chimeric antigen receptor (CAR) modified expanded natural killer (NK) cells significantly mediate Burkitt lymphoma (BL) regression and improve survival in human BL xenografted NSG mice. *Blood (ASH Annual Meeting Abstracts)* 2013;**22**:3263.

61 Carella AM, Cavaliere M, Lerma E *et al.* Autografting followed by nonmyeloablative immunosuppressive chemotherapy and allogeneic peripheral-blood hematopoietic stem-cell transplantation as treatment of resistant Hodgkin's disease and non-Hodgkin's lymphoma. *J Clin Oncol* 2000;**18**:3918–24.

62 Crocchiolo R, Castagna L, Furst S *et al.* Tandem autologous-allo-SCT is feasible in patients with high-risk relapsed non-Hodgkin's lymphoma. *Bone Marrow Transplant* 2013;**48**:249–52.

63 Shimoni A, Avivi I, Rowe JM *et al.* A randomized study comparing yttrium-90 ibritumomab tiuxetan (Zevalin) and high-dose BEAM chemotherapy versus BEAM alone as the conditioning regimen before autologous stem cell transplantation in patients with aggressive lymphoma. *Cancer* 2012;**118**:4706–14.

CHAPTER 5

Preparative regimens for lymphoma: autologous hematopoietic stem cell transplantation

Taiga Nishihori, Karma Z. Salem, Ernesto Ayala and Mohamed A. Kharfan-Dabaja

Rationale for chemotherapy dose intensification for disease eradication

Preclinical studies performed decades earlier demonstrated a dose-dependent sensitivity of leukemia and lymphoma cells to radiotherapy and chemotherapy [1–3]. Subsequently, animal studies demonstrated that autologous bone marrow can restore hematopoiesis after lethal irradiation [4–6]. The realization of critical chemotherapy dose intensification [7] and the understanding of basic biology of myeloablation followed by bone marrow rescue paved the way for the development of clinical hematopoietic cell transplantation (HCT). In general, conditioning regimens were developed considering the antitumor effects of the individual chemotherapy agent and the combined dose-limiting organ toxicities.

Conditioning regimens for HCT were first developed in the context of allogeneic bone marrow graft transplantation in order to achieve both myeloablation and immusuppression. In general, myelotoxic chemotherapeutic agents used in conditioning regimens were dose-escalated to the maximally tolerated nonhematologic toxicity to optimize antineoplastic cytotoxicity. These myeloablative regimens were then extrapolated to the clinical autologous HCT setting.

Stem cell rescue provides substantial dose escalation of cytotoxic chemotherapy or chemoradiotherapy, and so the ability of chemotherapy to eradicate tumor cells is maximized. High-dose therapy (HDT) followed by autologous HCT has become the major curative option for high-risk or relapsed chemosensitive lymphoid malignancies.

Traditional preparative regimens

HDT followed by autologous HCT has been utilized for the past few decades to improve progression-free survival (PFS) and overall survival (OS) in patients with relapsed and/or refractory aggressive lymphomas [8]. Through an international collaboration, Philip *et al.* [8] reported the outcomes of 100 intermediate- to high-grade non-Hodgkin lymphoma (NHL) patients who were treated with either high-dose chemotherapy or high-dose chemotherapy plus total body irradiation (TBI) with bone marrow transplantation. The actuarial 3-year disease-free survival was 36% for the sensitive-relapse group compared with 14% for the resistant-relapse group. In a retrospective analysis, the Group d'Etudes des Lymphomes de l'Adulte (GELA) showed that high-dose chemotherapy followed by autologous HCT resulted in longer OS and freedom from progression in 44 chemotherapy-sensitive relapsed or primary refractory aggressive NHL patients compared to salvage chemotherapy alone [9].

A prospective randomized landmark study, the Parma trial, demonstrated the superiority of autologous HCT in NHL patients (intermediate or high grade based on Working Formulation classification) who had chemotherapy-sensitive disease in first or second relapse without bone marrow involvement at relapse, compared with chemotherapy (DHAP: dexamethasone, cisplatin, and cytarabine) [10]. Those who achieved either a complete or partial response after two cycles of DHAP chemotherapy were randomized to either additional DHAP chemotherapy (four cycles) plus radiation (35 Gy) or high-dose BEAC (carmustine, etoposide, cytarabine, cyclophosphamide and mesna) conditioning and autologous transplantation [10]. Both arms received involved field radiotherapy to sites of bulky disease. At 5 years, the autologous HCT arm had a significantly improved event-free survival (EFS) of 46% versus 12% ($P = 0.0001$) and OS of 53% versus 32% ($P = 0.038$) vis-à-vis the chemotherapy arm, respectively [10]. This study established the key role of high-dose chemotherapy followed by stem cell support as the standard treatment of relapsed/refractory aggressive NHL.

There are several preparative regimens for autologous HCT. Many chemotherapeutic agents have the ability to cross the blood–brain barrier in a dose-dependent manner [11,12]. In practice, there are some variations in chemotherapy (or radiotherapy whenever applicable) dosing based on the institutional experience; and the choice of particular conditioning regimen may be related to physician familiarity and center preference as well as existing institutional treatment algorithms for various lymphoma subtypes.

The most commonly used preparative regimens for autografting in patients with lymphoma include BEAM (BCNU, etoposide, cytarabine and melphalan), CBV (cyclophosphamide, BCNU and VP-16), BEAC (BCNU, etoposide, cytarabine and cyclophosphamide) [10], Cy/VP-16/TBI (cyclophosphamide, etoposide and TBI) [13–17], and BuCy (busulfan, cyclophosphamide) [18–21]. The details of chemotherapy dosing and schedule variations have been reviewed elsewhere [11]. BEAM regimen consists of BCNU (300 mg/m² for 1 day), etoposide (100–200 mg/m² daily or 100 mg/m² twice a day for 4 days), cytarabine (100–200 mg/m² daily or 100 mg/m² twice a day for 4 days), and melphalan (140 mg/m² for 1 day) [22,23]. CBV consists of cyclophosphamide (1500 mg/m² daily for 4 days), BCNU 300 mg/m² for 1 day), and VP-16 (250 mg/m² daily for 4 days) [24,25]. Augmented CBV entails cyclophosphamide (100 mg/kg for 1 day), BCNU (15 mg/kg or 450–550 mg/m² for 1 day), and VP-16 (60 mg/kg for 1 day) [13–15,26].

Alkylating agents such as cyclophosphamide, melphalan, busulfan and carmustine (BCNU), topoisomerase inhibitors (such as etoposide), and platinum agents (cisplatin and carboplatin) constitute the backbone of preparative regimens based on their antitumor activity and preclinical data supporting their ability to overcome chemotherapy resistance with dose escalation. Nonhematologic dose-limiting toxicities for chemotherapy agents commonly used in preparative agents have been reviewed by others [11]. Dose-limiting toxicities for commonly used preparative regimen chemotherapeutics are as follows: BCNU – pulmonary, hepatic; cyclophosphamide – mucosal, urothelial; etoposide – mucosal; melphalan – mucosal. As the main toxicity of alkylating agents is predominantly hematologic, their dose can be intensified. Less commonly used regimens include melphalan plus etoposide and melphalan plus mitoxantrone [27,28]. Other preparative regimens combining carboplatin and ifosfamide have been developed [29,30].

Many transplant preparative regimens for lymphoma consist of only chemotherapeutic agents. Lymphoma cells are also sensitive to radiation-induced cytotoxicity. Moreover, radiation therapy can potentially reach sanctuary sites such as central nervous system and testes. Chemotherapy resistance can also be overcome by radiation therapy. However, there have been no prospective randomized controlled trials comparing chemotherapy with TBI-based preparative regimens in lymphoid malignancies. Use of TBI as part of preparative regimens for lymphoma transplant appears to be used less often nowadays [31].

In a retrospective study from Stanford where the outcomes for HDT followed by autologous HCT for lymphoma were examined, there were no differences in relapse rates between TBI-based and chemotherapy-only groups [15]. Other studies also did not find any significant advantage of using TBI-based regimens [8,32–34]. In a registry study by the Center for International Blood and Marrow Transplant Research (CIBMTR) where recent activities on autologous HCT have been reviewed including over 20,000 lymphoma patients from 1995 to 2005, a limited number of autologous HCTs were performed using cyclophosphamide/TBI or other TBI-based regimens [31]. TBI-based regimens are usually avoided in lymphoma patients who received prior radiation therapy due in part to significant toxicity concerns, particularly for the development of interstitial pneumonitis [35,36]. Choice of TBI-based regimens, over chemotherapy-based ones, is likely based on center preference. A future randomized controlled trial comparing TBI- with chemotherapy-based regimens for autografting is unlikely to be performed.

In a recent retrospective registry study by CIBMTR, outcomes of commonly used autologous HCT preparative regimens in 4917 lymphoma patients from 1995 to 2008 were compared [37]. The cohorts differed in age, histology, and year of HCT. There was no significant difference in outcomes with BEAM, CBV^{low} (BCNU dose <375 mg/m^2), busulfan plus cyclophosphamide (BuCy), and TBI-based regimens for NHL. However, NHL patients treated with CBV^{high} (BCNU dose >375 mg/m^2) had a worse progression rate as well as higher transplant-associated mortality. For patients with Hodgkin lymphoma (HL), BuCy- and TBI-based regimens were associated with higher rates of progression and shorter survival compared to BEAM. Additionally, a Phase II multicenter study of 184 lymphoma patients conditioned with a busulfan, cyclophosphamide and etoposide (BuCyE) regimen from 2010 to 2012 compared the results with recipients of BEAM regimen registered to CIBMTR in a matched-pair analysis [38]. The 2-year OS and transplant-related mortality were the same for both groups (younger than 65 years old with NHL); however, in a subset of HL patients the risk of progression was higher and consequently PFS was lower with the BuCyE regimen. These studies suggest that there are no significant differences in outcomes for autologous HCT in NHL based on preparative regimens with the exception of CBV^{high}, and BEAM appears to be the most widely used and better regimen for autologous HCT in HL.

Incorporation of monoclonal antibodies in autologous HCT preparative regimens

Use of monoclonal antibodies either as monotherapy or as part of chemoimmunotherapy regimens has become the standard therapy for various lymphoid malignancies [39–42]. In the setting of HDT and autologous HCT, addition of monoclonal antibodies is aimed at improving the anti-malignancy efficacy of the preparative regimen [43]. Here we summarize the published literatures pertaining to the use of rituximab as well as anti-CD20 radioimmunoconjugate monoclonal antibodies which have been evaluated as part of preparative regimens for autologous HCT.

Rituximab

Rituximab is a chimeric anti-CD20 monoclonal antibody approved for the treatment of various subtypes of B-cell NHL. Rituximab has been shown to be feasible when combined with conditioning regimens for autologous HCT. However, randomized controlled trials that demonstrate the superiority of adding rituximab to conventional high-dose conditioning regimens (compared to without rituximab) are lacking.

Moreover, rituximab has been shown to be feasible to use in the pre-mobilization phase aiming at elimination of disease from the stem cell product (*in vivo* purging) [44–50]. This strategy does not appear to affect engraftment kinetics after transplantation. However, no randomized data exist evaluating the ultimate benefit (or lack thereof) of this strategy to our knowledge. Also, other questions remain unanswered, including the best timing of administration of rituximab and whether there is a dose-effect for more effective purging.

Incorporating rituximab in the peri- and post-conditioning phase has also been shown to be feasible and, again, did not appear to affect engraftment kinetics. A retrospective multicenter study from the Gruppo Italiano Terapie Innovative nei Linfomi showed that addition of rituximab did not worsen transplant-associated mortality (2.8% vs. 3.3%; *P*-value, not significant) but resulted in better 5-year EFS (61% vs. 51%, *P* < 0.001) and OS (69% vs. 60%, *P* < 0.001) [51]. These and other studies are summarized in Table 5.1 [44,45,51–53].

It is important to keep in mind the potential concerns with use of rituximab in this setting, especially prolonged B-cell depletion with hypogammaglobulinemia, increased risk of opportunistic infections, and occurrence of late cytopenias [54,55].

Monoclonal antibodies conjugated to radionuclide

The ability of radioimmunoconjugates to deliver targeted radiation with relatively low organ toxicity provided the rationale to develop radioimmunotherapy (RIT)-based preparative regimens for autografting. Two anti-CD20 monoclonal antibodies, ibritumomab and tositumomab conjugated to either yttrium-90 or iodine-131, are currently in clinical use for treatment of indolent CD20-expressing lymphomas [56,57]. Several small single-arm studies have demonstrated encouraging results using RIT whether alone or

Table 5.1 Selected studies of rituximab addition to conditioning regimens for autologous HCT.

Study	Study type	N	Dose of rituximab	Conditioning regimen	Survival
Flinn et al. (2000) [47]	Phase II, single arm	25	Day 1 of mobilization chemotherapy at 375 mg/m^2 After engraftment at 375 mg/m^2	Cy/TBI	N/A
Voso et al. (2000) [49]	Pilot study	18	Day −1 of mobilization chemotherapy at 375 mg/m^2 Day −1 of TBI	Cy/TBI	N/A
Flohr et al. (2002) [44]	Phase II, single arm	27	Day 1 of mobilization chemotherapy at 375 mg/m^2 With conditioning regimens days −10 and −3 at 375 mg/m^2	Cy/TBI, BEAM or BEAC	PFS, 77% OS, 95% (at 16 months)
Khouri et al. (2005) [45]	Phase II, single arm	67	With mobilization chemotherapy at 375 mg/m^2 on day −1 and at 1000 mg/m^2 on day 7 With conditioning at 1000 mg/m^2 on days +1 and +8	BEAM	DFS, 67% OS, 80% (2-year)
Tarella et al. (2008) [51]	Retrospective	349	Four doses before PBSC collection Two doses after autologous HCT	Mitoxantrone/ melphalan or BEAM	OS 69% vs. 60% without rituximab (5-year)
Hicks et al. (2008) [53]	Phase II, single arm	23	At 375 mg/m^2 before or during G-CSF mobilization Post-transplantation maintenance: two 4-week courses with 375 mg/m^2 at 8 and 24 weeks after autologous HCT	CBV	PFS, 59% OS, 78% (5-year)
Vose et al. (2011) [79]	Phase III, randomized multicenter	112	Days −19 and −12 of conditioning at 375 mg/m^2	BEAM	PFS, 48.6% OS, 65.5% (2-year)

BEAC, BCNU, etoposide, cytarabine, and cyclophosphamide; BEAM, BCNU, etoposide, cytarabine, and melphalan; CBV, cyclophosphamide, BCNU, and VP-16 (etoposide); Cy, cyclophosphamide; DFS, disease-free survival; G-CSF, granulocyte-colony stimulating factor; HCT, hematopoietic cell transplantation; N/A, not available; OS, overall survival; PBSC, peripheral blood stem cells; PFS, progression-free survival; TBI, total body irradiation.

by incorporating them into conventional preparative regimens for autologous HCT for CD20-expressing lymphomas. Investigators at the Fred Hutchinson Cancer Research Center pioneered the use of myeloablative RIT conditioning for autologous HCT. A phase I study of ^{131}I-tositumomab conditioning showed that the maximum tolerated dose of radiation was 27 Gy [58], and further dosage escalation was limited by cardiopulmonary toxicities [58]. Several small phase II studies using high-dose RIT with ^{131}I-tositumomab alone, mainly in patients with chemosensitive relapsed B-cell NHL, demonstrated 4-year PFS of 40% and OS of 65% with tolerable toxicities [59–61]. High-dose ^{131}I-tositumomab (delivering radiation doses up to 27 Gy to normal organs) combined with high-dose therapy as conditioning before autologous HCT also appears to be feasible [62,63], with 3-year PFS and OS approaching 60–65% and 80–90%, respectively; these results compare favorably with outcomes with high-dose RIT conditioning alone [59–61]. Because ^{131}I-tositumomab emits gamma radiation, its administration is cumbersome, requiring prolonged patient isolation, caregiver/

healthcare worker exposure precautions, special infusion equipment, and complex dosimetry facilities.

Nademanee et al. [64] combined ^{90}Y-ibritumomab tiuxetan with HDT for autologous HCT in patients with B-cell NHL and reported, in a phase I/II study, 2-year PFS of 78% and OS of 92%. Other investigators have also reported encouraging outcomes in B-cell NHL with high-dose ^{90}Y-ibritumomab tiuxetan-based conditioning, with or without HDT [65–69]. While these studies demonstrate the feasibility of using high-dose RIT conditioning in autologous HCT, data are limited by small sample sizes and heterogeneous NHL histologies, among other reasons.

Standard doses of RIT have been combined with conventional conditioning regimens for autologous HCT [70–78]. While single-arm phase II studies mostly from single institutions have shown encouraging results (Table 5.2), the only multicenter phase III study completed so far conducted by the Blood and Marrow Transplant Clinical Trial Network (BMT CTN), which compared addition of ^{131}I-tositumomab at conventional dose to BEAM with rituximab-BEAM, failed to show

Table 5.2 Radioimmunotherapy (RIT) as conditioning regimen for autologous hematopoietic cell transplantation (HCT).

Study	Study type	N	Agent and dose	Conditioning regimen	Survival
High-dose RIT					
Press et al. (1993) [58]	Phase I	24	234–777 mCi	^{131}I-tositumomab	OS, 21 months (median)
Press et al. (2000) [62]	Phase I/II	52	20–27 Gy (1.7 mg/kg)	^{131}I-tositumomab + Cy/VP-16	PFS, 68% OS, 83% (2-year)
Behr et al. (2002) [97]	Pilot study	7	261–495 mCi (protein dose = 2.5 mg/kg)	^{131}I-rituximab	N/A
Gopal et al. (2002) [63]	Phase II	16	20–25 Gy (1.7 mg/kg); median dose – 510 mCi	^{131}I-tositumomab + Cy/VP-16	PFS, 61% OS, 93% (3-year)
Nademanee et al. (2005) [64]	Phase I/II	31	<1000 cGy; median dose = 71.6 mCi	^{90}Y-ibritumomab + Cy/VP-16	PFS, 78% OS, 92% (2-year)
Ferrucci et al. (2007) [67]	Phase I	13	0.8, 1.2 or 1.5 mCi/kg	^{90}Y-ibritumomab	N/A
Devizzi et al. (2008) [65]	Phase II	30	0.8 mCi/kg (13 patients) and 1.2 mCi/kg (17 patients)	^{90}Y-ibritumomab	OS, 87% PFS, 69% (2.5-year)
Winter et al. (2009) [66]	Phase I	44	15 Gy MTD	^{90}Y-ibritumomab + BEAM	PFS, 43% OS, 60% (3-year)
Hohloch et al. (2011) [68]	Phase II	16	8.6–13 GBq	BEAM for first autologous HCT ^{131}I-rituximab for second autologous HCT	PFS, 64% OS, 67% (4-year)
Gopal et al. (2011) [98]	Phase I	36	27 Gy (0.4 mCi/kg)	^{131}I-tositumomab + fludarabine	PFS, 53% OS, 54% (3-year)
Standard-dose RIT					
Vose et al. (2005) [70]	Phase I	23	0.75 Gy	^{131}I-tositumomab + BEAM	PFS, 39% OS, 55% (3-year)
Shimoni et al (2007) [71]	Phase II	23	0.4 mCi/kg	^{90}Y-ibritumomab + BEAM	PFS, 52% OS, 67% (2-year)
Krishnan et al. (2008) [74]	Phase II	41	0.4 mCi/kg	^{90}Y-ibritumomab + BEAM	PFS, 70% OS, 89% (2-year)
Decaudin et al. (2011) [75]	Phase II	77	0.3–0.4 mCi/kg	^{90}Y-ibritumomab + BEAM	PFS, 63% OS, 97% (2-year)
Zipp et al. (2011) [77]	Phase II	36	0.4 mCi/kg	^{90}Y-ibritumomab + BEAM	PFS, 60–78% OS, 60–76% (5-year)
Vose et al. (2011) [79]	Phase III	224	5 mCi on day –19 and 0.75 Gy on day –12	^{131}I-tositumomab + BEAM vs. rituximab-BEAM	PFS, 48% vs. 49% OS, 60% vs. 66% (2-year)
Shimoni et al. (2012) [72]	Phase III	22 vs. 21 (total 43)	0.4 mCi/kg	^{90}Y-ibritumomab + BEAM vs. BEAM	PFS, 59% vs. 37% OS, 91% vs. 62% (2-year)

(continued)

Table 5.2 *(continued)*

Study	Study type	N	Agent and dose	Conditioning regimen	Survival
Arne *et al.* (2012) [78]	Phase II	161	0.4 mCi/kg	^{90}Y-ibritumomab + BEAM or BEAC	PFS, 55% OS, 71% (5-year)
Briones *et al.* (2012) [99]	Phase II	30	0.4 mCi/kg	^{90}Y-ibritumomab + BEAM	PFS, 63% OS, 65% (2-year)
Vose *et al.* (2013) [73]	Phase II	40	75 cGy	^{131}I-tositutmomab + BEAM	PFS, 70% OS, 72% (5-year)

BEAC, BCNU, etoposide, cytarabine, and cyclophosphamide; BEAM, BCNU, etoposide, cytarabine, and melphalan; cGy, centigray; Cy, cyclophosphamide; GBq, gigabecquerel; Gy, gray; mCi, millicurie; MTD, maximum tolerated dose; N/A, not available; OS, overall survival; PFS, progression-free survival; VP-16, etoposide.

survival benefits (PFS and OS) or decreased relapse risk in patients with chemotherapy-sensitive relapsed diffuse large B-cell lymphoma (DLBCL) [79]. At present, using an RIT-based conditioning regimen is not considered standard therapy and should be performed in the context of clinical trials.

Novel agents used in preparative regimens

Relapse after HDT and autologous HCT remains a major challenge, particularly with primary refractory disease or high-risk features at relapse [80,81]. Ongoing efforts exist to develop novel preparative regimens to improve the outcomes of autologous HCT for various lymphoid malignancies. Using pharmacokinetic targeting of intravenous busulfan dosing to avoid excessive toxicities, a preparative regimen of busulfan plus melphalan (Bu/Mel) has been examined in advanced lymphoid malignancies [82]. The Bu/Mel regimen was well tolerated and appears to have comparable anti-lymphoma effect to BEAM [82]. Gemcitabine, a nucleoside analog, has been demonstrated to inhibit DNA damage repair caused by prior exposure to alkylating agents [83]. Gemcitabine has also been shown to have clinical anti-tumor activity against HL and NHL [84–87]. The M.D. Anderson Cancer Center has developed a combination preparative regimen of gemcitabine, busulfan, and melphalan (Gem/Bu/Mel); gemcitabine was given at different dose levels, busulfan was given at AUC (area under

the curve) of 4000 μmol/min daily for 4 days, and melphalan was given at 60 mg/m^2 daily for 2 days [88]. High anti-lymphoma activity was described in heavily pretreated and refractory cases. The group at Stanford University conducted a phase I/II trial of conditioning regimen with gemcitabine (escalating dose), vinorelbine, BCNU, etoposide, and cyclophosphamide (GN-BVC) with the aim of reducing BCNU dose and toxicity in recurrent/refractory HL [89]. The regimen resulted in decreased BCNU toxicity and encouraging disease control. With further refinement and incorporation of targeted agents, future autologous HCT regimens for lymphoid malignancies may evolve to disease-specific and/or patient-specific conditioning.

Future directions

To improve the outcomes of autologous HCT several approaches have been evaluated in the context of peri- or post-autologous HCT. The Collaborative Trial in Relapsed Aggressive Lymphoma (CORAL) randomized patients with relapsed or refractory DLBCL to either rituximab maintenance or observation following autologous HCT. There were no differences in 4-year EFS between the groups [90]. However, there was a difference in EFS between women and men, which may be partly due to enhanced clearance in men resulting in decreased efficacy of rituximab because of a shorter half-life [90,91]. The European Society for Blood and Marrow Transplantation (EBMT) conducted a randomized study where patients with relapsed follicular lymphoma were randomly assigned to maintenance rituximab (375 mg/m^2 every 2 months for four infusions) or observation [92]. Ten-year PFS was significantly better in the maintenance group (54% vs. 37%, P = 0.012), but OS was not improved with maintenance [92]. Other agents that are currently being considered for similar adjunctive therapy to improve autologous HCT outcomes include ibrutinib and anti-CD22 immunoconjugate inotuzumab ozogamicin [93,94].

Another strategy entails altering the immune checkpoint in the post-autologous HCT setting. PD-1 (Programmed Death-1) is a member of the B7 receptor family and with its primary ligands (PD-L1 and PD-L2) works as an immune checkpoint to limit the T-cell response in peripheral tissues. PD-L1 is aberrantly expressed on tumor-infiltrating lymphocytes and neoplastic cells in lymphoid malignancies, and may inhibit the host antitumor response by causing T-cell exhaustion [95]. Pharmacologic targeting of the PD-1/PD-L1 pathway may be an opportunity to restore antitumor immunity after autologous HCT. Pidilizumab, an anti-PD-1 humanized IgG1 monoclonal antibody, was administered to patients with DLBCL after autologous HCT in a Phase II study, with 16-month PFS of 72% [96]. The overall response rate after pidilizumab treatment was 51% for patients with measurable disease after autologous HCT, with 34% achieving complete response. This promising activity of PD-1 blockade after autologous HCT expands the therapeutic opportunity and may herald the evolution of autologous HCT for lymphoid malignancies. Further research is needed to augment antitumor response with immunotherapy after autologous HCT utilizing tumor vaccines and immune checkpoint targeting.

References

1 Hewitt HB, Wilson CW. A survival curve for mammalian leukaemia cells irradiated in vivo (implications for the treatment of mouse leukaemia by whole-body irradiation). *Br J Cancer* 1959;**13**:69–75.

2 Bush RS, Bruce WR. The radiation sensitivity of transplanted lymphoma cells as determined by the spleen colony method. *Radiat Res* 1964;**21**:612–21.

3 Bruce WR, Meeker BE, Valeriote FA. Comparison of the sensitivity of normal hematopoietic and transplanted lymphoma colony-forming cells to chemotherapeutic agents administered in vivo. *J Natl Cancer Inst* 1966;**37**:233–45.

4 Mannick JA, Lochte HL, Thomas ED, Ferrebee JW. In vitro and in vivo assessment of the viability of dog marrow after storage. *Blood* 1960;**15**:517–24.

5 Cavins JA, Kasakura S, Thomas ED, Ferrebee JW. Recovery of lethally irradiated dogs following infusion of autologous marrow stored at low temperature in dimethylsulphoxide. *Blood* 1962;**20**:730–4.

6 Buckner CD, Storb R, Dillingham LA, Thomas ED. Low temperature preservation of monkey marrow in dimethyl sulfoxide. *Cryobiology* 1970;**7**:136–40.

7 Frei E, Canellos GP. Dose: a critical factor in cancer chemotherapy. *Am J Med* 1980;**69**:585–94.

8 Philip T, Armitage JO, Spitzer G *et al.* High-dose therapy and autologous bone marrow transplantation after failure of conventional chemotherapy in adults with intermediate-grade or high-grade non-Hodgkin's lymphoma. *N Engl J Med* 1987;**316**:1493–8.

9 Bosly A, Coiffier B, Gisselbrecht C *et al.* Bone marrow transplantation prolongs survival after relapse in aggressive-lymphoma patients treated with the LNH-84 regimen. *J Clin Oncol* 1992;**10**:1615–23.

10 Philip T, Guglielmi C, Hagenbeek A *et al.* Autologous bone marrow transplantation as compared with salvage chemotherapy in relapses of chemotherapy-sensitive non-Hodgkin's lymphoma. *N Engl J Med* 1995;**333**:1540–5.

11 Mounier N, Gisselbrecht C. Conditioning regimens before transplantation in patients with aggressive non-Hodgkin's lymphoma. *Ann Oncol* 1998;**9**(Suppl 1):S15–21.

12 Fernandez H, Escalón M, Pereira D, Lazarus H. Autotransplant conditioning regimens for aggressive lymphoma: are we on the right road? *Bone Marrow Transplant* 2007;**40**:505–13.

13 Stiff PJ, Dahlberg S, Forman SJ *et al.* Autologous bone marrow transplantation for patients with relapsed or refractory diffuse aggressive non-Hodgkin's lymphoma: value of augmented preparative regimens. A Southwest Oncology Group trial. *J Clin Oncol* 1998;**16**:48–55.

14 Nademanee A, Molina A, O'Donnell MR *et al.* Results of high-dose therapy and autologous bone marrow/stem cell transplantation during remission in poor-risk intermediate- and high-grade lymphoma: international index high and high-intermediate risk group. *Blood* 1997;**90**:3844–52.

15 Stockerl-Goldstein KE, Horning SJ, Negrin RS *et al.* Influence of preparatory regimen and source of hematopoietic cells on outcome of autotransplantation for non-Hodgkin's lymphoma. *Biol Blood Marrow Transplant* 1996;**2**:76–85.

16 Horning SJ, Negrin RS, Chao JC, Long GD, Hoppe RT, Blume KG. Fractionated total-body irradiation, etoposide, and cyclophosphamide plus autografting in Hodgkin's disease and non-Hodgkin's lymphoma. *J Clin Oncol* 1994;**12**:2552–8.

17 Weaver CH, Petersen FB, Appelbaum FR *et al.* High-dose fractionated total-body irradiation, etoposide, and cyclophosphamide followed by autologous stem-cell support in patients with malignant lymphoma. *J Clin Oncol* 1994;**12**:2559–66.

18 Lazarus HM, Carreras J, Boudreau C *et al*. Influence of age and histology on outcome in adult non-Hodgkin lymphoma patients undergoing autologous hematopoietic cell transplantation (HCT): a report from the Center For International Blood and Marrow Transplant Research (CIBMTR). *Biol Blood Marrow Transplant* 2008;**14**:1323–33.

19 Lazarus HM, Zhang MJ, Carreras J *et al*. A comparison of HLA-identical sibling allogeneic versus autologous transplantation for diffuse large B cell lymphoma: a report from the CIBMTR. *Biol Blood Marrow Transplant* 2010;**16**:35–45.

20 Avalos BR, Klein JL, Kapoor N, Tutschka PJ, Klein JP, Copelan EA. Preparation for marrow transplantation in Hodgkin's and non-Hodgkin's lymphoma using Bu/CY. *Bone Marrow Transplant* 1993;**12**:133–8.

21 Escalon MP, Stefanovic A, Venkatraman A *et al*. Autologous transplantation for relapsed non-Hodgkin's lymphoma using intravenous busulfan and cyclophosphamide as conditioning regimen: a single center experience. *Bone Marrow Transplant* 2009;**44**:89–96.

22 Mills W, Chopra R, McMillan A, Pearce R, Linch DC, Goldstone AH. BEAM chemotherapy and autologous bone marrow transplantation for patients with relapsed or refractory non-Hodgkin's lymphoma. *J Clin Oncol* 1995;**13**:588–95.

23 Gaspard MH, Maraninchi D, Stoppa AM *et al*. Intensive chemotherapy with high doses of BCNU, etoposide, cytosine arabinoside, and melphalan (BEAM) followed by autologous bone marrow transplantation: toxicity and antitumor activity in 26 patients with poor-risk malignancies. *Cancer Chemother Pharmacol* 1988;**22**:256–62.

24 Haioun C, Lepage E, Gisselbrecht C *et al*. Comparison of autologous bone marrow transplantation with sequential chemotherapy for intermediate-grade and high-grade non-Hodgkin's lymphoma in first complete remission: a study of 464 patients. Groupe d'Etude des Lymphomes de l'Adulte. *J Clin Oncol* 1994;**12**:2543–51.

25 Wheeler C, Antin JH, Churchill WH *et al*. Cyclophosphamide, carmustine, and etoposide with autologous bone marrow transplantation in refractory Hodgkin's disease and non-Hodgkin's lymphoma: a dose-finding study. *J Clin Oncol* 1990;**8**:648–56.

26 Nademanee A, Schmidt GM, O'Donnell MR *et al*. High-dose chemoradiotherapy followed by autologous bone marrow transplantation as consolidation therapy during first complete remission in adult patients with poor-risk aggressive lymphoma: a pilot study. *Blood* 1992;**80**:1130–4.

27 Prince HM, Crump M, Imrie K *et al*. Intensive therapy and autotransplant for patients with an incomplete response to front-line therapy for lymphoma. *Ann Oncol* 1996;**7**:1043–9.

28 Gianni AM, Bregni M, Siena S *et al*. High-dose chemotherapy and autologous bone marrow transplantation compared with MACOP-B in aggressive B-cell lymphoma. *N Engl J Med* 1997;**336**:1290–7.

29 Kleiner S, Kirsch A, Schwaner I *et al*. High-dose chemotherapy with carboplatin, etoposide and ifosfamide followed by autologous stem cell rescue in patients with relapsed or refractory malignant lymphomas: a phase I/II study. *Bone Marrow Transplant* 1997;**20**:953–9.

30 Wilson WH, Jain V, Bryant G *et al*. Phase I and II study of high-dose ifosfamide, carboplatin, and etoposide with autologous bone marrow rescue in lymphomas and solid tumors. *J Clin Oncol* 1992;**10**:1712–22.

31 McCarthy PL, Hahn T, Hassebroek A *et al*. Trends in use of and survival after autologous hematopoietic cell transplantation in North America, 1995–2005: significant improvement in survival for lymphoma and myeloma during a period of increasing recipient age. *Biol Blood Marrow Transplant* 2013;**19**:1116–23.

32 Vose JM, Anderson JR, Kessinger A *et al*. High-dose chemotherapy and autologous hematopoietic stem-cell transplantation for aggressive non-Hodgkin's lymphoma. *J Clin Oncol* 1993;**11**:1846–51.

33 Petersen FB, Appelbaum FR, Hill R *et al*. Autologous marrow transplantation for malignant lymphoma: a report of 101 cases from Seattle. *J Clin Oncol* 1990;**8**:638–47.

34 Rapoport AP, Lifton R, Constine LS *et al*. Autotransplantation for relapsed or refractory non-Hodgkin's lymphoma (NHL): long-term follow-up and analysis of prognostic factors. *Bone Marrow Transplant* 1997;**19**:883–90.

35 Appelbaum FR, Sullivan KM, Buckner CD *et al*. Treatment of malignant lymphoma in 100 patients with chemotherapy, total body irradiation, and marrow transplantation. *J Clin Oncol* 1987;**5**:1340–7.

36 Pecego R, Hill R, Appelbaum FR *et al*. Interstitial pneumonitis following autologous bone marrow transplantation. *Transplantation* 1986;**42**:515–17.

37 Lane AA, Chen Y-B, Logan BR *et al*. Impact of conditioning regimen on outcomes for patients with lymphoma undergoing high-dose therapy with autologous hematopoietic cell transplantation (AutoHCT). *Biol Blood Marrow Transplant* 2014;**20**(2 Suppl):S45–6. http://www.ncbi.nlm.nih.gov/pubmed/25687795 (accessed April 23, 2015).

38 Pasquini MC, Le Rademacher J, Flowers C *et al*. Matched pair comparison of busulfan/cyclophosphamide/etoposide (BuCyE) to carmustine/etoposide/cytarabine/melphalan (BEAM) conditioning regimen prior to autologous hematopoietic cell transplantation (autoHCT) for lymphoma. *Biol Blood Marrow Transplant* 2014;**20**(2 Suppl):S162.

39 Coiffier B, Lepage E, Briere J *et al*. CHOP chemotherapy plus rituximab compared with CHOP alone in elderly patients with diffuse large-B-cell lymphoma. *N Engl J Med* 2002;**346**:235–42.

40 Récher C, Coiffier B, Haioun C *et al*. Intensified chemotherapy with ACVBP plus rituximab versus standard CHOP plus rituximab for the treatment of diffuse large B-cell lymphoma (LNH03-2B): an open-label randomised phase 3 trial. *Lancet* 2011;**378**:1858–67.

41 Kharfan-Dabaja MA, Fahed R, Hussein M, Santos ES. Evolving role of monoclonal antibodies in the treatment of chronic lymphocytic leukemia. *Expert Opin Investig Drugs* 2007;**16**:1799–815.

42 Kharfan-Dabaja MA, Wierda WG, Cooper LJ. Immunotherapy for chronic lymphocytic leukemia in the era of BTK inhibitors. *Leukemia* 2014;**28**:507–17.

43 Kharfan-Dabaja MA, Nishihori T, Otrock ZK, Haidar N, Mohty M, Hamadani M. Monoclonal antibodies in conditioning regimens for hematopoietic cell transplantation. *Biol Blood Marrow Transplant* 2013;**19**:1288–300.

44 Flohr T, Hess G, Kolbe K *et al*. Rituximab in vivo purging is safe and effective in combination with CD34-positive selected autologous stem cell transplantation for salvage therapy in B-NHL. *Bone Marrow Transplant* 2002;**29**:769–75.

45 Khouri IF, Saliba RM, Hosing C *et al*. Concurrent administration of high-dose rituximab before and after autologous stem-cell transplantation for relapsed aggressive B-cell non-Hodgkin's lymphomas. *J Clin Oncol* 2005;**23**:2240–7.

46 Hess G, Flohr T, Derigs HG. Rituximab as in vivo purging agent in autologous stem cell transplantation for relapsed B-NHL. *Ann Hematol* 2002;**81**(Suppl 2):S54–5.

47 Flinn I, O'Donnell P, Goodrich A *et al*. Immunotherapy with rituximab during peripheral blood stem cell transplantation for non-Hodgkin's lymphoma. *Biol Blood Marrow Transplant* 2000;**6**:628–32.

48 Buckstein R, Imrie K, Spaner D *et al*. Stem cell function and engraftment is not affected by "in vivo purging" with rituximab for autologous stem cell treatment for patients with low-grade non-Hodgkin's lymphoma. *Semin Oncol* 1999;**26**(5 Suppl 14):115–22.

49 Voso MT, Pantel G, Weis M *et al*. In vivo depletion of B cells using a combination of high-dose cytosine arabinoside/mitoxantrone and rituximab for autografting in patients with non-Hodgkin's lymphoma. *Br J Haematol* 2000;**109**:729–35.

50 Magni M, Di Nicola M, Devizzi L *et al*. Successful in vivo purging of CD34-containing peripheral blood harvests in mantle cell and indolent lymphoma: evidence for a role of both chemotherapy and rituximab infusion. *Blood* 2000;**96**:864–9.

51 Tarella C, Zanni M, Magni M *et al*. Rituximab improves the efficacy of high-dose chemotherapy with autograft for high-risk follicular and diffuse large B-cell lymphoma: a multicenter Gruppo Italiano Terapie Innnovative nei linfomi survey. *J Clin Oncol* 2008;**26**:3166–75.

52 Flinn IW, O'Donnell PV, Goodrich A *et al*. Immunotherapy with rituximab during peripheral blood stem cell transplantation for non-Hodgkin's lymphoma. *Biol Blood Marrow Transplant* 2000;**6**:628–32.

53 Hicks LK, Woods A, Buckstein R *et al*. Rituximab purging and maintenance combined with auto-SCT: long-term molecular remissions and prolonged hypogammaglobulinemia in relapsed follicular lymphoma. *Bone Marrow Transplant* 2009;**43**:701–8.

54 Tesfa D, Gelius T, Sander B *et al*. Late-onset neutropenia associated with rituximab therapy: evidence for a maturation arrest at the (pro)myelocyte stage of granulopoiesis. *Med Oncol* 2008;**25**:374–9.

55 McIver Z, Stephens N, Grim A, Barrett AJ. Rituximab administration within 6 months of T cell-depleted allogeneic SCT is associated with prolonged life-threatening cytopenias. *Biol Blood Marrow Transplant* 2010;**16**:1549–56.

56 Vose JM, Wahl RL, Saleh M *et al*. Multicenter phase II study of iodine-131 tositumomab for chemotherapy-relapsed/refractory low-grade and transformed low-grade B-cell non-Hodgkin's lymphomas. *J Clin Oncol* 2000;**18**:1316–23.

57 Witzig TE, Gordon LI, Cabanillas F *et al*. Randomized controlled trial of yttrium-90-labeled ibritumomab tiuxetan radioimmunotherapy versus rituximab immunotherapy for patients with relapsed or refractory low-grade, follicular, or transformed B-cell non-Hodgkin's lymphoma. *J Clin Oncol* 2002;**20**:2453–63.

58 Press OW, Eary JF, Appelbaum FR *et al*. Radiolabeled-antibody therapy of B-cell lymphoma with autologous bone marrow support. *N Engl J Med* 1993;**329**:1219–24.

59 Press OW, Eary JF, Appelbaum FR *et al*. Phase II trial of 131I-B1 (anti-CD20) antibody therapy with autologous stem cell transplantation for relapsed B cell lymphomas. *Lancet* 1995;**346**:336–40.

60 Liu SY, Eary JF, Petersdorf SH *et al*. Follow-up of relapsed B-cell lymphoma patients treated with iodine-131-labeled anti-CD20 antibody and autologous stem-cell rescue. *J Clin Oncol* 1998;**16**:3270–8.

61 Kaminski MS, Zasadny KR, Francis IR *et al*. Iodine-131-anti-B1 radioimmunotherapy for B-cell lymphoma. *J Clin Oncol* 1996;**14**:1974–81.

62 Press OW, Eary JF, Gooley T *et al*. A phase I/II trial of iodine-131-tositumomab (anti-CD20), etoposide, cyclophosphamide, and autologous stem cell transplantation for relapsed B-cell lymphomas. *Blood* 2000;**96**:2934–42.

63 Gopal AK, Rajendran JG, Petersdorf SH *et al*. High-dose chemoradioimmunotherapy with autologous stem cell support for relapsed mantle cell lymphoma. *Blood* 2002;**99**:3158–62.

64 Nademanee A, Forman S, Molina A *et al*. A phase 1/2 trial of high-dose yttrium-90-ibritumomab tiuxetan in combination with high-dose etoposide and cyclophosphamide followed by autologous stem cell transplantation in patients with poor-risk or relapsed non-Hodgkin lymphoma. *Blood* 2005;**106**:2896–902.

65 Devizzi L, Guidetti A, Tarella C *et al*. High-dose yttrium-90-ibritumomab tiuxetan with tandem stem-cell reinfusion: an outpatient preparative regimen for autologous hematopoietic cell transplantation. *J Clin Oncol* 2008;**26**:5175–82.

66 Winter JN, Inwards DJ, Spies S *et al*. Yttrium-90 ibritumomab tiuxetan doses calculated to deliver up to 15 Gy to critical organs may be safely combined with high-dose BEAM and autologous transplantation in relapsed or refractory B-cell non-Hodgkin's lymphoma. *J Clin Oncol* 2009;**27**:1653–9.

67 Ferrucci PF, Vanazzi A, Grana CM *et al*. High activity 90Y-ibritumomab tiuxetan (Zevalin) with peripheral blood progenitor cells support in patients with refractory/resistant B-cell non-Hodgkin lymphomas. *Br J Haematol* 2007;**139**:590–9.

68 Hohloch K, Sahlmann CO, Lakhani VJ *et al.* Tandem high-dose therapy in relapsed and refractory B-cell lymphoma: results of a prospective phase II trial of myeloablative chemotherapy, followed by escalated radioimmunotherapy with (131)I-anti-CD20 antibody and stem cell rescue. *Ann Hematol* 2011;**90**:1307–15.

69 Gopal AK, Gooley T, Rajendran J *et al.* A Phase I study of myeloablative I-131-anti CD-20 (tositumomab) radioimmunotherapy with escalating doses of fludarabine followed by autologous hematopoietic stem cell transplantation (ASCT) for adults ≥60 years of age with high-risk or relapsed/refractory B-cell lymphoma. *Blood (ASH Annual Meeting Abstracts)* 2011;**118**:Abstract 663.

70 Vose JM, Bierman PJ, Enke C *et al.* Phase I trial of iodine-131 tositumomab with high-dose chemotherapy and autologous stem-cell transplantation for relapsed non-Hodgkin's lymphoma. *J Clin Oncol* 2005;**23**:461–7.

71 Shimoni A, Zwas ST, Oksman Y *et al.* Yttrium-90-ibritumomab tiuxetan (Zevalin) combined with high-dose BEAM chemotherapy and autologous stem cell transplantation for chemo-refractory aggressive non-Hodgkin's lymphoma. *Exp Hematol* 2007;**35**:534–40.

72 Shimoni A, Avivi I, Rowe JM *et al.* A randomized study comparing yttrium-90 ibritumomab tiuxetan (Zevalin) and high-dose BEAM chemotherapy versus BEAM alone as the conditioning regimen before autologous stem cell transplantation in patients with aggressive lymphoma. *Cancer* 2012;**118**:4706–14.

73 Vose JM, Bierman PJ, Loberiza FR *et al.* Phase II trial of 131-Iodine tositumomab with high-dose chemotherapy and autologous stem cell transplantation for relapsed diffuse large B cell lymphoma. *Biol Blood Marrow Transplant* 2013;**19**:123–8.

74 Krishnan A, Nademanee A, Fung HC *et al.* Phase II trial of a transplantation regimen of yttrium-90 ibritumomab tiuxetan and high-dose chemotherapy in patients with non-Hodgkin's lymphoma. *J Clin Oncol* 2008;**26**:90–5.

75 Decaudin D, Mounier N, Tilly H *et al.* (90)Y ibritumomab tiuxetan (Zevalin) combined with BEAM (Z-BEAM) conditioning regimen plus autologous stem cell transplantation in relapsed or refractory low-grade CD20-positive B-cell lymphoma. A GELA phase II prospective study. *Clin Lymphoma Myeloma Leuk* 2011;**11**:212–18.

76 Briones J, Novelli S, García-Marco JA *et al.* Autologous stem cell transplantation after conditioning with yttrium-90 ibritumomab tiuxetan plus BEAM in refractory non-Hodgkin diffuse large B-cell lymphoma: results of a prospective, multicenter, phase II clinical trial. *Haematologica* 2014;**99**:505–10.

77 Zipp L, Saliba RM, Valverde R *et al.* Mature results of BEAM/high-dose rituximab vs BEAM/yttrium-90 ibritumomab tiuxetan (Zevalin®) and autologous stem cell transplantation (ASCT) for relapsed CD20⁺ follicular and diffuse large B-cell lymphoma: survival outcomes and risk of secondary malignancies. *Blood (ASH Annual Meeting Abstracts)* 2011; **118**:Abstract 2005.

78 Arne K, Laurell A, Jerkeman M *et al.* Nordic MCL3 Study: Zevalin combined with high-dose chemotherapy followed by autologous stem cell support as late intensification for mantle cell lymphoma (MCL) patients <66 years not in CR after induction chemoimmunotherapy: no benefit of Zevalin. *Blood (ASH Annual Meeting Abstracts)* 2012;**120**:Abstract 747.

79 Vose JM, Carter S, Burns LJ *et al.* Phase III randomized study of rituximab/carmustine, etoposide, cytarabine, and melphalan (BEAM) compared with iodine-131 tositumomab/BEAM with autologous hematopoietic cell transplantation for relapsed diffuse large B-cell lymphoma: results from the BMT CTN 0401 Trial. *J Clin Oncol* 2013;**31**:1662–8.

80 Lazarus H, Loberiza FJ, Zhang M *et al.* Autotransplants for Hodgkin's disease in first relapse or second remission: a report from the Autologous Blood and Marrow Transplant Registry (ABMTR). *Bone Marrow Transplant* 2001;**27**:387–96.

81 Vose JM, Zhang MJ, Rowlings PA *et al.* Autologous transplantation for diffuse aggressive non-Hodgkin's lymphoma in patients never achieving remission: a report from the Autologous Blood and Marrow Transplant Registry. *J Clin Oncol* 2001;**19**:406–13.

82 Kebriaei P, Madden T, Kazerooni R *et al.* Intravenous busulfan plus melphalan is a highly effective, well-tolerated preparative regimen for autologous stem cell transplantation in patients with advanced lymphoid malignancies. *Biol Blood Marrow Transplant* 2011;**17**:412–20.

83 Plunkett W, Huang P, Searcy CE, Gandhi V. Gemcitabine: preclinical pharmacology and mechanisms of action. *Semin Oncol* 1996;**23**(5 Suppl 10):3–15.

84 Bartlett NL, Niedzwiecki D, Johnson JL *et al.* Gemcitabine, vinorelbine, and pegylated liposomal doxorubicin (GVD), a salvage regimen in relapsed Hodgkin's lymphoma: CALGB 59804. *Ann Oncol* 2007;**18**:1071–9.

85 Santoro A, Bredenfeld H, Devizzi L *et al.* Gemcitabine in the treatment of refractory Hodgkin's disease: results of a multicenter phase II study. *J Clin Oncol* 2000;**18**:2615–19.

86 Ng M, Waters J, Cunningham D *et al.* Gemcitabine, cisplatin and methylprednisolone (GEM-P) is an effective salvage regimen in patients with relapsed and refractory lymphoma. *Br J Cancer* 2005;**92**:1352–7.

87 Crump M, Baetz T, Couban S *et al.* Gemcitabine, dexamethasone, and cisplatin in patients with recurrent or refractory aggressive histology B-cell non-Hodgkin lymphoma: a Phase II study by the National Cancer Institute of Canada Clinical Trials Group (NCIC-CTG). *Cancer* 2004;**101**:1835–42.

88 Nieto Y, Thall P, Valdez B *et al.* High-dose infusional gemcitabine combined with busulfan and melphalan with autologous stem-cell transplantation in patients with refractory lymphoid malignancies. *Biol Blood Marrow Transplant* 2012;**18**:1677–86.

89 Arai S, Letsinger R, Wong RM *et al.* Phase I/II trial of GN-BVC, a gemcitabine and vinorelbine-containing conditioning regimen for autologous hematopoietic cell transplantation in recurrent and refractory Hodgkin lymphoma. *Biol Blood Marrow Transplant* 2010;**16**:1145–54.

90 Gisselbrecht C, Schmitz N, Mounier N *et al*. Rituximab maintenance therapy after autologous stem-cell transplantation in patients with relapsed CD20(+) diffuse large B-cell lymphoma: final analysis of the collaborative trial in relapsed aggressive lymphoma. *J Clin Oncol* 2012;**30**:4462–9.

91 Carella AM, de Souza CA, Luminari S *et al*. Prognostic role of gender in diffuse large B-cell lymphoma treated with rituximab containing regimens: a Fondazione Italiana Linfomi/Grupo de Estudos em Moléstias Onco-Hematológicas retrospective study. *Leukemia Lymphoma* 2013;**54**:53–7.

92 Pettengell R, Schmitz N, Gisselbrecht C *et al*. Rituximab purging and/or maintenance in patients undergoing autologous transplantation for relapsed follicular lymphoma: a prospective randomized trial from the Lymphoma Working Party of the European Group for Blood and Marrow Transplantation. *J Clin Oncol* 2013;**31**:1624–30.

93 Aalipour A, Advani RH. Bruton tyrosine kinase inhibitors: a promising novel targeted treatment for B cell lymphomas. *Br J Haematol* 2013;**163**:436–43.

94 Advani A, Coiffier B, Czuczman MS *et al*. Safety, pharmacokinetics, and preliminary clinical activity of inotuzumab ozogamicin, a novel immunoconjugate for the treatment of B-cell non-Hodgkin's lymphoma: results of a phase I study. *J Clin Oncol* 2010;**28**:2085–93.

95 Chen BJ, Chapuy B, Ouyang J *et al*. PD-L1 expression is characteristic of a subset of aggressive B-cell lymphomas and virus-associated malignancies. *Clin Cancer Res* 2013;**19**: 3462–73.

96 Armand P, Nagler A, Weller EA *et al*. Disabling immune tolerance by programmed death-1 blockade with pidilizumab after autologous hematopoietic stem-cell transplantation for diffuse large B-cell lymphoma: results of an international phase II trial. *J Clin Oncol* 2013;**31**:4199–206.

97 Behr TM, Griesinger F, Riggert J *et al*. High-dose myeloablative radioimmunotherapy of mantle cell non-Hodgkin lymphoma with the iodine-131-labeled chimeric anti-CD20 antibody C2B8 and autologous stem cell support. Results of a pilot study. *Cancer* 2002;**94**(4 Suppl):1363–72.

98 Gopal AK, Gooley TA, Rajendran JG *et al*. Myeloablative I-131-tositumomab with escalating doses of fludarabine and autologous hematopoietic transplantation for adults age ≥60 years with B cell lymphoma. *Biol Blood Marrow Transplant* 2014;**20**:770–5.

99 Briones J, Novelli S, Marco JAG *et al*. Autologous stem cell transplantation with yttrium-90-ibritumomab tiuxetan (Zevalin) plus BEAM conditioning in patients with refractory non-Hodgkin diffuse large B-cell lymphoma: results of a prospective, multicenter, phase II clinical trial. *Blood (ASH Annual Meeting Abstracts)* 2012;**120**(21):Abstract 1978.

CHAPTER 6

Preparative regimens for lymphoma: allogeneic hematopoietic stem cell transplantation

Mohamed A. Kharfan-Dabaja, Najla El-Jurdi, Mehdi Hamadani and Ernesto Ayala

Introduction

The past two decades have witnessed major advances in the treatment of Hodgkin lymphoma (HL) and non-Hodgkin lymphoma (NHL) [1,2]. Nowadays, the available repertoire of therapies includes monoclonal antibodies such as rituximab and brentuximab vedotin which target CD20 and CD30, respectively [2,3]. A new generation of type I monoclonal antibodies, namely ofatumumab, which targets the small loop of CD20, as well as type II monoclonal antibodies, namely obinutuzumab, which is known to have more antibody-dependent cell-mediated cytotoxicity and less complement-dependent cytotoxicity, have emerged and have already entered the clinical therapeutic arena in diseases such as chronic lymphocytic leukemia (CLL) [4,5]. Their efficacy in various subtypes of CD20-expressing NHL has been described in clinical trials [6–8]. Moreover, therapies targeting the B-cell receptor signaling pathway, namely ibrutinib [9], and the proteasome inhibitor bortezomib [10] have shown impressive clinical activity and are already being incorporated into the treatment armamentarium of mantle cell lymphoma. While responses induced by these therapies are more frequent and even more durable, achieving the ultimate cure remains the desirable goal.

Allogeneic hematopoietic cell transplantation (allo-HCT) is an effective treatment modality that can offer a possibility of cure for various subtypes of lymphomas [11–14]. This procedure eliminates the risk of infusing neoplastic cells present in an autologous collection, and its purported benefit is also derived from both the cytoreductive effect of chemotherapy, especially when used in myeloablative doses, combined with the adoptive immunotherapy mediated by donor T cells. Better understanding of the latter resulted in development of lesser ablative regimens, so called reduced-intensity conditioning (RIC) regimens [15]. Availability of RIC regimens has expanded the applicability of allo-HCT to patients of more advanced age and/or with associated comorbidities. An alternative terminology, i.e., nonmyeloablative (NMA) conditioning regimens, has been used to describe this type of reduced-toxicity regimen. While it is arguable that a spectrum of dose intensities exists within these reduced-toxicity regimens, we include NMA under the rubric of RIC regimens for the purposes of this review. Moreover, exploration of alternative donors for hematopoietic cell allografting has resulted in the use of unrelated donors (HLA-matched or mismatched), umbilical cord blood (UCB) and, more recently, haploidentical transplantation [16,17]. Here we summarize the conditioning regimens as well as the available donor sources for allo-HCT for lymphomas. This chapter also highlights integration of novel therapies as part of conditioning regimens for hematopoietic cell allografting [18].

Myeloablative conditioning regimens for lymphomas

Allo-HCT using myeloablative conditioning (MAC) doses of chemotherapy or chemoradiotherapy was commonly offered to patients with lymphoma in the past. Use of high doses of total body irradiation (TBI), generally in

Clinical Guide to Transplantation in Lymphoma, First Edition. Edited by Bipin N. Savani and Mohamad Mohty.

the range 5–12 Gy, represented the backbone on which various preparative regimens were developed, by combining TBI with cyclophosphamide or etoposide, among others [11,14,19–32]. Unfortunately, use of these regimens was associated with significant nonrelapse mortality (NRM), reported in up to 50% in some studies (Table 6.1) [19,22,23]. This prohibitive mortality resulted in a shift in practice, by favoring the use of less toxic RIC regimens. To our knowledge there is no prospective randomized study performed to date that compares MAC with RIC conditioning regimens for allo-HCT for lymphomas; however, several nonrandomized comparisons have failed to show a clear benefit in overall survival (OS) with dose intensification, whether using chemotherapy-based or TBI-based regimens. For instance, a retrospective comparative analysis of Center for International Blood and Marrow Transplant Research (CIBMTR) data of 396 subjects with diffuse large B-cell NHL showed that patients who underwent an allo-HCT following MAC regimens had lower risk of relapse, but significantly higher NRM compared with RIC allo-HCT [33]. In the case of mature T-cell lymphomas, a CIBMTR registry study failed to show a clear OS advantage when using MAC regimens in this group of diseases [32].

Offering myeloablative preparative regimens for allo-HCT for lymphomas should be restricted to patients with good performance status and low HCT comorbidity scores [34]. The potential benefit of using myeloablative (vs. RIC) regimens in lymphoma cases with persistent disease at the time of allografting remains to be better studied.

Reduced-intensity conditioning regimens

Traditional MAC regimens are associated with more frequent grade 3 and 4 toxicities and higher NRM. By reducing the intensity of the conditioning regimen, older patients and those with higher comorbidity scores can be offered the procedure more frequently [35]. Furthermore, the curative effect of allo-HCT depends in great proportion on the immune-mediated graft-versus-tumor effect. Lower risk of relapse compared with autologous transplantation and response to donor lymphocyte infusions or to tapering down of immunosuppression in few instances have been observed in various types of lymphoma and support the existence of

a strong graft-versus-lymphoma effect [36–39]. As a result, the last decade has seen a major shift in the conditioning regimens used for allo-HCT and currently over 60% of transplants are performed using RIC regimens [40].

RIC allo-HCT in diffuse large B-cell lymphoma

It remains unclear what the best conditioning regimen is for diffuse large B-cell lymphoma (DLBCL). Several relatively small series have shown that RIC regimens are an acceptable option, with reproducible long-term OS and disease-free survival (DFS) (Table 6.2). In a large retrospective registry analysis, 396 allograft recipients reported to the CIBMTR were evaluated according to conditioning intensity (MAC, 165; RIC/NMA, 231) [41]. Patients in the RIC and NMC groups were older, had more prior lines of therapy including auto-HCT, were transplanted more recently, and received TBI-based regimens less frequently [41]. The 5-year mortality was higher with MAC than with RIC and/or NMA (56% vs. 47% vs. 36%; $P = 0.007$). Relapse/progression was lower (26% vs. 38% vs. 40%; $P = 0.031$) [41]. The 5-year progression-free survival (PFS) and OS did not differ significantly between the cohorts. In multivariate analysis, NMA conditioning and more recent year of allografting were associated with lower NRM, whereas a lower Karnosfsky performance score, resistant disease, and unrelated donors were associated with higher NRM. RIC regimens induce long-term PFS in selected patients with DLBCL, with lower NRM but a higher risk of progression/relapse [41]. The benefit of conditioning intensity in patients with DLBCL is likely dependent on the remission status at transplant, age and comorbidities of the patient, and the level of expertise of the transplant center.

RIC allo-HCT for follicular lymphoma

Published literature shows that MAC allo-HCT is effective in patients with follicular lymphoma [27]. However, NRM limits its use mostly to young fit subjects. As follicular lymphoma has shown particular sensitivity to the graft-versus-lymphoma effect, RIC regimens have largely replaced MAC regimens. Several single and multicenter studies have reproducibly shown low NRM, low progression/relapse rates, and favorable OS and PFS [42–44]. Unfortunately, the only prospective randomized study comparing RIC allo-HCT with auto-HCT was prematurely closed due to low accrual [45]. The

Table 6.1 Selected studies evaluating myeloablative regimens for allogeneic HCT for various lymphomas.

Study	Study type	Disease(s)	N	Conditioning regimen(s)	Donor source (%)	Cell source	NRM	Survival
Appelbaum et al. (1987) [11]	Retrospective, single center	HL and NHL	HL, 11 NHL, 49	CY-TBI	Various	BM	NR	23% (5-year)
Anderson et al. (1993) [19]	Retrospective, multicenter	HL	53	NR	MRD, 83%	BM	49% (5-year)	OS, 20% EFS, 22% (5-year)
Ratanatharathorn et al. (1994) [20]	Prospective	NHL	31	CY-TBI or CVB	Various	BM	NR	PFS, 47% (median follow-up 14 months)
Van Besien et al. (1996) [21]	Retrospective, single center	NHL	64	TBI-based, 58%	MRD, 98%	BM	NR	NR
Gajewski et al. (1996) [22]	IBMTR registry	HL	100	TBI-based, 45%	MRD, 100%	BM	61% (3-year)	OS. 21% DFS, 15% (3-year)
Milpied et al. (1996) [23]	EBMT registry	HL	45	TBI-based, 35.5% (N = 16)	MRD, 100%	BM	48% (4-year)	OS, 25% PFS, 15% (4-year)
Juckett et al. (1998) [24]	Retrospective, single center	NHL	37	TBI + CY + cytarabine + methylprednisone*	MRD, 65%	BM	43%	OS, 45% (5-year)
Dhedin et al. (1999) [25]	SFGM French database	NHL	73	TBI-based, 87% (N = 64)	MRD, 99%	BM	44%	OS, 41% PFS, 40% (5-year)
Akpek et al. (2001) [26]	Retrospective, single center	HL	53	BUCY, 51% BU-CY-ETOP, 24.5% TBI-CY, 24.5%	MRD, 100%	BM	32% (100 days)	EFS, 26% OS, 30% (10-year)
Van Besien et al. (2003) [27]	IBMTR/ASBMT	NHL	176	TBI-based, 68%	MRD, 100%	BM, 77% PBSC, 23%	24% (1-year) 28% (3-year) 30% (5-year)	DFS, 48% OS, 54% (3-year)
Doocey et al. (2005) [28]	Retrospective, single center	NHL	44	TBI-based, 95%	MRD, 75%	PBSC	25% (1-year)	OS, 48% (5-year)
Kim et al. (2006) [29]	Retrospective, multicenter	NHL	233	TBI-based, 83%	MRD, 66%	PBSC	42%	PFS, 36% OS, 39% (5-year)
Sureda et al. (2008) [30]	EBMT	HL	79	TBI-CY or high-dose BU	Various	PBSC	28% (3-month) 46% (1-year)	PFS, 20% OS, 22% (5-year)
Claviez et al. (2009) [31]	EBMT	HL	40	TBI-based, 40%	Various	PBSC	21% (1-year)	NR
Hamadani et al. (2013) [14]	CIBMTR	NHL	74	TBI-CY, 53%	MRD, 68%	PBSC	33% (100-day)	PFS, 20% OS, 25% (3-year)
Smith et al. (2013) [32]	CIBMTR	Mature T-cell NHL	241[†]	Various	MRD, 60%[‡]	PBSC, 71%[‡]	MAC, 34% (3-year)[§]	OS[§] MAC, 43% (3-year)

* T-cell depleted.
[†] 126 underwent allogeneic HCT (myeloablative regimen, N = 74).
[‡] All allogeneic HCT.
[§] Patient beyond CR1 at time of allografting.
BM, bone marrow cells; BU, busulfan; CVB, cyclophosphamide/VP-16/BCNU; CY, cyclophosphamide; EFS, event-free survival; ETOP, etoposide; HL, Hodgkin lymphoma; MAC, myeloablative conditioning; MRD, matched-related donor; NHL, non-Hodgkin lymphoma; NR, not reported; NRM, nonrelaspe mortality; OS, overall survival; PBSC, peripheral blood stem cells; PFS, progression-free survival; TBI, total body irradiation.

Table 6.2 Selected studies evaluating reduced-intensity conditioning regimens for allogeneic HCT for various lymphomas.

Study	N	Histology	Median age (years)	Conditioning regimen	Median follow-up (months)	OS	PFS	NRM	Relapse
Sirvent et al. [88]	68	DLBCL	48	FluCy or Flu/TBI	48	49%	44%	23%	41%
Bacher et al. [41]	RIC, 143 NMA, 88	DLBCL	RIC, 54 NMA, 54	RIC: FluMel or FluBu NMC: FluCy or FluTBI	RIC, 41 NMA, 59	RIC, 20% NMA, 26%	RIC, 15% NMA, 25%	47% 36%	38% 40%
Armand et al. [89]	87	Several	46	Flu, low-dose Bu	26	53% (3-year)	29%	23%	49%
Khouri et al. [42]	47	Follicular	53	FluCy/rituximab	60	85%	83%	14%	4%
Rezvani et al. [44]	62	Follicular and transformed	54	FluTBI 2 Gy		43%	38%	42%	20%
Piñana et al. [43]	37	Follicular	50	FluMel	52	57%	55%	35%	8%
Robinson et al. [46]	149	Follicular	46	Several	59	68% (3-year)	62%	22%	17%
Khouri et al. [50]	18	MCL	56	FluCy/rituximab	26	85% (3-year)	82%	6%	12%
Maris et al. [51]	33	MCL	53	FluTBI 2 Gy	24	60% (2-year)	60%	24%	9%
Le Gouill et al. [90]	70	MCL	56	Several	24	53% (2-year)	50%	32%	NA
Fenske et al. [53]	50	Early MCL	54	Several	48	62%	55%	25%	15%
	88	Late MCL	58	Several	37	31% (3-year)	24%	17% (1 year)	38%
Sarina et al. [55]	122	HL	31	Several	48	66% (2-year)	39%	14%	32%
Anderlini et al. [57]	58	HL	32	FluMel ± ATG	24	62% (2-year)	32%	15%	55%
Robinson et al. [58]	285	HL	31	Several	26	43% (3-year)	25%	21%	53%

ATG, antithymocyte globulin; Cy, cyclophosphamide; DLBCL, diffuse large B-cell lymphoma; Flu, fludarabine; HL, Hodgkin lymphoma; MCL, mantle cell lymphoma; Mel, melphalan; NMA, nonmyeloablative conditioning; NRM, nonrelapse mortality; OS, overall survival; PFS, progression-free survival; RIC, reduced-intensity conditioning; TBI, total body irradiation.

Lymphoma Working Party of the European Society for Blood and Marrow Transplantation (EBMT) retrospectively compared 149 patients who underwent RIC allo-HCT with 726 who underwent autografting. NRM was significantly higher after RIC allo-HCT (15% vs. 3% at 1 year; $P < 0.001$) but progression was lower (20% vs. 47% at 5 years; $P < 0.001$). OS at 5 years was not significantly different (67% vs. 72%) [45]. Interestingly, PFS was not significantly different in the first 24 months, but later there was a significant advantage for RIC allo-HCT (57% vs. 48% at 5 years; $P < 0.001$) [46].

It is unlikely that a prospective comparison of RIC versus MAC allo-HCT for follicular lymphoma will be performed. A retrospective comparison on behalf of the

CIBMTR showed 3-year OS for MAC and RIC cohorts of 71% and 62%, respectively ($P = 0.15$) and PFS of 67% and 55%, respectively ($P = 0.07$) [47]. In multivariate analysis, an increased risk of progression was seen after RIC allo-HCT (relative risk 2.97, $P = 0.04$) [47]. In our opinion, RIC allo-HCT has become the standard approach for eligible follicular lymphoma.

RIC allo-HCT in mantle cell lymphoma

Allo-HCT using MAC regimens offers cure to mantle cell lymphoma (MCL) but at the cost of a high NRM [48,49]. As a result, RIC regimens were pursued by several groups with variable results [50,51]. Patients in remission at the time of allografting derived the highest benefit, with low relapse and NRM rates. Also, older patients were included in these series. Larger retrospective multicenter registry studies have been published more recently. One was presented on behalf of the British Society for Blood and Marrow Transplantation [52]. In this study, 70 patients underwent RIC allo-HCT, 57 of them with an alemtuzumab-containing regimen. NRM and relapse rates were 21% and 65%, respectively at 5 years. Donor lymphocyte infusion was used successfully in 14 patients [52]. In another study, the outcomes of 381 patients who underwent first auto-HCT were compared with 138 patients who underwent RIC allo-HCT [53]. Patients who underwent HCT early (no more than two lines of therapy) had the greatest benefit, with similar OS (auto-HCT 61% vs. RIC-allo-HCT 62%, $P = 0.95$) and PFS (auto-HCT 52% vs. RIC allo-HCT 55%, $P = 0.746$) at 5 years. NRM was higher but relapse rates were lower in the RIC allo-HCT group. No relapses were seen in the early allo-HCT cohort after 2 years [53]. At this time, auto-HCT remains the preferred option in MCL, although RIC allo-HCT may be considered in relapsed or primary refractory disease as well as in patients with high-risk first remission (high MIPI score) in our opinion.

RIC allo-HCT in Hodgkin lymphoma

Because of the high NRM associated with MAC allo-HCT in HL, the role of allo-HCT in patients relapsing after an auto-HCT has been a matter of debate and controversy for several years [22,54]. A retrospective analysis based on donor availability [55] and a second one based on historical controls [56] showed improved OS and PFS in patients who underwent RIC allo-HCT compared with conventional therapy. Furthermore, a large retrospective registry study from EBMT evaluating 189 subjects with relapsed HL showed a significant decrease in NRM with RIC compared to those who received a MAC allo-HCT (hazard ratio, 2.05; 95% CI 1.27–3.29; $P = 0.04$). This reduction in NRM resulted in improved OS and PFS [30]. Performance score and disease status at transplant are strong prognostic factors associated with outcome [57,58]. A multicenter prospective study from the GEL/TAMO group confirmed these findings [59]. As NRM has decreased, relapse has emerged as the main cause of failure [59].

Currently, RIC allo-HCT has become the treatment of choice for relapsed HL after auto-HCT. Efforts should be made to attain a complete response before proceeding with RIC allo-HCT. New agents such as brentuximab vedotin are showing promise in this particular setting [60].

Incorporating monoclonal antibodies in preparative regimens for allo-HCT

Addition of rituximab to allo-HCT preparative regimens aiming at improving anti-lymphoma efficacy as well as potentially reducing incidence and severity of acute graft-versus-host disease (GVHD) has been shown to be feasible [12,18,42,61,62]. Prolonged and profound cytopenias associated with administration of rituximab as well as consequent risk of serious infections merit serious consideration when adding rtixumab to preparative allo-HCT, whether MAC or RIC [63]. Moreover, the optimal dose and schedule of rituximab remain important unanswered questions. Several studies have shown that combining the ^{90}Y-labeled anti-CD20 monoclonal antibody ibritumomab tiuxetan with RIC regimens is a feasible approach [64–66], but data are limited to small single-institution non-randomized trials. One particular challenge that limits wider applicability of this approach is related to the level of expertise required to administer this agent. At present, addition of ibritumomab tiuxetan or others should be offered in the context of clinical trials.

In contrast, in T-cell NHL, targeted therapies with monoclonal antibodies have had a more limited impact regarding disease control. Alemtuzumab, a humanized anti-CD52 monoclonal antibody, is used primarily as a GVHD preventive strategy [67,68]. Recently, brentuximab vedotin, an anti-CD30 drug conjugate, has demonstrated impressive efficacy in CD30-expressing malignancies, namely HL and anaplastic T-cell NHL [2], and is presently used to decrease disease burden in patients being considered for an allo-HCT [60,69].

Alternative donor sources

Less than 40% of allo-HCT eligible patients have an HLA-matched (sibling or adult unrelated) donor available. In recent years, the advent of single or double UCB and haploidentical (from parents, siblings, or children) transplantation have in theory expanded the allo-HCT option to nearly all medically fit patients. To date, no prospective studies have evaluated the optimal type and intensity of conditioning regimens for alternative donor allografting in patients with lymphoid malignancies.

Umbilical cord blood cells

UCB is widely used as an alternative source of hematopoietic cell support for allogeneic transplantation. It offers several advantages, such as immediate availability, absence of risk for donors, lower risk of acute GVHD, and a less stringent requirement for HLA matching [70]. Novel strategies, such as the use of double UCB units, cotransplantation with accessory cells, and *ex vivo* expansion of UCB progenitor cells, and others have to a certain extent overcome the cell-dose limitations inherent to cord blood units in adult allograft recipients [70]. RIC regimens are most commonly used for UCB transplantation for lymphoid malignancies, owing to frequently advanced age and associated comorbid conditions in such patients.

An NMA regimen developed at the University of Minnesota consisting of cyclophosphamide (50 mg/kg on day −6), fludarabine (40 mg/m^2 on days −6 to −2) and TBI (2 Gy) is a commonly used preparative regimen for UCB transplantation. In a report of 65 patients with HL or NHL, this regimen resulted in an NRM of 15% at 3 years. The PFS and OS were 34% and 55% at 3 years, respectively [71]. The EBMT registry analyzed outcomes of 104 lymphoma patients undergoing UCB transplantation, relative to the type of conditioning regimen used [72]. The majority of the patients undergoing NMA UCB transplantation received the University of Minnesota regimen while a variety of regimens were used for myeloablative transplantation (e.g., busulfan/fludarabine/thiotepa; busulfan/cyclophosphamide ± others; or cyclophosphamide/TBI ± fludarabine). In this analysis a significantly lower NRM and better PFS and OS rates were seen in patients who received low-dose TBI (a possible surrogate marker for the University of Minnesota approach). RIC regimens not incorporating low-dose TBI resulted in inferior outcomes comparable to those of myeloablative therapies [72]. Limited data also suggest the feasibility of RIC with fludarabine/melphalan for UCB transplantation in lymphoproliferative disorders [73]. Acknowledging the lack of data from prospective studies, cyclophosphamide/fludarabine/2-Gy TBI appears to be a reasonable NMA conditioning regimen for UCB transplantation, while myeloablative UCB allografts should preferably be reserved for clinical trials.

Haploidentical transplantation

The feasibility and reliable engraftment of haploidentical allografts using immunosuppressive and myeloablative conditioning (e.g., cyclophosphamide/TBI/thiotepa ± antithymocyte globulin) followed by infusion of mega-doses of T-cell-depleted hematopoietic progenitor cells (with, for example, soybean agglutination and E-rosetting techniques) in acute leukemia has been known for several years [74,75]. However, the application of such intensive conditioning approaches coupled with technically cumbersome T-cell depletion has been limited in lymphoid malignancies, particularly in the elder group. This situation is further confounded by the fact that a sizeable proportion of lymphoma patients undergo an allograft after a failed prior autograft, a scenario where application of MAC approaches is associated with prohibitive rates of NRM.

Recently, an alternative approach to myeloablative haploidentical transplantation was developed with the addition of post-transplant cyclophosphamide to prevent GVHD and graft rejection, using marrow allografts after RIC with fludarabine (30 mg/m^2 on days −6 to −2), cyclophosphamide (14.5 mg/kg on days −6 and −5), and 2-Gy TBI (on day −1) [76,77]. This approach has demonstrated promising results, including low rates of NRM in single- and multi-institution studies, and appears to provide patients with lymphoid malignancies an improved event-free survival compared to those with myelogenous malignancies ($P = 0.02$) [77]. However, rates of disease relapse with this regimen approach 50% at 1 year. Variations including MAC (fludarabine 25 mg/m^2 on days −6 to −2, busulfan 110–130 mg/m^2 on days −7 to −4, and cyclophosphamide 14.5 mg/kg on days −3 and −2) and use of peripheral blood grafts with post-transplant cyclophosphamide treatment are being studied in prospective trials [78]. With more intense conditioning regimens, 2-year relapse rates are approximately 30%, but data specifically relating to lymphoid malignancies are not presently available. Consistent engraftment is not reliably seen with all RIC approaches, with report of high rates of immunologic graft rejection with regimens consisting of fludarabine/busulfan and alemtuzumab [79].

In the context of alternative donor transplantation, continued research is needed to better define the optimal conditioning regimen intensity and the preferred method and amount of necessary T-cell depletion, address the high relapse rates with haploidentical transplantation, and also enhance the delayed immune reconstitution inherent to such transplant programs. A potential method to mitigate relapse risk following haploidentical transplantation is planned donor-cell infusions post transplantation, aimed at augmenting graft-versus-tumor effects. The groups at the Fred Hutchinson Cancer Center and Medical College of Wisconsin are investigating the role of post haploidentical transplant planned donor NK-cell infusions to reduce the risk of disease relapse (www.clinicaltrials.gov; NCT00789776). The Bone Marrow Transplantation Clinical Trials Network's (BMT CTN) two parallel multicenter Phase II trials (BMT-CTN 0603 and BMT-CTN 0604) showed comparable 1-year OS and PFS with RIC double UCB (54% and 46%, respectively) and haploidentical bone marrow transplantation (62% and 48%, respectively) in hematologic malignancies [80]. These trials have paved the way for the ongoing BMT-CTN 1101 trial (NCT01745913) randomizing patients with hematologic malignancies to either haploidentical transplantation or double UCB transplantation. This study will hopefully guide us further in choosing the optimal alternative donor source, at least in the RIC setting.

Vaccine strategies in allo-HCT

The rationale for considering antitumor vaccines in the setting of allo-HCT appears logical, especially as improvements in post-transplant outcomes following RIC regimens have mostly resulted from decrease in NRM without a major impact or even in some cases at the expense of higher relapse rates. Incorporation of vaccine strategies has the potential to further augment the graft-versus-lymphoma effect observed with adoptive immunotherapy in lymphoid maligancies [81]. Investigators at the Dana Farber Cancer Institute reported the feasibility of incorporating a vaccine strategy consisting of irradiated host CLL cells admixed with granulocyte–macrophage colony-stimulating factor (GM-CSF)-secreting bystander cells following allo-HCT for this particular disease. Interestingly, the authors reported that only CD8+ T cells from vaccinated subjects reacted against autologous CLL manifesting as increased secretion of interferon gamma [82]. Other groups have described encouraging results using other antigen targets in various hematologic diseases [83–85]. As advances in cancer immunology in lymphoid

malignancies continue to develop, we anticipate that more effective vaccines will evolve which might ultimately be used to synergize the anti-lymphoma effect of alloreactive donor T cells. This could potentially improve curability of allo-HCT without added toxicity.

Discussion and future direction

A better understanding of the key role of donor T cells in eradication of disease, lymphoid or myeloid, following hematopoietic cell allografting has resulted in a shift in practice favoring the use of RIC preparative regimens. Use of these regimens has broadened applicability of allo-HCT to patients who might have been deemed ineligible in the past. RIC regimens have resulted in lesser toxicity from the procedure and, consequently, a lower NRM, but has not translated into a clear survival advantage when compared to traditional myeloablative regimens probably due to a higher risk of disease relapse. Better supportive therapies after allo-HCT has favorably contributed to lowering the mortality associated with the procedure [86,87]. Availability of alternative donor sources, namely UCB and haploidentical transplantation, has expanded the number of eligible patients, with lymphoid or other malignancies, to be considered for allo-HCT. Further improvements in NRM would also necessitate development of more effective strategies for prophylaxis against GVHD as well as better therapies to treat it.

Disease relapse continues to be a serious concern and a major factor limiting post-transplant outcomes. Early referral of eligible subjects to be evaluated for their candidacy for allo-HCT is an important determinant of outcome as the number of pretransplant therapies is inversely correlated with NRM and OS in most of the studies. Additionally, strategies aimed at incorporating novel disease-specific therapies such as monoclonal antibodies or others in the peri- or post-transplant phase coupled with better tools to assess residual disease after allografting are necessary to continue to improve outcomes in our opinion. Incorporating such therapies needs to be carefully evaluated to avoid overlapping toxicities. Moreover, improvements in early detection of residual disease or relapse might allow a more timely therapeutic intervention. This could prove to be an effective strategy, especially as adoptive immunotherapy takes time to become fully established and its success depends in part on the kinetics of disease growth and proliferation. We anticipate that development of more effective antitumor vaccines will continue to evolve and ultimately will be incorporated in the allo-HCT setting to improve cure.

References

1 Coiffier B, Lepage E, Briere J *et al.* CHOP chemotherapy plus rituximab compared with CHOP alone in elderly patients with diffuse large-B-cell lymphoma. *N Engl J Med* 2002;**346**:235–42.

2 Younes A, Bartlett NL, Leonard JP *et al.* Brentuximab vedotin (SGN-35) for relapsed CD30-positive lymphomas. *N Engl J Med* 2010;**363**:1812–21.

3 Recher C, Coiffier B, Haioun C *et al.* Intensified chemotherapy with ACVBP plus rituximab versus standard CHOP plus rituximab for the treatment of diffuse large B-cell lymphoma (LNH03-2B): an open-label randomised phase 3 trial. *Lancet* 2011;**378**:1858–67.

4 Wierda WG, Kipps TJ, Mayer J *et al.* Ofatumumab as single-agent CD20 immunotherapy in fludarabine-refractory chronic lymphocytic leukemia. *J Clin Oncol* 2010;**28**:1749–55.

5 Goede V, Fischer K, Busch R *et al.* Obinutuzumab plus chlorambucil in patients with CLL and coexisting conditions. *N Engl J Med* 2014;**370**:1101–10.

6 Matasar MJ, Czuczman MS, Rodriguez MA *et al.* Ofatumumab in combination with ICE or DHAP chemotherapy in relapsed or refractory intermediate grade B-cell lymphoma. *Blood* 2013;**122**:499–506.

7 Coiffier B, Lepretre S, Pedersen LM *et al.* Safety and efficacy of ofatumumab, a fully human monoclonal anti-CD20 antibody, in patients with relapsed or refractory B-cell chronic lymphocytic leukemia: a phase 1-2 study. *Blood* 2008;**111**:1094–100.

8 Santos ES, Kharfan-Dabaja MA, Ayala E, Raez LE. Current results and future applications of radioimmunotherapy management of non-Hodgkin's lymphoma. *Leukemia Lymphoma* 2006;**47**:2453–76.

9 Wang ML, Rule S, Martin P *et al.* Targeting BTK with ibrutinib in relapsed or refractory mantle-cell lymphoma. *N Engl J Med* 2013;**369**:507–16.

10 O'Connor OA, Wright J, Moskowitz C *et al.* Phase II clinical experience with the novel proteasome inhibitor bortezomib in patients with indolent non-Hodgkin's lymphoma and mantle cell lymphoma. *J Clin Oncol* 2005;**23**:676–84.

11 Appelbaum FR, Sullivan KM, Buckner CD *et al.* Treatment of malignant lymphoma in 100 patients with chemotherapy, total body irradiation, and marrow transplantation. *J Clin Oncol* 1987;**5**:1340–7.

12 Kharfan-Dabaja MA, Anasetti C, Fernandez HF *et al.* Phase II study of CD4⁺-guided pentostatin lymphodepletion and pharmacokinetically targeted busulfan as conditioning for hematopoietic cell allografting. *Biol Blood Marrow Transplant* 2013;**19**:1087–93.

13 Hamadani M, Saber W, Ahn KW *et al.* Impact of pretransplantation conditioning regimens on outcomes of allogeneic transplantation for chemotherapy-unresponsive diffuse large B cell lymphoma and grade III follicular lymphoma. *Biol Blood Marrow Transplant* 2013;**19**:746–53.

14 Hamadani M, Saber W, Ahn KW *et al.* Allogeneic hematopoietic cell transplantation for chemotherapy-unresponsive mantle cell lymphoma: a cohort analysis from the Center for International Blood and Marrow Transplant Research. *Biol Blood Marrow Transplant* 2013;**19**:625–31.

15 Bacigalupo A, Ballen K, Rizzo D *et al.* Defining the intensity of conditioning regimens: working definitions. *Biol Blood Marrow Transplant* 2009;**15**:1628–33.

16 Rodrigues CA, Rocha V, Dreger P *et al.* Alternative donor hematopoietic stem cell transplantation for mature lymphoid malignancies after reduced-intensity conditioning regimen: similar outcomes with umbilical cord blood and unrelated donor peripheral blood. *Haematologica* 2014;**99**:370–7.

17 Raiola A, Dominietto A, Varaldo R *et al.* Unmanipulated haploidentical BMT following non-myeloablative conditioning and post-transplantation CY for advanced Hodgkin's lymphoma. *Bone Marrow Transplant* 2014;**49**:190–4.

18 Kharfan-Dabaja MA, Nishihori T, Otrock ZK, Haidar N, Mohty M, Hamadani M. Monoclonal antibodies in conditioning regimens for hematopoietic cell transplantation. *Biol Blood Marrow Transplant* 2013;**19**:1288–300.

19 Anderson JE, Litzow MR, Appelbaum FR *et al.* Allogeneic, syngeneic, and autologous marrow transplantation for Hodgkin's disease: the 21-year Seattle experience. *J Clin Oncol* 1993;**11**:2342–50.

20 Ratanatharathorn V, Uberti J, Karanes C *et al.* Prospective comparative trial of autologous versus allogeneic bone marrow transplantation in patients with non-Hodgkin's lymphoma. *Blood* 1994;**84**:1050–5.

21 van Besien KW, Mehra RC, Giralt SA *et al.* Allogeneic bone marrow transplantation for poor-prognosis lymphoma: response, toxicity and survival depend on disease histology. *Am J Med* 1996;**100**:299–307.

22 Gajewski JL, Phillips GL, Sobocinski KA *et al.* Bone marrow transplants from HLA-identical siblings in advanced Hodgkin's disease. *J Clin Oncol* 1996;**14**:572–8.

23 Milpied N, Fielding AK, Pearce RM, Ernst P, Goldstone AH. Allogeneic bone marrow transplant is not better than autologous transplant for patients with relapsed Hodgkin's disease. European Group for Blood and Bone Marrow Transplantation. *J Clin Oncol* 1996;**14**:1291–6.

24 Juckett M, Rowlings P, Hessner M *et al.* T cell-depleted allogeneic bone marrow transplantation for high-risk non-Hodgkin's lymphoma: clinical and molecular follow-up. *Bone Marrow Transplant* 1998;**21**:893–9.

25 Dhedin N, Giraudier S, Gaulard P *et al.* Allogeneic bone marrow transplantation in aggressive non-Hodgkin's lymphoma (excluding Burkitt and lymphoblastic lymphoma): a series of 73 patients from the SFGM database. Societ Francaise de Greffe de Moelle. *Br J Haematol* 1999;**107**:154–61.

26 Akpek G, Ambinder RF, Piantadosi S *et al.* Long-term results of blood and marrow transplantation for Hodgkin's lymphoma. *J Clin Oncol* 2001;**19**:4314–21.

27 van Besien K, Loberiza FR Jr, Bajorunaite R *et al.* Comparison of autologous and allogeneic hematopoietic stem cell transplantation for follicular lymphoma. *Blood* 2003;**102**:3521–9.

28 Doocey RT, Toze CL, Connors JM *et al.* Allogeneic haematopoietic stem-cell transplantation for relapsed and refractory aggressive histology non-Hodgkin lymphoma. *Br J Haematol* 2005;**131**:223–30.

29 Kim SW, Tanimoto TE, Hirabayashi N *et al.* Myeloablative allogeneic hematopoietic stem cell transplantation for non-Hodgkin lymphoma: a nationwide survey in Japan. *Blood* 2006;**108**:382–9.

30 Sureda A, Robinson S, Canals C *et al.* Reduced-intensity conditioning compared with conventional allogeneic stem-cell transplantation in relapsed or refractory Hodgkin's lymphoma: an analysis from the Lymphoma Working Party of the European Group for Blood and Marrow Transplantation. *J Clin Oncol* 2008;**26**:455–62.

31 Claviez A, Canals C, Dierickx D *et al.* Allogeneic hematopoietic stem cell transplantation in children and adolescents with recurrent and refractory Hodgkin lymphoma: an analysis of the European Group for Blood and Marrow Transplantation. *Blood* 2009;**114**:2060–7.

32 Smith SM, Burns LJ, van Besien K *et al.* Hematopoietic cell transplantation for systemic mature T-cell non-Hodgkin lymphoma. *J Clin Oncol* 2013;**31**:3100–9.

33 Bacher U, Klyuchnikov E, Carreras J *et al.* Conditioning intensity in allogeneic hematopoietic cell transplantation (alloHCT) for diffuse large B-cell lymphoma (DLBCL). *Blood (ASH Annual Meeting Abstracts)* 2011;**118**:Abstract 501.

34 Sorror ML, Maris MB, Storb R *et al.* Hematopoietic cell transplantation (HCT)-specific comorbidity index: a new tool for risk assessment before allogeneic HCT. *Blood* 2005;**106**:2912–19.

35 Sorror ML, Maris MB, Storer B *et al.* Comparing morbidity and mortality of HLA-matched unrelated donor hematopoietic cell transplantation after nonmyeloablative and myeloablative conditioning: influence of pretransplantation comorbidities. *Blood* 2004;**104**:961–8.

36 Butcher BW, Collins RH Jr. The graft-versus-lymphoma effect: clinical review and future opportunities. *Bone Marrow Transplant* 2005;**36**:1–17.

37 Bishop MR, Dean RM, Steinberg SM *et al.* Clinical evidence of a graft-versus-lymphoma effect against relapsed diffuse large B-cell lymphoma after allogeneic hematopoietic stem-cell transplantation. *Ann Oncol* 2008;**19**:1935–40.

38 Thomson KJ, Morris EC, Milligan D *et al.* T-cell-depleted reduced-intensity transplantation followed by donor leukocyte infusions to promote graft-versus-lymphoma activity results in excellent long-term survival in patients with multiply relapsed follicular lymphoma. *J Clin Oncol* 2010;**28**:3695–700.

39 Khouri IF, Lee MS, Romaguera J *et al.* Allogeneic hematopoietic transplantation for mantle-cell lymphoma: molecular remissions and evidence of graft-versus-malignancy. *Ann Oncol* 1999;**10**:1293–9.

40 Schmitz N, Dreger P, Glass B, Sureda A. Allogeneic transplantation in lymphoma: current status. *Haematologica* 2007;**92**:1533–48.

41 Bacher U, Klyuchnikov E, Le-Rademacher J *et al.* Conditioning regimens for allotransplants for diffuse large B-cell lymphoma: myeloablative or reduced intensity? *Blood* 2012;**120**:4256–62.

42 Khouri IF, McLaughlin P, Saliba RM *et al.* Eight-year experience with allogeneic stem cell transplantation for relapsed follicular lymphoma after nonmyeloablative conditioning with fludarabine, cyclophosphamide, and rituximab. *Blood* 2008;**111**:5530–6.

43 Pinana JL, Martino R, Gayoso J *et al.* Reduced intensity conditioning HLA identical sibling donor allogeneic stem cell transplantation for patients with follicular lymphoma: long-term follow-up from two prospective multicenter trials. *Haematologica* 2010;**95**:1176–82.

44 Rezvani AR, Storer B, Maris M *et al.* Nonmyeloablative allogeneic hematopoietic cell transplantation in relapsed, refractory, and transformed indolent non-Hodgkin's lymphoma. *J Clin Oncol* 2008;**26**:211–17.

45 Tomblyn MR, Ewell M, Bredeson C *et al.* Autologous versus reduced-intensity allogeneic hematopoietic cell transplantation for patients with chemosensitive follicular non-Hodgkin lymphoma beyond first complete response or first partial response. *Biol Blood Marrow Transplant* 2011;**17**:1051–7.

46 Robinson SP, Canals C, Luang JJ *et al.* The outcome of reduced intensity allogeneic stem cell transplantation and autologous stem cell transplantation when performed as a first transplant strategy in relapsed follicular lymphoma: an analysis from the Lymphoma Working Party of the EBMT. *Bone Marrow Transplant* 2013;**48**:1409–14.

47 Hari P, Carreras J, Zhang MJ *et al.* Allogeneic transplants in follicular lymphoma: higher risk of disease progression after reduced-intensity compared to myeloablative conditioning. *Biol Blood Marrow Transplant* 2008;**14**:236–45.

48 Kasamon YL, Jones RJ, Diehl LF *et al.* Outcomes of autologous and allogeneic blood or marrow transplantation for mantle cell lymphoma. *Biol Blood Marrow Transplant* 2005;**11**:39–46.

49 Ganti AK, Bierman PJ, Lynch JC, Bociek RG, Vose JM, Armitage JO. Hematopoietic stem cell transplantation in mantle cell lymphoma. *Ann Oncol* 2005;**16**:618–24.

50 Khouri IF, Lee MS, Saliba RM *et al.* Nonablative allogeneic stem-cell transplantation for advanced/recurrent mantle-cell lymphoma. *J Clin Oncol* 2003;**21**:4407–12.

51 Maris MB, Sandmaier BM, Storer BE *et al.* Allogeneic hematopoietic cell transplantation after fludarabine and 2 Gy total body irradiation for relapsed and refractory mantle cell lymphoma. *Blood* 2004;**104**:3535–42.

52 Cook G, Smith GM, Kirkland K *et al.* Outcome following reduced-intensity allogeneic stem cell transplantation (RIC AlloSCT) for relapsed and refractory mantle cell lymphoma (MCL): a study of the British Society for Blood and Marrow Transplantation. *Biol Blood Marrow Transplant* 2010;**16**: 1419–27.

53 Fenske TS, Zhang MJ, Carreras J *et al.* Autologous or reduced-intensity conditioning allogeneic hematopoietic cell transplantation for chemotherapy-sensitive mantle-cell lymphoma: analysis of transplantation timing and modality. *J Clin Oncol* 2014;**32**:273–81.

54 Kharfan-Dabaja MA, Hamadani M, Sibai H, Savani BN. Managing Hodgkin lymphoma relapsing after autologous hematopoietic cell transplantation: a not-so-good cancer after all! *Bone Marrow Transplant* 2014;**49**:599–606.

55 Sarina B, Castagna L, Farina L *et al.* Allogeneic transplantation improves the overall and progression-free survival of Hodgkin lymphoma patients relapsing after autologous transplantation: a retrospective study based on the time of HLA typing and donor availability. *Blood* 2010;**115**:3671–7.

56 Thomson KJ, Peggs KS, Smith P *et al.* Superiority of reduced-intensity allogeneic transplantation over conventional treatment for relapse of Hodgkin's lymphoma following autologous stem cell transplantation. *Bone Marrow Transplant* 2008;**41**:765–70.

57 Anderlini P, Saliba R, Acholonu S *et al.* Fludarabine–melphalan as a preparative regimen for reduced-intensity conditioning allogeneic stem cell transplantation in relapsed and refractory Hodgkin's lymphoma: the updated M.D. Anderson Cancer Center experience. *Haematologica* 2008;**93**:257–64.

58 Robinson SP, Sureda A, Canals C *et al.* Reduced intensity conditioning allogeneic stem cell transplantation for Hodgkin's lymphoma: identification of prognostic factors predicting outcome. *Haematologica* 2009;**94**:230–8.

59 Sureda A, Canals C, Arranz R *et al.* Allogeneic stem cell transplantation after reduced intensity conditioning in patients with relapsed or refractory Hodgkin's lymphoma. Results of the HDR-ALLO study: a prospective clinical trial by the Grupo Espanol de Linfomas/Trasplante de Medula Osea (GEL/TAMO) and the Lymphoma Working Party of the European Group for Blood and Marrow Transplantation. *Haematologica* 2012;**97**:310–17.

60 Garciaz S, Coso D, Peyrade F *et al.* Brentuximab vedotin followed by allogeneic transplantation as salvage regimen in patients with relapsed and/or refractory Hodgkin's lymphoma. *Hematol Oncol* 2014;**32**:187–191.

61 Michallet M, Socie G, Mohty M *et al.* Rituximab, fludarabine, and total body irradiation as conditioning regimen before allogeneic hematopoietic stem cell transplantation for advanced chronic lymphocytic leukemia: long-term prospective multicenter study. *Exp Hematol* 2013;**41**:127–33.

62 Pidala J, Roman-Diaz J, Kim J *et al.* Targeted IV busulfan and fludarabine followed by post-allogeneic hematopoietic cell

transplantation rituximab demonstrate encouraging activity in CD20⁺ lymphoid malignancies without increased risk of infectious complications. *Int J Hematol* 2011;**93**:206–12.

63 McIver Z, Stephens N, Grim A, Barrett AJ. Rituximab administration within 6 months of T cell-depleted allogeneic SCT is associated with prolonged life-threatening cytopenias. *Biol Blood Marrow Transplant* 2010;**16**:1549–56.

64 Shimoni A, Zwas ST, Oksman Y *et al.* Ibritumomab tiuxetan (Zevalin) combined with reduced-intensity conditioning and allogeneic stem-cell transplantation (SCT) in patients with chemorefractory non-Hodgkin's lymphoma. *Bone Marrow Transplant* 2008;**41**:355–61.

65 Bethge WA, Lange T, Meisner C *et al.* Radioimmunotherapy with yttrium-90-ibritumomab tiuxetan as part of a reduced-intensity conditioning regimen for allogeneic hematopoietic cell transplantation in patients with advanced non-Hodgkin lymphoma: results of a phase 2 study. *Blood* 2010;**116**: 1795–802.

66 Khouri IF, Saliba RM, Erwin WD *et al.* Nonmyeloablative allogeneic transplantation with or without 90yttrium ibritumomab tiuxetan is potentially curative for relapsed follicular lymphoma: 12-year results. *Blood* 2012;**119**:6373–8.

67 Mead AJ, Thomson KJ, Morris EC *et al.* HLA-mismatched unrelated donors are a viable alternate graft source for allogeneic transplantation following alemtuzumab-based reduced-intensity conditioning. *Blood* 2010;**115**:5147–53.

68 Marsh JC, Gupta V, Lim Z *et al.* Alemtuzumab with fludarabine and cyclophosphamide reduces chronic graft-versus-host disease after allogeneic stem cell transplantation for acquired aplastic anemia. *Blood* 2011;**118**:2351–7.

69 Chen R, Palmer JM, Thomas SH *et al.* Brentuximab vedotin enables successful reduced-intensity allogeneic hematopoietic cell transplantation in patients with relapsed or refractory Hodgkin lymphoma. *Blood* 2012;**119**:6379–81.

70 Bashir Q, Robinson SN, de Lima MJ, Parmar S, Shpall E. Umbilical cord blood transplantation. *Clin Adv Hematol Oncol* 2010;**8**:786–801.

71 Brunstein CG, Cantero S, Cao Q *et al.* Promising progression-free survival for patients low and intermediate grade lymphoid malignancies after nonmyeloablative umbilical cord blood transplantation. *Biol Blood Marrow Transplant* 2009;**15**:214–22.

72 Rodrigues CA, Sanz G, Brunstein CG *et al.* Analysis of risk factors for outcomes after unrelated cord blood transplantation in adults with lymphoid malignancies: a study by the Eurocord-Netcord and Lymphoma Working Party of the European Group for Blood and Marrow Transplantation. *J Clin Oncol* 2009;**27**:256–63.

73 Sawada A, Inoue M, Koyama-Sato M *et al.* Umbilical cord blood as an alternative source of reduced-intensity hematopoietic stem cell transplantation for chronic Epstein–Barr virus-associated T or natural killer cell lymphoproliferative diseases. *Biol Blood Marrow Transplant* 2014;**20**:214–21.

74 Aversa F, Tabilio A, Terenzi A *et al*. Successful engraftment of T-cell-depleted haploidentical "three-loci" incompatible transplants in leukemia patients by addition of recombinant human granulocyte colony-stimulating factor-mobilized peripheral blood progenitor cells to bone marrow inoculum. *Blood* 1994;**84**:3948–55.

75 Aversa F, Tabilio A, Velardi A *et al*. Treatment of high-risk acute leukemia with T-cell-depleted stem cells from related donors with one fully mismatched HLA haplotype. *N Engl J Med* 1998;**339**:1186–93.

76 O'Donnell PV, Luznik L, Jones RJ *et al*. Nonmyeloablative bone marrow transplantation from partially HLA-mismatched related donors using posttransplantation cyclophosphamide. *Biol Blood Marrow Transplant* 2002;**8**: 377–86.

77 Luznik L, O'Donnell PV, Symons HJ *et al*. HLA-haploidentical bone marrow transplantation for hematologic malignancies using nonmyeloablative conditioning and high-dose, posttransplantation cyclophosphamide. *Biol Blood Marrow Transplant* 2008;**14**:641–50.

78 Bashey A, Zhang X, Sizemore CA *et al*. T-cell-replete HLA-haploidentical hematopoietic transplantation for hematologic malignancies using post-transplantation cyclophosphamide results in outcomes equivalent to those of contemporaneous HLA-matched related and unrelated donor transplantation. *J Clin Oncol* 2013;**31**:1310–16.

79 Kanda J, Long GD, Gasparetto C *et al*. Reduced-intensity allogeneic transplantation using alemtuzumab from HLA-matched related, unrelated, or haploidentical related donors for patients with hematologic malignancies. *Biol Blood Marrow Transplant* 2014;**20**:257–63.

80 Brunstein CG, Fuchs EJ, Carter SL *et al*. Alternative donor transplantation after reduced intensity conditioning: results of parallel phase 2 trials using partially HLA-mismatched related bone marrow or unrelated double umbilical cord blood grafts. *Blood* 2011;**118**:282–8.

81 El-Jurdi N, Reljic T, Kumar A *et al*. Efficacy of adoptive immunotherapy with donor lymphocyte infusion in relapsed lymphoid malignancies. *Immunotherapy* 2013;**5**: 457–66.

82 Burkhardt UE, Hainz U, Stevenson K *et al*. Autologous CLL cell vaccination early after transplant induces leukemia-specific T cells. *J Clin Invest* 2013;**123**:3756–65.

83 McLarnon A, Piper KP, Goodyear OC *et al*. CD8(+) T-cell immunity against cancer-testis antigens develops following allogeneic stem cell transplantation and reveals a potential mechanism for the graft-versus-leukemia effect. *Haematologica* 2010;**95**:1572–8.

84 Rezvani K, Yong AS, Mielke S *et al*. Lymphodepletion is permissive to the development of spontaneous T-cell responses to the self-antigen PR1 early after allogeneic stem cell transplantation and in patients with acute myeloid leukemia undergoing WT1 peptide vaccination following chemotherapy. *Cancer Immunol Immunother* 2012;**61**:1125–36.

85 Teshima T, Mach N, Hill GR *et al*. Tumor cell vaccine elicits potent antitumor immunity after allogeneic T-cell-depleted bone marrow transplantation. *Cancer Res* 2001;**61**: 162–71.

86 Herbrecht R, Denning DW, Patterson TF *et al*. Voriconazole versus amphotericin B for primary therapy of invasive aspergillosis. *N Engl J Med* 2002;**347**:408–15.

87 Zaia JA, Schmidt GM, Chao NJ *et al*. Preemptive ganciclovir administration based solely on asymptomatic pulmonary cytomegalovirus infection in allogeneic bone marrow transplant recipients: long-term follow-up. *Biol Blood Marrow Transplant* 1995;**1**:88–93.

88 Sirvent A, Dhedin N, Michallet M *et al*. Low nonrelapse mortality and prolonged long-term survival after reduced-intensity allogeneic stem cell transplantation for relapsed or refractory diffuse large B cell lymphoma: report of the Société Française de Greffe de Moelle et de Thérapie Cellulaire. *Biol Blood Marrow Transplant* 2010;**16**:78–85.

89 Armand P, Kim HT, Ho VT *et al*. Allogeneic transplantation with reduced-intensity conditioning for Hodgkin and non-Hodgkin lymphoma: importance of histology for outcome. *Biol Blood Marrow Transplant* 2008;**14**:418–25.

90 Le Gouill S, Kröger N, Dhedin N *et al*. Reduced-intensity conditioning allogeneic stem cell transplantation for relapsed/refractory mantle cell lymphoma: a multicenter experience. *Ann Oncol* 2012;**23**:2695–703.

Pretransplantation evaluation, comorbidities, and nondisease-related eligibility criteria for transplantation in lymphoma

Melissa Logue

Introduction

Hematologic malignancies account for approximately 10% of new cancer diagnoses in the United States [1]. For some, chemotherapy alone gives a high chance of cure. However, those diseases that cannot be cured with chemotherapy alone must often proceed to hematopoietic stem cell transplantation (HCT). HCT provides curative therapy for a variety of diseases. Over the past several decades, significant advances have been made in the field of HCT and allogeneic (allo)-HCT has now become an integral part of treatment for a variety of hematologic malignancies and nonmalignant diseases [2,3]. Advances in transplantation technology and supportive care measures have resulted in a significant decrease in early mortality, resulting in continued growth in the number of long-term HCT survivors [3–6].

Since the first three cases of successful allo-HCT in 1968, the number of allo-HCTs performed annually has increased steadily over the past three decades [3]. It is estimated that by 2015 more than 100,000 patients will receive HCT (combined allogeneic and autologous) annually throughout the world, and numbers are increasing rapidly. Long-term survival after HCT has improved significantly since its inception over 40 years ago due to improved supportive care and early recognition of long-term complications [7,8]. With broadening indications, more options for HCT and improvement in survival, by 2020 there may be up to 1 million long-term survivors after HCT worldwide. In order to offer the curative allo-HCT treatment option in most patients, safer regimens with acceptable graft-versus-host disease (GVHD)-associated morbidity and transplant-related mortality (TRM) are preferred. A recently published study from the M.D. Anderson Cancer Center showed an excellent overall survival and progression-free survival (85% and 83%, respectively, after median follow-up of 60 months) for relapsed follicular lymphoma after fludarabine, cyclophosphamide, and rituximab reduced-intensity conditioning (RIC) allo-HCT [9]. Similarly, many disease-specific transplant regimens are in development to improve transplant outcome after HCT.

In this era, a stem cell source can be found for virtually all patients who have an indication to receive allo-HCT. Since 2007, more allo-HCT procedures have been performed using stem cells from alternative donor sources, such as volunteer unrelated donors or cord blood, than those from related donors [4]. RIC haploidentical related donor or cord blood transplantations have emerged as alternatives to fill the gap for those patients who do not have matched related donor or unrelated donor [10–12] and the outcome of these types of transplantation are expected to be better than chemotherapy alone or even better than autologous HCT for selected indications.

Being a most effective therapy for many hematologic diseases creates an obligation to educate referring physicians on timely referral for HCT and coordination of pretransplantation care to further improve transplant outcomes. Many physicians are not aware of procedures

Clinical Guide to Transplantation in Lymphoma, First Edition. Edited by Bipin N. Savani and Mohamad Mohty.

involved in the transplant process after an initial referral discussion with a transplant physician and the goal of this chapter is to walk through the basic steps to HCT.

Initial steps

Once it is determined that a patient should consider HCT, several key steps are involved in progress toward this objective. A patient should be referred to a transplant center to undergo a detailed evaluation. It is optimal to refer early as some pretransplant treatments could alter a patient's anticipated transplant course.

Once a patient is referred to a transplant center, many internal steps begin. Prior to the patient's first visit, the clinic staff will obtain outside records (Table 7.1). These would include baseline and cumulative laboratory results, clinic notes, hospital admission and discharge notes, chemotherapy infusion records, radiation records, and imaging reports. Pathology will also be requested for review at the transplant center for confirmation of diagnosis.

Preparation for transplant center evaluation

Generally a referral appointment with the transplant center occurs within 1–2 weeks of initial request. At the first visit the physician team will review patient's history. This review will include diagnostic work-up, treatment completed, and tolerance to the treatment. The team will also ask the patient numerous other questions to determine their eligibility for transplant. Key information to obtain will be past medical history, past surgical history, family history, substance use (prior and current), and social support.

Patients being considered for allogeneic stem cell transplant will also be asked about potential family donors. Potential donors would primarily include full siblings, but may not be limited to these. They would also be questioned about children, parents, and double first cousins. It is important for patients to be aware of the healthcare concerns of family members that might preclude them from donation, such as heart disease or oncologic history. If it is determined that there is a

Table 7.1 Data review during different stages of the transplant evaluation process.

Discussion/testing	Initial transplant center (pre-evaluation) visit	Pretransplant evaluation	Per referring hematologist/ oncologist
Diagnosis			×
Confirm diagnosis, review pathology	×		
PMH review for consults needed (for clearance)	×	×	×
Question regarding potential related donors	×		×
Initial HLA typing	×		
Confirmatory HLA typing		×	
Question regarding substance use	×	×	×
Obtain negative substance screens	×	×	×
Review transplant goals	×	×	×
Review transplant complications (i.e., infection, GVHD)	×	×	
Review transplant long-term follow-up	×	×	
Review dental requirements	×	×	
Review organ function requirements	×		
Review time required near transplant center	×	×	
Review need for 24-hour caregiver during transplant	×	×	
Final disease testing		×	
Final organ function testing and lab work	×	×	
Donor testing (if applicable)		×	
Psychosocial evaluation		×	
Outside department referrals for transplant clearance	×	×	

GVHD, graft-versus-host disease; HLA, human leukocyte antigen; PMH, past medical history.

suitable candidate or candidates, the physician team will request HLA typing on the patient and family member(s). HLA typing results are typically available within 1 week.

During the initial visit, patients are also counseled regarding the transplant procedure. For patients who will be proceeding to an autologous HCT, the discussion will focus on the process of stem cell collection followed by high-dose chemotherapy and stem cell rescue. They will be asked to stay near the transplant center for approximately 1 month after the transplant. Patients proceeding to allo-HCT will be counseled on high-dose chemotherapy followed by stem cell rescue from an allogeneic donor. They will be asked to stay near the transplant center for approximately 3 months after the transplant. These patients are at risk for GVHD. Discussions regarding GVHD begin at this visit. Patients will also be told at this visit of their dental requirements and the need for a 24-hour caregiver during the acute transplant course.

After the initial visit, the patient is instructed to follow up with their local oncologist. Any recommendations for further treatment prior to transplant will be communicated by the staff at the transplant center. Treatment recommendations may focus on disease debulking or maintenance therapy while a donor is selected (for allo-HCT patients). The local oncologist is asked to communicate with the transplant center once the requested disease control is obtained or if there is difficulty achieving this goal. Extension or a change in treatment may be recommended for the latter scenario. The transplant center, in turn, will also communicate with the referring oncologist once the patient and family members' HLA typing is complete. If no suitable donor is found, an unrelated donor search may be initiated.

Also, after the patient's initial visit with the transplant center, their primary hematologist will present the patient's case to the transplant board. This board consists of both transplant and nontransplant physicians. Each case is discussed in detail with a recommendation to follow. If a patient is approved to proceed to either an autologous or allogeneic HCT, the patient is placed on the physician's waiting list until all identified pending criteria are met. The results of this discussion are reviewed with the patient and referring physician along with what criteria must be met before proceeding to transplant.

Transplant center evaluation

Once a patient has met the criteria to move ahead with transplant and a donor has been identified (self, related, or unrelated), he or she is referred internally from the transplant center's hematologist to the actual transplant program. The patient's insurance company is contacted to gain initial clearance to proceed with further testing to ensure eligibility. The patient will be contacted by the transplant nurse practitioner to set up a thorough transplant evaluation.

During the evaluation, patients will undergo disease and organ function testing as well as a teaching session [13]. Disease testing may include hematology, bone marrow biopsy, radiological scans, and possibly a lumbar puncture. Organ function testing will include electrocardiogram, chest X-ray, echocardiogram, and a pulmonary function test. Other blood work beyond disease testing will include a comprehensive metabolic panel, cholesterol and triglyceride levels, viral testing, urinalysis, drug and nicotine screens. Women will have hormone levels tested along with a pregnancy test. Men will have prostate-specific antigen checked. Allo-HCT patients will also see physical therapy and have a baseline bone density scan performed. If any of the evaluation work-up is abnormal or if a patient is known to have health concerns, additional referrals will be made at this time. Referrals may include cardiology, urology, pulmonology, or infectious disease, for example. These referrals may require additional visits to the transplant center.

During the transplant evaluation, patients will be counseled further about the need for a 24-hour caregiver during transplant. They will be asked to submit their dental clearance and must have a tuberculosis skin test completed. Patients will have a visit with the financial counselor during the evaluation as well as meet with a research team member to assess if they are eligible for any current transplant-related clinical trials. Patients will also meet with a social worker. The social worker will assist with securing local housing for the transplant, but will also screen for any psychosocial concerns that may cause barriers to transplant. The social workers also help inform patients of charities and programs that can assist patients throughout the transplant.

Transplant education is a significant portion of the evaluation. A mid-level provider will meet with the patient and caregiver(s) to not only review his or her in-depth history but also to inform the patient of the anticipated course along with the risks and benefits of the transplant. Items discussed will be proposed treatment dates, central line placement, treatment regimen (chemotherapy and/or radiation), nutrition, need for transfusions, infection risk, GVHD, and long-term complications. Patients will also be informed of TRM, along with other alternatives to transplant management.

Post-evaluation review and final pretransplant process

For patients proceeding directly to transplant, a calendar will be reviewed with them. Patients awaiting dates from an unrelated donor (through the National Marrow Donor Program) will be asked to continue routine follow-up with their referring physician and possibly receive interim therapy. After the evaluation, it typically takes a full week for all results to become available. Once these data are obtained, the patient's insurance company is again contacted, this time for final approval to proceed. Insurance approval typically occurs within 1 week. Therefore, most patients will begin transplant about 2 weeks after initial evaluation, provided no additional work-up is needed. Patients undergoing transplants from unrelated donors usually wait about 6 weeks between evaluation and transplant.

For those patients with related donors, the donor will undergo simultaneous work-up. Donors will be asked to come to the transplant center for their evaluation. Their evaluation will include blood work, tuberculosis testing, electrocardiogram, and chest X-ray. They will also undergo questioning regarding medical history and potential exposures which might present a risk to the recipient. Physical examination, along with the above-mentioned studies, will help determine any risks to the donors themselves. Donors will also be counseled regarding the procedure and their individual risk.

After all testing is complete and insurance approval has been obtained, the recipient will undergo a final day of evaluation just prior to the start date for the transplant. This is to ensure no significant changes have occurred since evaluation that might place a patient at greater risk after transplant. This evaluation includes a physical examination, blood work, and questioning regarding current health status. Multiple physicians will review all the patient (and donor if applicable) information. If all data are unchanged and no heightened risk is identified, the patient will then proceed to central line placement and chemotherapy in preparation for the transplant. A handover procedure is in place to ensure smooth transition to the post-transplant team that will then assume care. Referring physicians will be sent periodic updates as well as end of treatment notifications and recommendations.

References

1 Siegel R, Naishadham D, Jemal A. Cancer statistics, 2012. *CA Cancer J Clin* 2012;**62**:10–29.

2 Thomas ED. A history of bone marrow transplantation. In: Appelbaum FR, Forman SJ, Negrin RS, Blume KG, eds. *Thomas' Hematopoietic Cell Transplantation*. Chichester, UK: Wiley-Blackwell, 2009:3–7.

3 Horowitz MM. Uses and growth of hematopoietic cell transplantation. In: Appelbaum FR, Forman SJ, Negrin RS, Blume KG, eds. *Thomas' Hematopoietic Cell Transplantation*. Chichester, UK: Wiley-Blackwell, 2009:15–21.

4 Pasquini MC, Wang Z. Current use and outcome of hematopoietic stem cell transplantation: CIBMTR Summary Slides, 2010. Available at http://www.cibmtr.org

5 Majhail NS, Rizzo JD, Lee SJ et al. Recommended screening and preventive practices for long-term survivors after hematopoietic cell transplantation. *Bone Marrow Transplant* 2012;**47**:337–41.

6 Majhail NS, Rizzo JD. Surviving the cure: long term followup of hematopoietic cell transplant recipients. *Bone Marrow Transplant* 2013;**48**:1145–51.

7 Savani BN. How can we improve life expectancy and quality of life in long-term survivors after allogeneic stem cell transplantation? *Semin Hematol* 2012;**49**:1–3.

8 Savani BN, Griffith ML, Jagasia S, Lee SJ. How I treat late effects in adults after allogeneic stem cell transplantation. *Blood* 2011;**117**:3002–9.

9 Khouri IF, McLaughlin P, Saliba RM et al. Eight-year experience with allogeneic stem cell transplantation for relapsed follicular lymphoma after nonmyeloablative conditioning with fludarabine, cyclophosphamide, and rituximab. *Blood* 2008;**111**:5530–6.

10 Savani BN. Transplantation in AML CR1. *Blood* 2010;**116**:1822–3.

11 Nishiwaki S, Atsuta Y, Tanaka J. Allogeneic hematopoietic cell transplantation from alternative sources for adult Philadelphia chromosome-negative ALL: what should we

choose when no HLA-matched related donor is available? *Bone Marrow Transplant* 2013;**48**:1369–76.

12 Bacigalupo A, Marsh JC. Unrelated donor search and unrelated donor transplantation in the adult aplastic anaemia patient aged 18–40 years without an HLA-identical sibling and failing immunosuppression. *Bone Marrow Transplant* 2013;**48**:198–200.

13 Hamadani M, Craig M, Awan FT, Devine SM. How we approach patient evaluation for hematopoietic stem cell transplantation. *Bone Marrow Transplant* 2010;**45**:1259–68.

CHAPTER 8

Stem cell mobilization in lymphoma patients

Tarah Ballinger, Bipin N. Savani and Mohamad Mohty

Introduction

Autologous hematopoietic stem cell transplant aims to restore normal bone marrow function after high-dose chemotherapy using an individual's own stem cells, with the ideal source for collection being the peripheral blood. Because of low concentrations in the peripheral blood at steady state, it is necessary to recruit hematopoietic stem cells (HSCs) from the bone marrow to the peripheral circulation in a process termed "stem cell mobilization." Collection of peripheral blood stem cells (PBSCs) has largely replaced bone marrow collection due to more efficient engraftment, shorter hospital stays, improved patient outcomes, and lower costs. However, methods of mobilization and collection vary widely across institutions and depend on multiple variables, including patient safety, efficacy, physician familiarity, cost-effectiveness, and availability of multidisciplinary coordination across departments.

Historically, PBSCs were mobilized using chemotherapy after it was observed that high-dose chemotherapy increases the concentration of circulating stem cells [1]. Currently, methods for mobilization rely on either growth factor cytokines, such as granulocyte colony-stimulating factor (G-CSF, or filgrastim), or chemotherapy plus G-CSF. Stem cells are anchored to the stromal network of the bone marrow by numerous adhesion molecules, and these bonds can be loosened in order to mobilize stem cells into the peripheral circulation [2]. Following the observation that G-CSF receptors on stem cells are not necessary for mobilization, it is believed that G-CSF leads to granulocyte activation and the release of proteases, which cleave the adhesion molecules that hold stem cells in the bone marrow [2,3]. In addition, a clinically useful target called stromal-derived factor (SDF)-1 is expressed by stromal cells and binds to CXCR4, a receptor found on CD34-positive stem cells [4]. The interaction regulates stem cell homing and migration, and its disruption results in the release of stem cells into the circulation. This is the target of the reversible chemokine receptor antagonist plerixafor (Mozobil), which is approved for use in combination with G-CSF in autologous stem cell transplant for patients with lymphoma and multiple myeloma [5].

Previously, no clear standard approach or recommendations for autologous stem cell mobilization had been defined; however, guidelines were released in early 2014 by a panel of experts for both the American Society for Blood and Marrow Transplantation and the European Group for Blood and Marrow Transplantation [6–8]. These consensus guidelines will help guide clinical practice for choosing methods of mobilization and address difficult situations, such as how to approach poor mobilization, special populations, and possible complications of mobilization and collection.

Methods for mobilization

The current methods for mobilization of PBSCs in auto-stem cell transplant are shown in Figure 8.1. The present preferred method is G-CSF monotherapy, or steady-state mobilization. G-CSF has been shown to be superior to sargramostim, or granulocyte–macrophage

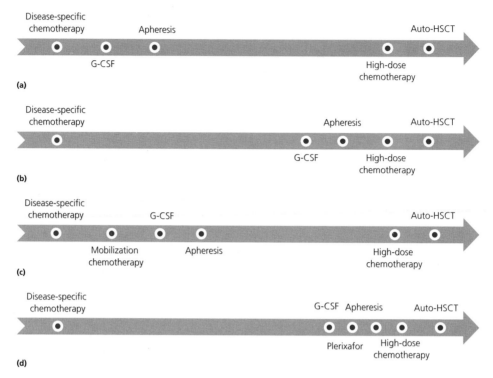

Figure 8.1 Current mobilization strategies for autologous hematopoietic stem cell transplant (HSCT): **a)** steady-state mobilization with growth factor alone, **b)** chemotherapy-based mobilization with disease-specific chemotherapy or **c)** separate mobilization chemotherapy, and **d)** plerixafor plus G-CSF.

colony-stimulating factor (GM-CSF), as well as the combination of G-CSF and GM-CSF [9–11]. Other formulations of G-CSF include lenograstim (glycosylated G-CSF) and the longer-acting pegfilgrastim (pegylated G-CSF). Lenograstim has been shown to be of equivalent efficacy to filgrastim, while pegfilgrastim remains more expensive with possibly higher toxicities and is not routinely used [12]. However, emerging data indicate that pegfilgrastim may have similar efficacy, with the advantage of a single longer-acting injection, and therefore may be more widely used as familiarity increases [13–15].

The recommended dosing of both filgrastim and lenograstim is 10 μg/kg daily, with leukapheresis on the fifth day. The majority of centers administer this as a once-daily subcutaneous injection, as higher doses of 12–16 μg/kg daily or split dosing of 5 μg/kg twice daily have been shown to result in more efficient collection but higher toxicity profiles, cost, and inconvenience [16–18]. It is recommended that filgrastim be administered for 5–7 days consecutively, and lenograstim for 4–6 days consecutively [2,6]. Leukapheresis is performed on the final

day, the specific guidelines for which are discussed in the following section. Studies have shown improved efficacy of stem cell collection when G-CSF is given 3 hours before apheresis, compared to the evening prior [19].

G-CSF monotherapy has the inherent advantages of low cost, minimal toxicity, and predictable kinetics to enable easier calculation of apheresis timing. However, the addition of chemotherapy to G-CSF, termed "chemomobilization," can increase the yield of CD34-positive stem cells at the time of collection and has the added benefit of a possible further decrease in tumor burden [20]. Chemotherapy for mobilization can be administered during the disease-specific initial induction or salvage therapies, or later as a separate monotherapy. It is generally preferred to administer G-CSF along with chemotherapy as part of disease-specific therapy, especially in heavily pretreated patients, in an effort to minimize the need for additional mobilization. Treatment regimens that include mobilization in the initial cycles of induction or salvage chemotherapy have been shown to possibly reduce collection failure rates to less than 3% [6]. In addition, chemotherapy for mobilization apart from disease-specific therapy is more costly and toxic than G-CSF alone. The majority of chemomobilization regimens include cyclophosphamide or etoposide, with some evidence showing improved yields with etoposide-containing regimens [21,22]. There is no clear consensus on chemotherapy dosing, as increased doses show better stem cell yield and engraftment, but with additional toxicity and cost [23]. It was hypothesized that chemomobilization would reduce graft contamination and therefore improve long-term response rates, but this has not been confirmed. Compared with G-CSF alone, chemomobilization is associated with increased overall cost, increased episodes of neutropenic fever, and more patient hospital stays, but no difference has been found for mortality, overall survival, or long-term risk of secondary malignancy [24]. G-CSF added to myelosuppressive chemotherapy is given at a recommended dose of 5–10 µg/kg daily for 1–5 days after the completion of chemotherapy until the time of leukapheresis [8].

In 2008, the novel agent plerixafor was approved for use in patients with non-Hodgkin lymphoma and multiple myeloma and is currently used most commonly in conjunction with G-CSF. It may be used for delayed remobilization after patients fail initial mobilization, or as a "preemptive" measure along with G-CSF or chemomobilization in patients with low pre-apheresis counts or predicted failure. Plerixafor has a quicker onset of action than G-CSF, with peak mobilization of CD34-positive cells in just 4–10 hours, and has a more sustained effect, decreasing difficulties with apheresis timing [5]. Recommended dosing is 240 µg/kg subcutaneously on the day of apheresis, following four prior days of G-CSF therapy. Patients with creatinine clearance less than 50 mL/min tolerate a reduced dose of 160 µg/kg [25]. Studies have shown that initial addition of plerixafor to G-CSF leads to increased yield, fewer days of apheresis, and lower failure rates compared to G-CSF monotherapy or G-CSF plus chemotherapy [26,27]. In addition, plerixafor plus G-CSF has been shown to effectively mobilize patients who have previously failed G-CSF monotherapy or chemomobilization [28]. Given its current high relative cost, most centers reserve the addition of plerixafor to those patients who are known or predicted poor mobilizers at high risk for failure of adequate collection [29–31]. Monitoring of pre- apheresis CD34-positive cell counts may aid in detecting patients at risk for poor

mobilization. Many published reports from centers which have adopted a protocol for the addition of plerixafor in patients with low peripheral blood CD34$^+$ counts prior to apheresis have found failure rates less than 10%. Some have shown that despite the additional cost of plerixafor, the decreased failure rates result in an overall optimization of resources [31,32]. Studies on the effects of combining all three methods (G-CSF, chemomobilization, and plerixafor) are ongoing [33].

Stem cell collection and apheresis

Collection of CD34-positive stem cells must be adequate in order for hematopoietic recovery to occur. A dose of 2×10^6 cells/kg is generally considered adequate for engraftment, but many studies suggest that the optimal dose is at least 5×10^6 cells/kg. More appears to be better, with increasing doses showing more robust recovery and improved overall survival in so-called "supermobilizers" [34–36]; however, these data have not yet been collected in well-controlled patient populations. A peripheral blood CD34-positive cell count of more than 20/µL by flow cytometry generally allows for a goal collection of more than 2×10^6 cells/kg, but this continues to be debated [37]. Given that CD34-positive cells peak around 4–6 days after beginning G-CSF, it is recommended to begin monitoring pre-apheresis counts on day 4 or 5. The same is true for the addition of plerixafor. Leukapheresis is then generally initiated on day 5. For patients undergoing chemomobilization plus G-CSF, cell counts peak later at around 8–10 days, so monitoring should begin around day 8. The peak time for leukapheresis is less predictable for chemomobilization and is generally guided by a threshold cell count [6,8].

Stem cell collection has been shown to be more efficient at larger volumes of at least four times the patient's blood volume. Higher volumes are especially recommended for those patients felt to be poor mobilizers [38]. This is not recommended for those at risk for cardiac issues, as increased volumes and increased dimethyl sulfoxide content in the infusion product are associated with cardiac side effects [39]. Large-volume apheresis is generally safe, with additional risks including more exposure to anticoagulant, higher levels of citrate causing muscle cramping, and worsened thrombocytopenia [40]. It is recommended that up to four leukapheresis sessions are practical. Additional sessions add increased cost and are rarely successful. Higher volumes should not be obtained at the cost of increasing the number of leukapheresis sessions.

Poor mobilizers and mobilization failure

Predicting patients who will be difficult to mobilize can help determine the best initial method for mobilization. Attempting to prevent initial failure can save the extensive utilization of resources such as growth factor and transfusion support, antibiotics, apheresis days, and hospital admissions associated with failure and remobilization attempts [41]. However, despite the establishment of predictive models and the knowledge of characteristics that increase the likelihood of failure, predictions of who will mobilize poorly remain less than accurate. One strategy is to preemptively use plerixafor as an initial mobilization technique in patients who are at high risk for failure based on their clinical history. Factors that have been described as predictive of a high risk for failure are listed in Table 8.1 and include older age, time from diagnosis to transplant, more advanced disease, lower bone marrow cellularity, higher number of prior treatment regimens, previous radiation therapy or certain chemotherapy drugs, history of prior stem cell transplant, lower platelet count prior to mobilization, and lower PBSC counts prior to apheresis. Number of prior chemotherapy cycles and PBSC counts seem to be the most consistent predictors of poor mobilization [42–46]. Monitoring actual pre-apheresis peripheral blood CD34-positive cell counts is another strategy that can identify who is at risk for poor mobilization, as these counts have been shown to correlate with the number of CD34-positive stem cells

Table 8.1 Risk factors associated with poor mobilization in autologous stem cell transplant [41–45].

Age greater than 60 years
Shorter time interval from diagnosis or prior treatment to transplant
Advanced or refractory disease
Increased number of prior chemotherapy regimens
Prior radiotherapy
Lower bone marrow cellularity or higher tumor infiltration of the bone marrow
Lower platelet count
Lower peripheral blood stem cell count

collected during apheresis [37]. Patients with low peripheral blood CD34-positive cell counts can then undergo salvage mobilization techniques and hopefully reduce the rate of failure. Retrospective analysis of patients with Hodgkin or non-Hodgkin lymphoma and prior mobilization with G-CSF alone showed that ideal peripheral blood cell counts of less than $6/\mu L$ on day 4 or 5 was predictive of failure to collect at least 2×10^6 cells/kg, while a cell count less than $15/\mu L$ predicted failure to collect at least 4×10^6 cells/kg. This supports creating a peripheral blood CD34-positive cell count cut-off based on collection targets [47]. Both the preemptive and risk-adapted strategies have been shown to result in failure rates less than 10% in many studies [32,48].

Currently, many centers use algorithms that take into account both the pre-apheresis peripheral blood CD34-positive cell counts and other influential factors, such as number of prior treatment lines, in order to determine who should receive plerixafor prior to apheresis. The European Society for Blood and Marrow Transplantation (EBMT) issued recommendations in their 2014 position statement that call for the use of preemptive plerixafor if peripheral blood CD34-positive cell counts are below $10/\mu L$ (Figure 8.2). The EBMT recommend considering the patient's treatment history and predicted future transplant course to determine if plerixafor is appropriate for those that fall into the "gray zone" of 10–20 cells/μL. No plerixafor is needed for those patients with greater than 20 cells/μL prior to apheresis. The American Society for Blood and Marrow Transplantation also issued 2014 guidelines in which the use of preemptive plerixafor is supported and it is recommended that each institution develop an algorithim for determining poor mobilizers. The Gruppo Italiano Trapianto di Midollo Osseo working group proposed a definition of poor mobilizers in order to guide future trials and clinical practice, which they defined as circulating CD34-positive cell peak less than $20/\mu L$ up to 6 days after mobilization with G-CSF or up to 20 days after chemotherapy plus G-CSF, or yielding less than 2.0×10^6 CD34-positive cells per kilogram in up to three apheresis sessions. Patients were defined as predicted poor mobilizers if they failed a previous collection attempt, previously received extensive radiotherapy, or received full courses of therapy affecting stem cell mobilization, and they met two of the following criteria: advanced disease, refractory disease, extensive bone marrow involvement, cellularity less than 30% at the time of

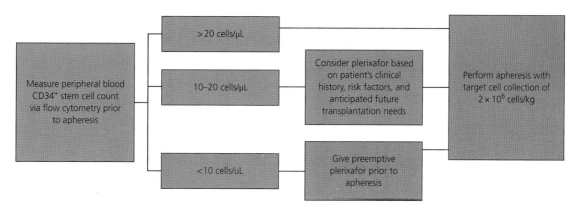

Figure 8.2 EBMT position statement algorithm for determining the use of preemptive plerixafor prior to apheresis for the rescue of poor mobilization. From Mohty *et al.* [7]. Reproduced with permission of Nature Publishing Group.

mobilization, or age 65 years and above. This definition has been supported retrospectively but has yet to undergo prospective validation [49,50].

In the event of initial failure, it is recommended to give patients a break of 2–4 weeks prior to attempting a remobilization strategy. Steady-state mobilization with G-CSF alone is not considered adequate for remobilization and is associated with a high repeat failure rate. Previously, chemomobilization was recommended as the initial remobilization strategy in patients who had failed prior G-CSF alone, but failure rates remain high [28,51]. Bone marrow harvest has also been a customary strategy for remobilization harvest, but is no longer typically performed due to increased costs, patient discomfort, increased risk of tumor contamination, and poor success rates in poor mobilizers. Currently, the recommended strategy for remobilization is G-CSF plus plerixafor, which has shown failure rates less than 30% in the majority of studies [28,52–54]. This strategy appears to be adequate even in patients who previously failed salvage therapy containing plerixafor [55]. The addition of plerixafor to chemotherapy increases success rates but has not been studied sufficiently to be recommended as a remobilization strategy and remains unpredictable.

Special populations

Obese

It has been suggested that the efficacy of stem cell mobilization is affected by the physiology and pharmacokinetics of a higher body mass index (BMI). Evidence from both autologous and allogeneic transplantation has shown that obese patients are likely to respond more to mobilization, possibly due to higher doses of chemotherapy or G-CSF, or due to some intrinsic physiologic mechanism. Unlike patients with normal BMI, obese patients do show a significant difference in efficacy with once-daily versus split dosing of G-CSF. Improved cell collection is seen after treatment with once-daily dosing compared to split dosing, likely due to differences in the pharmacokinetics of these patients [56]. In addition, plerixafor likely has impaired efficacy in obese patients due to a possible proinflammatory state that increases SDF-1. It has been shown that obese patients usually require an additional apheresis session and increased doses of plerixafor for mobilization, but the ability to collect stem cells is not impaired [57]. It is unclear whether obese patients should have cells collected with their actual or ideal body weight in mind as a goal. Thus far, studies have shown improved efficacy with increasing cell dose, but no difference between using ideal or actual body weight. Additional cost savings are likely with dosing by ideal body weight, but this has not yet become standard clinical practice [58].

Diabetes mellitus, a frequent complication of obesity, has also been shown to affect stem cell mobilization. It is suspected that the bone marrow is affected by microangiopathic injury in a similar manner as other microvascular complications of the disease. Through complex mechanisms, the presence of diabetes has been shown to downregulate proteases responsible for G-CSF stimulated mobilization. However, the ability to respond to plerixafor appears to remain intact, suggesting that this may be a better mobilization choice for those patients likely to be suffering from complications of type 1 or type 2 diabetes [59].

Children

Pediatric patients are generally mobilized in a manner similar to adults. G-CSF, usually in conjunction with disease-specific chemotherapy, is the recommended choice for initial mobilization, at a dose of 10 µg/kg daily for 1–5 days, with leukapheresis performed on the fifth day. As with adults, studies of higher growth factor dosing have shown slightly more efficacy but increased toxicity profiles [60]. Pegfilgrastim has also been recently studied in the pediatric population, showing early CD34-positive cell peaks and higher yields, even in those patients with heavy prior chemotherapy exposure [61]. It is not yet recommended for mobilization in pediatric patients, but Phase II and III studies support its use with similar efficacy to filgrastim, without any additional toxicities and the possible benefit of reduction in neutropenia and febrile neutropenia episodes [62,63]. The minimum goal dose of stem cells for sufficient engraftment is 2×10^6 cells/kg, as in adults. In heavily pretreated pediatric patients, mobilization with chemotherapy plus G-CSF may be unsuccessful. Strategies for poor mobilization include remobilization attempts and dose escalation of G-CSF. Plerixafor has been shown to be successful in pediatric patients who are difficult to mobilize in some case series, but is not yet routinely used [64,65].

Complications

The administration of growth factor or plerixafor for mobilization and the process of collection via apheresis both come with particular complications. G-CSF is relatively benign, with the most common side effect being musculoskeletal pain. More significant adverse effects, such as transient hypotension, worsening thrombocytopenia, elevated liver enzymes and uric acid, and splenomegaly, are infrequent and rarely cause discontinuation of the drug. Plerixafor does not commonly carry the side effect of bone pain, as its mechanism of action does not result from bone marrow hyperplasia. The most common side effects associated with the use of plerixafor include gastrointestinal upset and injection-site erythema. Similar to G-CSF, transient hypotension and worsening thrombocytopenia have also been reported [66,67]. As indicated previously, dose adjustment is recommended for those patients with renal failure as this is the primary route of excretion for the drug. Lower doses have been used successfully to mobilize patients with end-stage renal disease without an increase in toxicity [25,68]. Both drugs have similar side-effect profiles in elderly transplant patients, compared to those less than 60 years of age [66].

The majority of complications during mobilization are associated with the process of apheresis, which usually requires repetitive access of a central venous catheter. With this comes an inherent risk of infection, increased by the use of chemotherapy for mobilization. Hematologic complications resulting from apheresis include anemia and thrombocytopenia, sometimes requiring transfusion support. Thrombocytopenia combined with the need for anticoagulants in the extracorporeal circuit of the apheresis machine increases bleeding risk, especially in those patients with lower platelet counts before apheresis [69]. Patients may complain of muscle cramping or paresthesias associated with citrate and resulting hypocalcemia, which resolves with calcium administration. This reaction is more common in patients with underlying renal or liver dysfunction due to altered calcium homeostasis [70]. Hypocalcemia can be treated by slowing the rate of apheresis, increasing the blood to citrate ratio, and administering calcium replacement. Hypomagnesemia, hypokalemia, or metabolic alkalosis may also occur and can be treated with a slower rate and electrolyte replacement. Large shifts in volume during apheresis can result in hypovolemia and possible life-threating cardiac arrhythmias, so close attention should be paid to the patient's volume state, especially in those with underlying cardiac disease.

Future considerations

There are accumulating data indicating that early lymphocyte recovery is associated with outcomes of hematologic malignancies after autologous hematopoietic stem cell transplantation (HSCT). Early lymphocyte recovery, its composition and impact on outcome depends on a variety of factors; however, very limited information is available on the pattern of early lymphocyte recovery after different mobilization strategies (G-CSF vs. G-CSF plus high-dose chemotherapy vs. G-CSF plus plerixafor). Similarly, the findings from a recent study demonstrate that G-CSF plus plerixafor mobilization can affect the numbers and properties of immune competent cell subsets contained in the graft.

We have recently shown that grafts mobilized with G-CSF plus plerixafor exhibited major differences in graft composition and favorable post-transplant outcome compared with grafts mobilized with G-CSF alone or G-CSF plus high-dose chemotherapy after autologous HSCT. G-CSF plus plerixafor mobilization accelerates lymphocyte engraftment, even in heavily pretreated groups, compared to G-CSF alone or G-CSF plus high-dose chemotherapy. Recent data have also shown that plerixafor reduces pro-inflammatory cytokine/chemokine production and significantly improves animal survival when administered from day +2 post HSCT and this property might also reduce the risk of post-transplant mucositis; however, this remains to be studied in clinical trials.

Stem cell mobilization for autologous HSCT is a developing and progressing area of transplant medicine. Clinical practice varies widely across institutions depending on resource availability, patient population, and physician comfort. This chapter discusses current recommendations and most common practices for stem cell mobilization, pointing toward multiple areas for additional research and the evolving use of different mobilization agents.

References

1 Richman CM, Weiner RS, Yankee RA. Increase in circulating stem cells following chemotherapy in man. *Blood* 1976;**47**:1031–9.

2 Pusic I, DiPersio JF. The use of growth factors in hematopoietic stem cell transplantation. *Curr Pharm Des* 2008;**14**:1950–61.

3 Liu F, Poursine Laurent J, Link DC. Expression of the G-CSF receptor on hematopoietic progenitor cells is not required for their mobilization by G-CSF. *Blood* 2000;**95**:3025–31.

4 Petit I, Szyper-Kravitz M, Nagler A *et al.* G-CSF induces stem cell mobilization by decreasing bone marrow SDF-1 and up-regulating CXCR4. *Nat Immunol* 2002;**3**:687–94.

5 Devine SM, Flomenberg N, Vesole DH *et al.* Rapid mobilization of CD34+ cells following administration of the CXCR4 antagonist AMD3100 to patients with multiple myeloma and non-Hodgkin's lymphoma. *J Clin Oncol* 2004;**22**:1095–102.

6 Giralt S, Costa L, Schriber J *et al.* Optimizing autologous stem cell mobilization strategies to improve patient outcomes: consensus guidelines and recommendations. *Biol Blood Marrow Transplant* 2014;**20**:295–308.

7 Mohty M, Hubel K, Kroger N *et al.* Autologous haematopoietic stem cell mobilisation in multiple myeloma and lymphoma patients: a position statement from the European Group for Blood and Marrow Transplantation. *Bone Marrow Transplant* 2014;**49**:865–72.

8 Duong HK, Savani BN, Copelan E *et al.* Peripheral blood progenitor cell mobilization for autologous and allogeneic hematopoietic cell transplantation: guidelines from the American Society for Blood and Marrow Transplantation. *Biol Blood Marrow Transplant* 2014;**20**:1262–73.

9 Weaver CH, Schulman KA, Buckner CD. Mobilization of peripheral blood stem cells following myelosuppressive chemotherapy: a randomized comparison of filgrastim, sargramostim, or sequential sargramostim and filgrastim. *Bone Marrow Transplant* 2001;**27**(Suppl 2):S23–9.

10 Fischmeister G, Kurz M, Haas OA *et al.* G-CSF versus GM-CSF for stimulation of peripheral blood progenitor cells (PBPC) and leukocytes in healthy volunteers: comparison of efficacy and tolerability. *Ann Hematol* 1999;**78**:117–23.

11 Kim SN, Moon JH, Kim JG *et al.* Mobilization effects of G-CSF, GM-CSF, and darbepoetin-alpha for allogeneic peripheral blood stem cell transplantation. *J Clin Apher* 2009;**24**:173–9.

12 Perez-Lopez O, Martin-Sanchez J, Parody-Porras R *et al.* Lenograstim compared to filgrastim for the mobilization of hematopoietic stem cells in healthy donors. *Transfusion* 2013;**53**:3240–2.

13 Herbert KE, Gambell P, Link EK *et al.* Pegfilgrastim compared with filgrastim for cytokine-alone mobilization of autologous haematopoietic stem and progenitor cells. *Bone Marrow Transplant* 2013;**48**:351–6.

14 Costa LJ, Kramer C, Hogan KR *et al.* Pegfilgrastim- versus filgrastim-based autologous hematopoietic stem cell mobilization in the setting of preemptive use of plerixafor: efficacy and cost analysis. *Transfusion* 2012;**52**:2375–81.

15 Ria R, Reale A, Melaccio A, Racanelli V, Dammacco F, Vacca A. Filgrastim, lenograstim and pegfilgrastim in the mobilization of peripheral blood progenitor cells in patients with lymphoproliferative malignancies. *Clin Exp Med* 2014. doi: 10.1007/s10238-014-0282-9.

16 Kroger N, Renges H, Sonnenberg S *et al.* Stem cell mobilisation with 16 µg/kg vs 10 µg/kg of G-CSF for allogeneic transplantation in healthy donors. *Bone Marrow Transplant* 2002;**29**:727–30.

17 Komeno Y, Kanda Y, Hamaki T *et al.* A randomized controlled trial to compare once- versus twice-daily filgrastim for mobilization of peripheral blood stem cells from healthy donors. *Biol Blood Marrow Transplant* 2006;**12**:408–13.

18 Kroger N, Renges H, Kruger W *et al.* A randomized comparison of once versus twice daily recombinant human granulocyte colony-stimulating factor (filgrastim) for stem cell mobilization in healthy donors for allogeneic transplantation. *Br J Haematol* 2000;**111**:761–5.

19 Kim JE, Yoo C, Kim S *et al.* Optimal timing of G-CSF administration for effective autologous stem cell collection. *Bone Marrow Transplant* 2011;**46**:806–12.

20 Sung AD, Grima DT, Bernard LM *et al.* Outcomes and costs of autologous stem cell mobilization with chemotherapy plus G-CSF vs G-CSF alone. *Bone Marrow Transplant* 2013;**48**:1444–9.

21 Pavone V, Gaudio F, Guarini A *et al.* Mobilization of peripheral blood stem cells with high-dose cyclophosphamide or the

DHAP regimen plus G-CSF in non-Hodgkin's lymphoma. *Bone Marrow Transplant* 2002;**29**:285–90.

22 Hyun SY, Cheong JW, Kim SJ et al. High-dose etoposide plus granulocyte colony-stimulating factor as an effective chemomobilization regimen for autologous stem cell transplantation in patients with non-Hodgkin lymphoma previously treated with CHOP-based chemotherapy: a study from the Consortium for Improving Survival of Lymphoma. *Biol Blood Marrow Transplant* 2014;**20**:73–9.

23 Sizemore C, Laporte J, Holland HK et al. A comparison of toxicity and mobilization efficacy following two difference doses of cyclophosphamide for mobilization of hematopoietic stem cells in non-Hodgkin's lymphoma patients. *Biol Blood Marrow Transplant* 2010;**16**(Suppl 2):S206.

24 Mahindra A, Bolwell BJ, Rybicki L et al. Etoposide plus G-CSF priming compared with G-CSF alone in patients with lymphoma improves mobilization without an increased risk of secondary myelodysplasia and leukemia. *Bone Marrow Transplant* 2012;**47**:231–5.

25 MacFarland R, Hard ML, Scarborough R et al. A pharmacokinetic study of plerixafor in subjects with varying degrees of renal impairment. *Biol Blood Marrow Transplant* 2010;**16**:95–101.

26 Flomenberg N, Devine SM, Dipersio JF et al. The use of AMD3100 plus G-CSF for autologous hematopoietic progenitor cell mobilization is superior to G-CSF alone. *Blood* 2005;**106**:1867–74.

27 DiPersio JF, Micallef IN, Stiff P.I et al. Phase III prospective randomized double-blind placebo-controlled trial of plerixafor plus granulocyte colony-stimulating factor compared with placebo plus granulocyte colony-stimulating factor for autologous stem-cell mobilization and transplantation for patients with non-Hodgkin's lymphoma. *J Clin Oncol* 2009;**27**:4767–73.

28 Calandra G, McCarty J, McGuirk J et al. AMD3100 plus G-CSF can successfully mobilize CD34+ cells from non-Hodgkin's lymphoma, Hodgkin's disease and multiple myeloma patients previously failing mobilization with chemotherapy and/or cytokine treatment: compassionate use data. *Bone Marrow Transplant* 2008;**41**:331–8.

29 Micallef IN, Sinha S, Gastineau DA et al. Cost-effectiveness analysis of a risk-adapted algorithm of plerixafor use for autologous peripheral blood stem cell mobilization. *Biol Blood Marrow Transplant* 2013;**19**:87–93.

30 Abhyankar S, DeJarnette S, Aljitawi O et al. A risk-based approach to optimize autologous hematopoietic stem cell (HSC) collection with the use of plerixafor. *Bone Marrow Transplant* 2012;**47**:483–7.

31 Vishnu P, Roy V, Paulsen A et al. Efficacy and cost–benefit analysis of risk-adaptive use of plerixafor for autologous hematopoietic progenitor cell mobilization. *Transfusion* 2012;**52**:55–62.

32 Costa LJ, Alexander ET, Hogan KR et al. Development and validation of a decision-making algorithm to guide the use of plerixafor for autologous hematopoietic stem cell mobilization. *Bone Marrow Transplant* 2011;**46**:64–9.

33 Dugan MJ, Maziarz RT, Bensinger WI et al. Safety and preliminary efficacy of plerixafor (Mozobil) in combination with chemotherapy and G-CSF: an open-label, multicenter, exploratory trial in patients with multiple myeloma and non-Hodgkin's lymphoma undergoing stem cell mobilization. *Bone Marrow Transplant* 2010;**45**:39–47.

34 Bensinger W, Appelbaum F, Rowley S et al. Factors that influence collection and engraftment of autologous peripheral-blood stem cells. *J Clin Oncol* 1995;**13**:2547–55.

35 Bolwell BJ, Pohlman B, Rybicki L et al. Patients mobilizing large numbers of CD34+ cells ("super mobilizers") have improved survival in autologous stem cell transplantation for lymphoid malignancies. *Bone Marrow Transplant* 2007;**40**:437–41.

36 Yoon DH, Sohn BS, Jang G et al. Higher infused CD34+ hematopoietic stem cell dose correlates with earlier lymphocyte recovery and better clinical outcome after autologous stem cell transplantation in non-Hodgkin's lymphoma. *Transfusion* 2009;**49**:1890–900.

37 Elliott C, Samson DM, Armitage S et al. When to harvest peripheral-blood stem cells after mobilization therapy: prediction of CD34-positive cell yield by preceding day CD34-positive concentration in peripheral blood. *J Clin Oncol* 1996;**14**:970–3.

38 Abrahamsen JF, Stamnesfet S, Liseth K et al. Large-volume leukapheresis yields more viable CD34+ cells and colony-forming units than normal-volume leukapheresis, especially in patients who mobilize low numbers of CD34+ cells. *Transfusion* 2005;**45**:248–53.

39 Donmez A, Tombuloglu M, Gungor A et al. Clinical side effects during peripheral blood progenitor cell infusion. *Transfus Apher Sci* 2007;**36**:95–101.

40 Humpe A, Riggert J, Munzel U et al. A prospective, randomized, sequential crossover trial of large-volume versus normal-volume leukapheresis procedures: effects on serum electrolytes, platelet counts, and other coagulation measures. *Transfusion* 2000;**40**:368–74.

41 Gertz MA, Wolf RC, Micallef IN et al. Clinical impact and resource utilization after stem cell mobilization failure in patients with multiple myeloma and lymphoma. *Bone Marrow Transplant* 2010;**45**:1396–403.

42 Hosing C, Saliba RM, Ahlawat S et al. Poor hematopoietic stem cell mobilizers: a single institution study of incidence and risk factors in patients with recurrent or relapsed lymphoma. *Am J Hematol* 2009;**84**:335–7.

43 Wuchter P, Ran D, Bruckner T et al. Poor mobilization of hematopoietic stem cells: definitions, incidence, risk factors, and impact on outcome of autologous transplantation. *Biol Blood Marrow Transplant* 2010;**16**:490–9.

44 Sugrue MW, Williams K, Pollock BH et al. Characterization and outcome of "hard to mobilize" lymphoma patients undergoing autologous stem cell transplantation. *Leukemia Lymphoma* 2000;**39**:509–19.

45 Han X, Ma L, Zhao L et al. Predictive factors for inadequate stem cell mobilization in Chinese patients with NHL and

HL: 14-year experience of a single-center study. *J Clin Apher* 2012;**27**:64–74.

46 Perseghin P, Terruzzi E, Dassi M *et al.* Management of poor peripheral blood stem cell mobilization: incidence, predictive factors, alternative strategies and outcome. A retrospective analysis on 2177 patients from three major Italian institutions. *Transfus Apher Sci* 2009;**41**:33–7.

47 Sinha S, Gastineau D, Micallef I *et al.* Predicting PBSC harvest failure using circulating CD34 levels: developing target-based cutoff points for early intervention. *Bone Marrow Transplant* 2011;**46**:943–9.

48 Chen AI, Bains T, Murray S *et al.* Clinical experience with a simple algorithm for plerixafor utilization in autologous stem cell mobilization. *Bone Marrow Transplant* 2012;**47**:1526–9.

49 Olivieri A, Marchetti M, Lemoli R *et al.* Proposed definition of "poor mobilizer" in lymphoma and multiple myeloma: an analytic hierarchy process by ad hoc working group Gruppo Italiano Trapianto di Midollo Osseo. *Bone Marrow Transplant* 2012;**47**:342–51.

50 Piccirillo N, Vacca M, Lanti A *et al.* Poor mobilizer: a retrospective study on proven and predicted incidence according to GITMO criteria. *Transfus Apher Sci* 2012;**47**:217–21.

51 Pusic I, Jiang SY, Landua S *et al.* Impact of mobilization and remobilization strategies on achieving sufficient stem cell yields for autologous transplantation. *Biol Blood Marrow Transplant* 2008;**14**:1045–56.

52 Duarte RF, Shaw BE, Marin P *et al.* Plerixafor plus granulocyte CSF can mobilize hematopoietic stem cells from multiple myeloma and lymphoma patients failing previous mobilization attempts: EU compassionate use data. *Bone Marrow Transplant* 2011;**46**:52–8.

53 Perkins JB, Shapiro JF, Bookout RN *et al.* Retrospective comparison of filgrastim plus plerixafor to other regimens for remobilization after primary mobilization failure: clinical and economic outcomes. *Am J Hematol* 2012;**87**:673–7.

54 Micallef IN, Stiff PJ, DiPersio JF *et al.* Successful stem cell remobilization using plerixafor (Mozobil) plus granulocyte colony-stimulating factor in patients with non-Hodgkin lymphoma: results from the plerixafor NHL phase 3 study rescue protocol. *Biol Blood Marrow Transplant* 2009;**15**:1578–86.

55 Yuan S, Nademanee A, Krishnan A *et al.* Second time a charm? Remobilization of peripheral blood stem cells with plerixafor in patients who previously mobilized poorly despite using plerixafor as a salvage agent. *Transfusion* 2013;**53**:3244–50.

56 Cetin T, Arpaci F, Ozet A *et al.* Stem cell mobilization by G-CSF in solid and hematological malignancies: single daily dose is better than split dose in obese patients. *J Clin Apher* 2003;**18**:120–4.

57 Basak GW, Wiktor-Jedrzejczak W, Apperley JF *et al.* Higher BMI is not a barrier to stem cell mobilization with standard doses of plerixafor and G-CSF. *Bone Marrow Transplant* 2012;**47**:1003–5.

58 Waples JM, Moreb JS, Sugrue M *et al.* Comparison of autologous peripheral blood stem cell dosing by ideal vs actual body weight. *Bone Marrow Transplant* 1999;**23**:867–73.

59 Fadini GP, Albiero M, Vigili de Kreutzenberg S *et al.* Diabetes impairs stem cell and proangiogenic cell mobilization in humans. *Diabetes Care* 2013;**36**:943–9.

60 Sevilla J, Gonzalez-Vicent M, Madero L *et al.* Granulocyte colony-stimulating factor alone at 12 µg/kg twice a day for 4 days for peripheral blood progenitor cell priming in pediatric patients. *Bone Marrow Transplant* 2002;**30**:417–20.

61 Fritsch P, Schwinger W, Schwantzer G *et al.* Peripheral blood stem cell mobilization with pegfilgrastim compared to filgrastim in children and young adults with malignancies. *Pediatr Blood Cancer* 2010;**54**:134–7.

62 Cesaro S, Zanazzo AG, Frenos S *et al.* A Phase II study on the safety and efficacy of a single dose of pegfilgrastim for mobilization and transplantation of autologous hematopoietic stem cells in pediatric oncohematology patients. *Transfusion* 2011;**51**:2480–7.

63 Cesaro S, Nesi F, Tridello G *et al.* A randomized, non-inferiority study comparing efficacy and safety of a single dose of pegfilgrastim versus daily filgrastim in pediatric patients after autologous peripheral blood stem cell transplant. *PLOS ONE* 2013;**8**:e53252.

64 Emir S, Demir HA, Aksu T *et al.* Use of plerixafor for peripheral blood stem cell mobilization failure in children. *Transfus Apher Sci* 2014;**50**:214–18.

65 Vettenranta K, Mottonen M, Riikonen P. The use of plerixafor in harvesting autologous stem cells in the pediatric setting. *Pediatr Blood Cancer* 2012;**59**:197–8.

66 Micallef IN, Stiff PJ, Stadtmauer EA *et al.* Safety and efficacy of upfront plerixafor + G-CSF versus placebo + G-CSF for mobilization of CD34(+) hematopoietic progenitor cells in patients ≥60 and <60 years of age with non-Hodgkin's lymphoma or multiple myeloma. *Am J Hematol* 2013;**88**:1017–23.

67 Shaughnessy P, Uberti J, Devine S *et al.* Plerixafor and G-CSF for autologous stem cell mobilization in patients with NHL, Hodgkin's lymphoma and multiple myeloma: results from the expanded access program. *Bone Marrow Transplant* 2013;**48**:777–81.

68 Douglas KW, Parker AN, Hayden PJ *et al.* Plerixafor for PBSC mobilisation in myeloma patients with advanced renal failure: safety and efficacy data in a series of 21 patients from Europe and the USA. *Bone Marrow Transplant* 2012;**47**:18–23.

69 Sarkodee-Adoo C, Taran I, Guo C *et al.* Influence of preapheresis clinical factors on the efficiency of CD34+ cell collection by large-volume apheresis. *Bone Marrow Transplant* 2003;**31**:851–5.

70 Strauss RG. Mechanisms of adverse effects during hemapheresis. *J Clin Apher* 1996;**11**:160–4.

Allogeneic hematopoietic stem cell transplantation for lymphoma: stem cell source, donor, and HLA matching

Michael Green and Mitchell Horwitz

Historical perspective

For many years, hematopoietic stem cell transplantation (HSCT) has been a part of the treatment armament for a variety of both solid tumors and hematologic malignant conditions. High-dose chemotherapy followed by autologous HSCT has been used to treat solid tumors such as breast and testicular cancer. Both autologous and allogeneic HSCT is used to treat hematologic malignancies such as acute leukemia and lymphoma. While relatively rare in current practice for the management of solid tumors, HSCT continues to have utility in the management of high-risk hematologic malignancies. For lymphoma specifically, the autologous HSCT approach has historically been favored over allogeneic HSCT as the most commonly utilized stem cell transplant technique. As Jantunen and Sureda [1] report in their review "The evolving role of stem cell transplants in lymphomas," approximately 6000 autologous transplants are undertaken annually in Europe for lymphomas [1]. In the United States, lymphoma trails only multiple myeloma as the most common indication for autologous HSCT. According to the Center for International Blood and Marrow Transplant Research (CIBMTR), approximately 3000 autologous transplants were performed in the United States in 2011 for the treatment of non-Hodgkin lymphoma.

The role for allogeneic (hematopoietic stem cells derived from a healthy donor) transplantation in the treatment of lymphoma is less well established. The refinement of allogeneic transplantation techniques has led to an increased utilization of this therapy for patients with high-risk, relapsed or refractory lymphoma. In the past decade, the number of autologous transplants has remained relatively stable. In contrast, the number of allogeneic transplants over the same period has increased dramatically. The CIBMTR database details that from 1998 to 2004, only 20% of all transplants for major hematologic malignancies performed in adults over 50 years of age were allogeneic. This percentage increased to nearly 40% for the period from 2005 to 2011 [2].

Rationale for allogeneic transplantation

Autologous HSCT offers a potentially curative option for patients with relapsed/refractory and high-risk lymphomas. For autologous HSCT, the main therapeutic effect is derived from the chemotherapeutic agents, sometimes accompanied by radiation. In contrast, when using allogeneic transplantation, the donor-derived immune system that is reconstituted in the recipient leads to immune activation against residual tumor cells. This process is often referred to as the graft-versus-tumor response. While this graft-versus-tumor response is beneficial, a parallel but deleterious process in recipients of allogeneic transplants is termed graft-versus-host disease (GVHD), which is characterized by immune activation directed against normal recipient tissue. In this condition, the transplanted cells identify

Clinical Guide to Transplantation in Lymphoma, First Edition. Edited by Bipin N. Savani and Mohamad Mohty.

immune epitopes present in the recipient as foreign and mount an immune response (mainly T-cell mediated) against these antigens. The graft-versus-tumor theory is supported by evidence that patients with GVHD have a lower incidence of relapse. In a recent retrospective study of over 2000 patients with a variety of hematologic malignancies that underwent HSCT, patients who developed either acute or chronic GVHD had a reduced risk of late relapse when compared to patients who did not develop GVHD [3]. Donor T cells, natural killer (NK) cells, and possibly B cells are implicated in this reaction. In addition, it has also been demonstrated that infusion of additional donor lymphocytes following transplantation has the potential to augment the graft-versus-tumor response in leukemia patients, sometimes without inducing GVHD [4].

The proper role of allogeneic HSCT for treatment of lymphoma continues to be defined. For the purpose of this chapter, we will discuss lymphoma broadly. We will explore stem cell sources and the influence of donor and human leukocyte antigen (HLA) matching on a variety of outcome measures including but not limited to hematologic recovery, GVHD, and survival after allogeneic HSCT. However, the impact of allogeneic transplant may differ for the varying subtypes of lymphoma and subsequent chapters in this book cover disease-specific outcomes.

Stem cell source

Bone marrow

Until the early 1990s, bone marrow harvested directly from the posterior iliac crests of a donor was the only widely available source for a stem cell graft. This is typically performed either under general anesthesia or with a regional block paired with conscious sedation. Using this technique, approximately 700–1500 mL of aspirate must be extracted in order to obtain a sufficient number of stem cells to ensure engraftment in an adult recipient.

Mobilized peripheral blood

With the advent of stem cell mobilization techniques, stem cell collection from the peripheral blood became feasible via apheresis. Peripheral blood stem cell collection has replaced bone marrow harvests as the preferred stem cell source for autologous transplantation. Several techniques are available to mobilize stem and progenitor cells into the peripheral blood. The standard method is to treat the donor with granulocyte colony-stimulating factor (G-CSF) at a dose of 10–15 µg/kg daily, with peak mobilization occurring on day 5 of treatment. A large-volume leukapheresis procedure is then performed using peripheral or central venous catheters. For autologous stem cell collection, G-CSF is often used following a cycle of cytotoxic chemotherapy, resulting in peripheral blood stem and progenitor cell mobilization.

Umbilical cord blood

High concentrations of hematopoietic stem and progenitor cells contained within umbilical cord blood collected at the time of delivery has resulted in a third source of stem cells for transplantation. Allogeneic umbilical cord blood transplantation was first performed in 1988, confirming the presence of stem cells capable of long-term hematopoiesis. Since then, use of these cells for transplantation has steadily increased, first in the pediatric population and now in adults [5]. These cells are now being processed and cryopreserved in public and private cord blood banks throughout the world.

Stem cells collected from bone marrow, peripheral blood, or umbilical cord blood have each demonstrated the potential to facilitate reliable engraftment following transplantation. However, each graft source is associated with its own challenges. In general, as discussed in later sections, HLA-matched peripheral blood or bone marrow grafts are the first choice for adult recipients of allogeneic HSCT.

Allogeneic bone marrow versus mobilized peripheral blood transplantation

When comparing outcomes from transplants using bone marrow or peripheral blood stem cells as the source, much of the available data involves patients with acute myeloid leukemia, chronic myelogenous leukemia, aplastic anemia, and myelodysplastic syndromes. Robust lymphoma-specific data are not yet available. This section explores differences in outcome measures that are attributable to stem cell source, including likelihood of engraftment, disease relapse, speed of hematologic recovery, and incidence of GVHD.

The largest trial comparing bone marrow and peripheral blood stem cell transplantation is a retrospective analysis from the European Bone Marrow

Transplant registry comparing 536 adult patients (defined as 20 years of age or older) who underwent HLA-identical allogeneic HSCT using bone marrow with 288 adult patients who underwent HLA-identical sibling transplants using peripheral blood stem cells. Patients were transplanted for acute leukemia in first or second remission or chronic myelogenous leukemia in chronic or accelerated phase, after undergoing myeloablative conditioning (using total body irradiation, cyclophosphamide, busulfan, etc.). Recipients of peripheral blood stem cell transplantation had more rapid recovery of neutrophils (median 14 days vs. 19 days for bone marrow) and platelets (median 18 days vs. 25 days for bone marrow recipients). There was no statistically significant difference in acute GVHD. However, chronic GVHD was more prevalent after peripheral blood stem cell transplantation than after bone marrow stem cell transplantation. There was no difference in the incidence of relapse. Leukemia-free survival and overall survival had mixed results and depended on the disease type and the stage of disease [6]. This study compared outcomes for a large group of transplant recipients and it is generally accepted to also apply to patients with lymphoma.

These findings were validated in a prospective fashion by a randomized study comparing 172 patients (aged 12–55 years) with a variety of hematologic malignancies (including Hodgkin and non-Hodgkin lymphoma) who underwent HLA-identical allogeneic HSCT with either peripheral blood or bone marrow-derived stem cells following myeloablative conditioning. This study again demonstrated faster neutrophil and platelet count recovery in those patients who received peripheral blood HSCT compared to those who received bone marrow HSCT. However, unlike the previous study, there was no significant difference in the cumulative incidence of acute and chronic GVHD (for acute GVHD, 64% for peripheral blood HSCT vs. 57% for bone marrow HSCT, $P = 0.35$; for chronic GVHD, 15% for peripheral blood HSCT vs. 12% for bone marrow HSCT, $P = 0.57$). Transplant-related mortality for recipients of peripheral blood stem cells and bone marrow stem cells was 21% and 30% ($P = 0.24$), respectively. Disease-free survival at 2 years was significantly better in the group receiving peripheral blood stem cells (65%) compared to the recipients of bone marrow stem cells (45%). Relapse at 2 years in recipients of peripheral blood stem cells and recipients of bone marrow stem cells was 14%

and 25% ($P = 0.04$), respectively. There was a trend toward better survival in the recipients of peripheral blood stem cells (66% vs. 54%, $P = 0.06$) [7].

Despite a comparable degree of matching of major histocompatibility antigens, the degree of minor histocompatibility antigen mismatch is greater in recipients of unrelated donor compared to related donor grafts. GVHD is driven by donor-derived lymphocytes, and peripheral blood HSCT recipients receive more passively transferred donor-derived lymphocytes than bone marrow HSCT recipients. Thus, there is a theoretical potential for an increased risk of GVHD among peripheral blood HSCT recipients. In a prospective multicenter randomized study, 551 patients with a variety of hematologic malignancies (acute myeloid leukemia, chronic myeloid leukemia, chronic myelomonocytic leukemia, myelodysplasia, or myelofibrosis) were assigned to undergo either matched unrelated peripheral HSCT or matched unrelated bone marrow HSCT [8]. There was no significant difference in disease-free or overall survival between the two groups. The median time to neutrophil engraftment was 5 days shorter and platelet engraftment was 7 days shorter in the peripheral stem cell group. There was an increased incidence of graft failure in the bone marrow group of 6% compared with only 2% in the peripheral blood stem cell group. The rate of acute GVHD was similar within the two groups, although the incidence of chronic GVHD was 53% in the peripheral blood stem cell group and 41% in the bone marrow stem cell group, respectively (P = ~0.01).

In conclusion, with regard to matched allogeneic transplantation, these data suggest that peripheral blood stem cell transplantation leads to more rapid blood count recovery with increased risk of chronic GVHD. The effect of graft source on overall survival is less clear, but appears to be negligible. Extensive outcomes data for lymphoma are not yet available but are likely to be in line with these findings.

HLA matching

Selecting a donor is an important decision that affects the success of HSCT. Human leukocyte antigens are found on the surface of cells and allow an individual's immune system to distinguish self from non-self. Although this definition is overly simplified, the immune system's ability to recognize "self" is paramount to the understanding of allogeneic cellular therapy and the importance of donor selection to allogeneic HSCT. HLA classes are subdivided into two large categories: class I (A, B, and C) and class II (which includes the clinically significant transplant-related alleles DRB1 and DQB1). The nomenclatures as well as the techniques for determining HLA type have evolved with the discovery of additional HLA alleles and improved methods of typing. Until the 1990s serologic typing using cell-based assays was the only method available for antigen matching [9]. Consequently, when interpreting early transplant data the method for HLA testing must be considered. What were once believed to be, and therefore described in the literature as, perfectly matched donors would now be considered mismatched at multiple loci when analyzed with high-resolution assays. Advances in technologies for detection of HLA epitopes using molecular (both low and high resolution) DNA-based methods have helped to enhance matching, resulting in improved outcomes for transplant recipients [10]. There are a multitude of choices with regard to allogeneic transplantation donors, including HLA identical (syngeneic) from an identical twin, HLA matched or mismatched from a relative or nonrelative, or umbilical cord blood (Table 9.1). The degree of HLA matching ranges from 12 of 12 (with matches in HLA-A, -B, -C, -DRB1, -DQB1, and -DP1), 10 of 10 (with pairs matched for HLA-A, -B, -C, -DRB1, and -DQB1), 9 of 10 (with a single allele or antigen mismatch with HLA-A, -B, -C, -DRB1, or -DQB1), 8 of 8 (with matches in HLA-A, -B, -C, and -DRB1), 7 of 8 (with a single allele or antigen mismatch with HLA-A, -B, -C, and -DRB1), and 6 of 6 (i.e., HLA-A, -B, and -DRB1 at the allele level). Although complex, this process is of

the utmost importance because the degree of matching is an integral factor in predicting survival.

Graft source, HLA matching and impact on transplant outcome

HLA-matched donor allogeneic stem cell transplantation

Once a patient has been identified as a candidate for allogeneic HSCT, the search for an HLA-identical donor should begin immediately. An HLA-identical healthy sibling is the ideal stem cell donor. Each full sibling has a 25% chance of being a match. For those patients who do not have an HLA-identical sibling, it is common practice to try to secure a suitable unrelated donor using national donor registries. The largest US-based donor registry is the National Marrow Donor Program (NMDP), which is a nonprofit organization founded in the 1980s that works to connect unrelated donors with potential hematopoietic transplant recipients. Each year, the NMDP facilitates more than 6000 transplant procedures using stem cells collected from mobilized peripheral blood, bone marrow, or umbilical cord blood.

While, by definition, HLA-matched unrelated donors are matched at the major histocompatibility complex antigens, these donors are more discordant at minor histocompatibility complex loci when compared to HLA-matched sibling donors. As a consequence, there is an increased risk of GVHD. This increased risk of GVHD led to speculation that recipients of HSCT from unrelated donors would also translate into a more potent graft-versus-tumor response. To explore this idea, Ringden *et al.* [11] retrospectively analyzed data of outcomes from 4099 adult patients with myeloid and lymphoid leukemia receiving myeloablative chemotherapy. HSCT

Table 9.1 Donor source and HLA-matching combinations.

	HLA-matched*	Single antigen mismatch*	Multiple antigen mismatch*	Haploidentical (one haplotype) mismatch
Related donor	✓	✓	✗	✓
Unrelated donor	✓	✓	✗	✗
Unrelated umbilical cord blood	✗	✗	✓†	✗

*HLA-A, B, C and DRB1 using high-resolution molecular typing assays.
†Typically four to six antigen matches using low-resolution typing assays for HLA-A and B, and high-resolution assays for HLA-DRB1.

was from either related or unrelated donors there were reported to the CIBMTR. While the incidence of acute GVHD was higher (52%) in those with unrelated donors compared to those with related donors (34%), this analysis failed to demonstrate any reduced risk for relapse in unrelated donor transplant recipients.

HLA donor matching considerations for lymphoma patients

Many patients with relapsed lymphoma of all subtypes are treated with high-dose chemotherapy and autologous stem cell rescue. Patients who again relapse after autologous transplantation may then be considered candidates for an allogeneic procedure. Because it has been demonstrated that the risk of undergoing a second course of myeloablative chemotherapy is poorly tolerated among all age groups, most lymphoma patients who are candidates for allogeneic HCT receive nonmyeloablative or reduced-intensity conditioning regimens [12]. Nonmyeloablative and reduced-intensity conditioning regimens are better tolerated, but have reduced antitumor efficacy. Thus, a potent graft-versus-tumor effect is critical to providing a curative outcome.

Ho *et al.* [13] set out to determine whether the increased minor HLA antigen disparities that characterize unrelated donor grafts translated into a reduced risk of relapse following allogeneic HSCT using reduced-intensity conditioning. The authors analyzed the outcomes of 433 matched related and matched unrelated donor HSCTs whose data was reported to the CIBMTR. Unrelated donors were generally younger and provided larger stem cell products. The incidence of acute and chronic GVHD and 2-year nonrelapse mortality and overall survival were similar among the two groups. At 2 years, there was a lower incidence of relapse and more favorable progression-free survival in the unrelated donor group. The analysis included patients with a variety of hematologic malignancies including non-Hodgkin lymphoma.

With regard to patients with lymphoma specifically, more robust studies must be performed before a standard can be established. In the era of high-resolution molecular HLA typing, matched unrelated donor and matched sibling transplants provide comparable outcomes. An increased graft-versus-tumor response may counterbalance any increase in GVHD experienced by matched unrelated donor recipients. Based on the

currently available data, both matched unrelated and matched related are acceptable donor sources for lymphoma patients who are candidates for allogeneic HSCT.

Mismatched unrelated donors

Many patients will not have an available matched donor. This is particularly a problem for non-white patients. While the chance of finding a matched unrelated donor for patients of European descent is greater than 50%, the chance of finding a matched donor for North American ethnic minorities is less than 33%. Prior to recent advances in using alternative donor sources, allogeneic HSCT was not an option for patients without an HLA-matched sibling or matched unrelated donor. Increased HLA disparity results in increased risk of GVHD, graft rejection, and delayed immune recovery. However, over the past 20 years, great progress has been made in improving outcomes for HSCT using mismatched related donors or mismatched unrelated umbilical cord blood. In 2014, nearly all candidates for allogeneic HSCT, regardless of the underlying diagnosis, will have a suitable stem cell donor.

Identical matching for patients undergoing allogeneic HSCT remains ideal. However, this may not always be possible. For some, the unrelated donor registry search may reveal donors with a single mismatch at a class 1 or class 2 allele. Although many studies have demonstrated that the outcomes following single-antigen mismatched unrelated HSCT is inferior to fully matched transplants, the risk–benefit considerations may still favor the use of such a donor [14,15]. Thus, a single-antigen mismatched related or unrelated donor transplant is a viable option for some patients. In general, an unrelated donor with more than one mismatched allele is avoided due to the excessive risk of GVHD.

Haploidentical

Nearly all patients have a haploidentical related donor. Mismatched siblings, parents or children are potential donor candidates. In order to prevent rapidly lethal, severe acute GVHD, recipients of haploidentical donor grafts must receive additional anti-T cell therapy. Two commonly used techniques are either *in vivo* or *ex vivo* T-cell depletion of the donor graft. A third technique involves delivery of high-dose cyclophosphamide following the transplant to deplete host-reactive donor T cells.

A retrospective study analyzed 90 patients with relapsed or refractory Hodgkin lymphoma who underwent nonmyeloablative conditioning followed by HSCT with either HLA-matched related, HLA-matched unrelated, or haploidentical related donors. Interestingly, the progression-free survival was highest in the group that received the haploidentical donor graft. However, there was no statistical difference in overall survival among the groups (53%, 58%, and 58% for HLA-matched related, HLA-matched unrelated, and haploidentical related, respectively). Nonrelapse mortality was significantly lower for haploidentical recipients compared to HLA-matched related recipients ($P = 0.02$). Furthermore, relapse risk was lowest for haploidentical recipients compared to HLA-matched related ($P = 0.01$) and unrelated ($P = 0.03$) recipients. The incidence of acute grade III/IV and extensive chronic GVHD (acute GVHD/chronic GVHD) was 16%/50% for HLA-matched related HSCT recipients, 8%/63% for HLA-matched unrelated HSCT recipients, and 11%/35% for HLA haploidentical related HSCT recipients. While small and retrospective in nature, these data demonstrate the progress that is being made toward improving outcomes of recipients of alternative donor grafts [16].

Umbilical cord blood

There are multiple potential benefits of the use of umbilical cord blood as a stem cell graft source. These cells are harvested at delivery and then cryopreserved at multiple public cord blood banks throughout the world, making them readily accessible. Since the T cells contained within the umbilical cord blood unit are essentially naive to foreign antigens, they appear to be more permissive to coexisting in an HLA-discordant host. The first umbilical cord blood transplantation was performed in a child in 1988. Most umbilical cord blood transplant activity in the ensuing years was limited to the pediatric population. With expansion of the public cord blood banks and improved quality of the units, adult cord blood transplantation activity has steadily increased between 2000 and 2014 [17–19].

The Blood and Marrow Transplant Clinical Trials Network (BMT CTN), an HSCT-focused cooperative group, performed two parallel Phase II trials assessing the outcome of nonmyeloablative haploidentical and dual umbilical cord blood transplantation; 100 adult patients with leukemia or lymphoma were enrolled [20]. In patients who received umbilical cord blood derived HSCT, the cumulative incidence of neutrophil recovery was 94%. The median time to absolute neutrophil count above 500/µL was 15 days. The cumulative incidence of platelet recovery in this group was 82% at a median time of 38 days. The cumulative incidence of neutrophil recovery and platelet recovery for the haploidentical related HSCT recipients was 96% (median 16 days) and 98% (median 24 days), respectively. The incidence of acute GVHD in the umbilical cord blood HSCT recipients was 40% and of chronic GVHD was 25%. In haploidentical related HSCT recipients, acute GVHD incidence was 32% and chronic GVHD at 1 year was 13%. The 1-year nonrelapse mortality, relapse, and survival (at 6 months) were comparable between the two studies. These results were quite promising because they supported previously reported data from single-center studies. However, because the patients were not randomly assigned, the two groups cannot be directly compared [20]. A follow-up randomized Phase III BMT CTN study comparing nonmyeloablative dual cord blood HSCT and haploidentical related HSCT is currently accruing subjects.

Further evidence for the efficacy of umbilical cord blood HSCT is provided from a European study that analyzed 645 patients with lymphoid malignancies who received allogeneic HSCT with either matched unrelated donors or umbilical cord blood-derived stem cells [21]. The study included patients with Hodgkin lymphoma, non-Hodgkin lymphoma, and chronic lymphocytic leukemia who received reduced-intensity conditioning regimens. Patients who had matched unrelated donor HSCT had faster neutrophil recovery at both 30 days (95% vs. 67%) and 60 days (97% vs. 81%). Median time to platelet recovery was 14 days after matched unrelated donor HSCT and 35 days after cord blood HSCT. Although there was no statistically significant difference in acute GVHD, chronic GVHD was more prevalent in patients who received matched unrelated donor HSCT (52% vs. 26%). The cumulative incidence of relapse was similar in the two groups (~34%) and there was no difference in progression-free or overall survival.

Conclusion

The role of allogeneic stem cell transplantation for lymphoma is evolving rapidly. This chapter compiles data that are likely to find applicability in lymphoma studies and treatment. When evaluating stem cell source, donor, and HLA matching in the allogeneic transplant setting for lymphoma, one must take into account the changing landscape of treatment for lymphomas. With the advent of immunotherapy and targeted therapies, the proper role for allogeneic HSCT will need to be continuously reassessed. Further chapters in this book explore the utility of allogeneic HSCT for particular subtypes of lymphoma.

References

1 Jantunen E, Sureda A. The evolving role of stem cell transplants in lymphomas. *Biol Blood Marrow Transplant* 2012;**18**:660–73.

2 Pasquini MC, Wang Z. Current use and outcome of hematopoietic stem cell transplantation: CIBMTR summary slides, 2013. Available at http://www.cibmtr.org

3 Inamoto Y, Flowers ME, Lee SJ et al. Influence of immunosuppressive treatment on risk of recurrent malignancy after allogeneic hematopoietic cell transplantation. *Blood* 2011; **118**:456–63.

4 Claret EJ, Alyea EP, Orsini E et al. Characterization of T cell repertoire in patients with graft-versus-leukemia after donor lymphocyte infusion. *J Clin Invest* 1997;**100**:855–66.

5 Anasetti C, Aversa F, Brunstein CG. Back to the future: mismatched unrelated donor, haploidentical related donor, or unrelated umbilical cord blood transplantation? *Biol Blood Marrow Transplant* 2012;**18**(1 Suppl):S161–5.

6 Champlin RE, Schmitz N, Horowitz MM et al. Blood stem cells compared with bone marrow as a source of hematopoietic cells for allogeneic transplantation. IBMTR Histocompatibility and Stem Cell Sources Working Committee and the European Group for Blood and Marrow Transplantation (EBMT). *Blood* 2000;**95**:3702–9.

7 Bensinger WI, Martin PJ, Storer B et al. Transplantation of bone marrow as compared with peripheral-blood cells from HLA-identical relatives in patients with hematologic cancers. *N Engl J Med* 2001;**344**:175–81.

8 Anasetti C, Logan BR, Lee SJ et al. Peripheral-blood stem cells versus bone marrow from unrelated donors. *N Engl J Med* 2012;**367**:1487–96.

9 Eng HS, Leffell MS. Histocompatibility testing after fifty years of transplantation. *J Immunol Method* 2011;**369**:1–21.

10 Petersdorf EW. Optimal HLA matching in hematopoietic cell transplantation. *Curr Opin Immunol* 2008;**20**:588–93.

11 Ringden O, Pavletic SZ, Anasetti C et al. The graft-ersus-leukemia effect using matched unrelated donors is not superior to HLA-identical siblings for hematopoietic stem cell transplantation. *Blood* 2009;**113**:3110–18.

12 Bacigalupo A, Ballen K, Rizzo D et al. Defining the intensity of conditioning regimens: working definitions. *Biol Blood Marrow Transplant* 2009;**15**:1628–33.

13 Ho VT, Kim HT, Aldridge J et al. Use of matched unrelated donors compared with matched related donors is associated with lower relapse and superior progression-free survival after reduced-intensity conditioning hematopoietic stem cell transplantation. *Biol Blood Marrow Transplant* 2011;**17**: 1196–204.

14 Woolfrey A, Klein JP, Haagenson M et al. HLA-C antigen mismatch is associated with worse outcome in unrelated donor peripheral blood stem cell transplantation. *Biol Blood Marrow Transplant* 2011;**17**:885–92.

15 Loiseau P, Busson M, Balere ML et al. HLA association with hematopoietic stem cell transplantation outcome: the number of mismatches at HLA-A, -B, -C, -DRB1, or -DQB1 is strongly associated with overall survival. *Biol Blood Marrow Transplant* 2007;**13**:965–74.

16 Burroughs LM, O'Donnell PV, Sandmaier BM et al. Comparison of outcomes of HLA-matched related, unrelated, or HLA-haploidentical related hematopoietic cell transplantation following nonmyeloablative conditioning for relapsed or refractory Hodgkin lymphoma. *Biol Blood Marrow Transplant* 2008;**14**:1279–87.

17 Eapen M, Rubinstein P, Zhang MJ et al. Outcomes of transplantation of unrelated donor umbilical cord blood and bone marrow in children with acute leukaemia: a comparison study. *Lancet* 2007;**369**:1947–54.

18 Raiola A, Dominietto A, Varaldo R et al. Unmanipulated haploidentical BMT following non-myeloablative conditioning and post-transplantation CY for advanced Hodgkin's lymphoma. *Bone Marrow Transplant* 2014;**49**:190–4.

19 Rocha V, Cornish J, Sievers EL et al. Comparison of outcomes of unrelated bone marrow and umbilical cord blood transplants in children with acute leukemia. *Blood* 2001;**97**:2962–71.

20 Brunstein CG, Fuchs EJ, Carter SL et al. Alternative donor transplantation after reduced intensity conditioning: results of parallel phase 2 trials using partially HLA-mismatched related bone marrow or unrelated double umbilical cord blood grafts. *Blood* 2011;**118**:282–8.

21 Rodrigues CA, Rocha V, Dreger P et al. Alternative donor hematopoietic stem cell transplantation for mature lymphoid malignancies after reduced-intensity conditioning regimen: similar outcomes with umbilical cord blood and unrelated donor peripheral blood. *Haematologica* 2014;**99**: 370–7.

CHAPTER 10

Management of early and late toxicities of autologous hematopoietic stem cell transplantation

Sai Ravi Pingali and Yago Nieto

Introduction

Lymphoma is the second most common indication for autologous stem cell transplantation (ASCT) after multiple myeloma. With advances in hematopoietic transplantation strategies and supportive care, ASCT has become a feasible treatment option for elderly patients and patients with comorbidities [1–3]. Of all ASCT reported to the Center for International Blood and Marrow Transplant Research (CIBMTR) from 2007 to 2011, 39% of recipients were over 60 years and 70% were over 50 years of age [4]. Recurrent disease is the most common cause of treatment failure and remains more prevalent than non-relapse mortality until 8 years after ASCT [5]. ASCT recipients continue to have higher rates of mortality compared to the normal population until at least 10 years after transplantation and need periodic follow-up to assess toxicities [6,7]. With improvements in survival rates, the population at risk for long-term complications after ASCT is growing, which increases the need for more rigorous screening and surveillance [7–9].

Early toxicities

Early toxicities of ASCT are usually caused by high-dose chemotherapy (HDC), and mortality at day 100 is often used as a surrogate end point for treatment-related toxicity. Incidence and severity of toxicities depends on age, performance status, and comorbidities of patients [3,10–14]. Early studies, including total body irradiation (TBI)-based regimens, showed a 1-year treatment-related mortality (TRM) of 25–38%. However, with improvements in supportive care and HDC, TRM has decreased to less than 5% [9–12,15–17].

Infections

Infections after ASCT are common during pre-engraftment and the immediate post-engraftment period and account for 8% of deaths [4]. Risk factors include mucositis, prolonged neutropenia, poor cellular immunity, and organ dysfunction associated with HDC. Febrile neutropenia is common after ASCT in up to 90% of patients [18]. Fever of unknown origin is the most common cause of febrile neutropenia. A microbiological pathogen is detected in around 39% of cases, and pneumonia without an identified pathogen is seen in 9% of cases [18,19]. Complications and management of infections are summarized in Table 10.1.

Prophylaxis

Use of granulocyte colony-stimulating factor (G-CSF) has reduced the duration of neutropenia and, along with prophylactic antibiotics, has reduced the incidence of febrile neutropenia [20]. Most of the infections are from bacterial causes; viral and invasive fungal infections account for a small number of cases. Invasive fungal infections are rare after ASCT, occurring in about 1.5%, and two-thirds of these patients fully recover with antifungal therapy [21]. Prophylaxis for aspergillosis during the pre-engraftment period has not been shown to be effective, probably due to its low incidence [22]. Prophylaxis against *Candida* is most useful in ASCT patients who do not receive G-CSF

Clinical Guide to Transplantation in Lymphoma, First Edition. Edited by Bipin N. Savani and Mohamad Mohty.
© 2015 John Wiley & Sons, Ltd. Published 2015 by John Wiley & Sons, Ltd.

Table 10.1 Infectious complications.

	Pre-engraftment	Post-engraftment to 6 months	Prophylaxis
Viral	Herpes simplex	Varicella zoster Cytomegalovirus	Acyclovir, 6 months to 1 year
Bacterial	Gram-positive and Gram-negative		Flouroquinolones, pre-engraftment
Fungal	*Candida*		Fluconazole, pre-engraftment
Parasitic		*Pneumocystis jirovecii*	Trimethoprim/sulfamethoxazole*, post-engraftment to 6 months

*Dapsone, atovaquone and pentamidine are acceptable alternatives.

support or have mucositis, and fluconazole is the most commonly used agent [23]. After neutrophil engraftment the risk of candidiasis is minimal and prophylaxis can be safely discontinued. Prophylaxis for herpes simplex virus (HSV) with acyclovir or valacyclovir is recommended for all patients with HSV seropositivity. Varicella zoster prophylaxis with those drugs is usually given for 6 months to 1 year after ASCT [24]. Unlike allogeneic transplantation, cytomegalovirus reactivation is uncommon in ASCT patients. The true incidence of *Pneumocystis jirovecii* pneumonia in ASCT patients is unknown, but two recent retrospective studies reported an incidence of less than 0.5% with prophylaxis [25,26]. Prophylaxis with trimethoprim sulfamethoxazole is routinely started after engraftment and used until 6 months after ASCT.

Management of febrile neutropenia
Patients with febrile neutropenia should be started on empiric broad-spectrum antibiotics which have activity against *Pseudomonas*. Monotherapy with cefepime or carbapenems or piperacillin/tazobactam are as effective as multidrug combinations [22]. Additional coverage with vancomycin for suspected line infection or aminoglycosides in cases with hemodynamic instability is recommended.

Mucositis
Mucositis is a common side effect after ASCT, occurring in 71–100% of patients at various degrees of severity, and contributes to significant morbidity and mortality [27–29]. It is an end result of interactions between epithelial damage caused by chemotherapy, cytokine-mediated responses, and the bacterial flora of the oral cavity. The Sonis model describes five interdependent phases of initiation: primary damage response (I), upregulation/amplification (II/III), ulceration (IV), and healing (V) [30].

The oral mucositis assessment scale (OMAS) is a reproducible and effective tool for monitoring mucositis.

A 1-point increase in OMAS is associated with increase in number of days with fever, parenteral nutrition, intravenous antibiotics, and 100-day mortality from increased risk of infections. Higher OMAS is also associated with significantly higher healthcare costs [29]. Patients with mucositis are at high risk for *Streptococcus viridans* infections and patients with fever and mucositis should receive antibiotics with activity against this pathogen. The severity of mucositis increases with age and prolonged neutropenia. Patients with non-Hodgkin lymphoma, patients who had mobilization of stem cells, and patients who received prior radiation therapy tend to have worse mucositis post transplant [31].

Management of mucositis should begin with pretransplant dental evaluation. Oral hygiene with sterile water, normal saline, or sodium bicarbonate should be mandatory. Patient-controlled analgesia with opioids is recommended for symptom control. Keratinocyte growth factor-1 (palifermin) prophylaxis decreases the incidence and severity of mucositis in patients receiving TBI-based preparative regimen for ASCT [32]. However, its use in chemotherapy-only HDC is controversial: recent studies with melphalan alone or high-dose busulfan, cyclophosphamide, and etoposide did not show a significant benefit [33,34].

Agents like oral glutamine, supersaturated calcium/phosphate (Caphosol), and laser therapy have been tested with some benefit, although further confirmation is needed [35–38]. Systemic glutamine and amifostine are ineffective and not recommended [39].

Cardiovascular side effects
Although patients receive evaluation for adequate cardiac function prior to ASCT, early and long-term cardiac complications are common. Atrial fibrillation is the most common early cardiac complication, seen in 10–18% of patients younger than 65 years of age and in

up to 50% of patients over the age of 60 [40,41]. Often, it reverts rapidly and needs treatment only in the short term. Edema and hypotension are other common side effects more often seen in elderly patients [41].

Engraftment syndrome

Engraftment syndrome (ES) is a constellation of symptoms and signs occurring immediately around the time of neutrophil engraftment that are related to proinflammatory cytokines. It is characterized by noninfectious fever, maculopapular rash, pulmonary opacities, diarrhea, weight gain and, sometimes, neurologic manifestations [42–44]. The incidence of ES ranges from 7 to 13% [42,44–46]. Use of peripheral blood stem cells, female gender, and absence of intensive chemotherapy before ASCT seem associated with higher risk of ES [42].

The Spitzer diagnostic criteria of ES include symptoms, signs and laboratory findings categorized as major (noninfectious fever, erythema involving >25% of body surface area, and hypoxia with pulmonary infiltrates from noncardiogenic pulmonary edema) and minor (hepatic dysfunction, elevation of creatinine, weight gain, and transient encephalopathy). According to this model, all three major criteria or two major criteria and one or more minor criteria within 96 hours of engraftment establish a diagnosis of ES. Maiolino et al. [43] proposed simplified criteria, with noninfectious fever and one of skin rash, pulmonary infiltrates or diarrhea. Both sets of criteria require development of these symptoms within 1–5 days of neutrophil engraftment.

Though ES is usually self-limited, it results in longer hospital stays and duration of antibiotic therapy, and possibly higher TRM rates [43,44]. Brief systemic glucocorticoid therapy is sometimes required for patients with pulmonary compromise.

Pulmonary complications

Pulmonary complications after ASCT are common and seen in about 25% of patients within 1 year of transplantation [47]. Most of these complications are infections (14% of patients). Among noninfectious causes, pulmonary edema and idiopathic pneumonia syndrome are the most common causes.

Independent factors for development of pulmonary complications include the pre-ASCT diffusion capacity of lung for carbon monoxide (D_{LCO}) and the disease indication for ASCT. Factors predicting mortality from

pulmonary complications include previous lung disease, male gender, and disease status at the time of transplantation. Bacterial, fungal, and viral pneumonias develop in 14% of patients. An aggressive diagnostic approach with bronchoscopy and computerized tomography is needed for patients with infectious complications not responding to broad-spectrum antibiotics. Pulmonary edema can be cardiogenic or noncardiogenic. It is more common in patients receiving cyclophosphamide in the preparative regimen, in those with previous exposure to anthracycline, in those receiving mediastinal radiation, and in those with arrhythmias. Its treatment depends on the underlying etiology.

Idiopathic pneumonia syndrome (IPS) is a well-recognized complication of ASCT and is characterized by the pathologic findings of interstitial pneumonitis and/or diffuse alveolar damage [48]. Diagnostic criteria include multilobar infiltrates, increased alveolar–arterial gradient, and negative work-up for lower respiratory tract infections. The incidence of IPS is highly variable, ranging between 1 and 10%, and is more common with carmustine- or busulfan-based HDC regimens [47,49–54]. This syndrome usually occurs early in the course of ASCT and can be fatal in 50–80% of patients despite early treatment with glucocorticoids [51].

An aggressive clinical presentation of IPS is diffuse alveolar hemorrhage (DAH), which presents with rapid respiratory failure usually within the first 2 weeks of ASCT [55,56]. Hemoptysis occurs only in 15% of cases [56]. DAH is caused by bleeding into the alveolar space due to disruption of the alveolar capillary basement membrane and is classically confirmed by bronchoscopic findings of progressively bloodier bronchoalveolar lavage aliquots. Mortality from DAH is about 26–28% in patients receiving ASCT for lymphoma, although early initiation of high-dose glucocorticoids (methylprednisolone 0.5–1 g/day) may improve outcomes [56–59].

Renal toxicity

Acute kidney injury (AKI) is seen in up to 12–24% of ASCT patients, most commonly due to HDC, tumor lysis, nephrotoxic antibiotics, or sepsis during the early post-transplant period [60–63]. Patients with AKI needing dialysis have a higher risk of TRM, up to 6% in the first 100 days [64]. Early intervention with hydration, dose adjustment of medications to creatinine clearance, avoidance of nephrotoxic agents if possible, and early consultation with a nephrologist are required.

Liver toxicity

Liver toxicity in seen in 45–61% of ASCT recipients, with drug toxicity and sepsis as the most common causes [65–67]. Liver toxicity is usually reversible with withdrawal of the offending drug. Patients with liver toxicity have a higher incidence of TRM when associated with sepsis and AKI, but fatal fulminant hepatic failure is rare.

Hepatic venoocclusive disease

Hepatic venoocclusive disease (VOD) or sinusoidal obstruction syndrome is characterized by painful hepatomegaly, jaundice, and weight gain from ascites. A hepatic venous pressure gradient of 10 mmHg is highly predictive of VOD and transjugular liver biopsy is the gold standard [68]. VOD is characterized by sinusoidal endothelial injury in zone 3 of the liver acinus. Early changes include deposition of fibrinogen, factor VIII and erythrocytes, leading to progressive venular occlusion, zonal disruption, and centrilobular hemorrhagic necrosis. It used to occur in 5–9% of ASCT [69,70], but fortunately its incidence has decreased dramatically with the advent of the intravenous formulation of busulfan, which decreases pharmacokinetic variability and avoids hepatic first-pass metabolism [71–73]. Treatment for VOD is challenging; small Phase II studies suggested improved outcomes with defibrotide [75,76]. A multicenter study which evaluated use of defibrotide in 88 patients with pathologically confirmed diagnosis of VOD showed 36% complete resolution without any significant hemorrhage or other toxicities [75]. Prospective studies are needed to confirm these findings and identify predictors of response or failure.

Neurologic toxicity

The incidence of neurologic toxicity among ASCT patients has varied from 3% to 39% in different reports [77,78]. Often these neurologic symptoms are reversible and are related to drug toxicity, metabolic abnormalities, or infections. HDC regimens containing busulfan, carmustine, cytarabine, etoposide, ifosfamide, carboplatin, or thiotepa can cause neurotoxicity [79]. Busulfan causes seizures in up to 10% of patients without the usual prophylactic antiepileptics [80,81]. Subdural

hemorrhage can present during thrombocytopenia as severe headaches or mental status changes.

Late toxicities

HDC puts ASCT recipients at risk for several long-term toxic effects (Table 10.2). Patients who are in remission 2 years after ASCT are likely to be long-term survivors, but at a higher mortality rate compared to the general population until at least 10 years from transplantation, mainly due to tumor relapse [6,7]. Secondary cancers and organ toxicities are the leading causes of nonrelapse mortality among survivors. Compared to siblings, ASCT survivors have significantly higher frequency of cataracts, dry mouth, hypothyroidism, bone disease, congestive heart failure, neurosensory impairments, inability to attend full-time work, and poor overall health [82,83].

Secondary malignancies

Secondary malignancies after ASCT are well-recognized late effects and occur in up to 17% of patients at 10 years after transplant using TBI [6,84,85]. The most common secondary malignancy is myelodysplastic syndrome/acute myelogenous leukemia (t-MDS/AML), with an incidence of about 4%, and accounts for two-thirds of deaths from secondary malignancies [6,86]. Median time to onset of t-MDS/AML is 2.5 years and the risk increases with intensity of pretransplantation use of alkylating agents and prior radiation therapy [87]. t-MDS/AML is classically associated with exposure to alkylating agents and topoisomerase II inhibitors The risk for alkylating agent-related t-MDS/AML is dose-dependent, with a latency of 3–5 years after exposure to alkylating agents. Alkylator-related t-MDS/AML is associated with abnormalities involving chromosomes 5 (−5/del[5q]) and 7 (−7/del[7q]). Topoisomerase II inhibitor-related t-AML presents as overt leukemia without preceding myelodysplasia, usually after a latency of 6 months to 3 years, and is associated with balanced translocations involving chromosome bands 11q23 or 21q22. Solid tumors, especially breast cancer, sarcoma and thyroid cancer, are common among patients who received radiation therapy.

Patients must be educated regarding the risks of second infections and the importance of avoiding high-risk lifestyles, such as smoking, unprotected sun exposure and excessive use of alcohol, as well as routine annual screening for secondary cancers. Screening mammograms

Table 10.2 Long-term toxicities.

Organ system	Incidence	Follow-up recommendations
Second cancers [85,86]	16.7% (at 10 years)	Annual screening examinations
MDS/AML	4%	Patient counseling
		Monthly self-breast examination in women
		Monthly self-scrotal examination in men
		Smoking cessation
Cardiovascular [88–90]	22–43%	Annual screening examinations
Cardiomyopathy		More specific screening in high-risk patients*
Coronary artery disease		Smoking cessation
		Control of risk factors: diabetes, hypertension, hyperlipidemia and obesity
Pulmonary [93–96]	38% (often asymptomatic)	Symptom screening annually
		Follow-up pulmonary function tests in symptomatic patients
Endocrine [83,86,98]	23%	Screening for endocrine symptoms annually
Hypothyroidism	5–19%	Thyroid function tests with dose adjustments
Infertility	18% men; 29% women	Fertility expert input prior to ASCT
Osteoporosis	4–6%	Vitamin D, calcium supplementation. Bone density scan after 1 year and as required
Renal [98]	11%†	Good risk factor control: hypertension, diabetes
Neurologic [82,83,100]	19%	Expert evaluation as needed
Tinnitus		
Taste abnormalities		
Smell abnormalities		
Cognitive deficits		
Psychosocial [82,83,86]	Unknown	Routine screening
		Early identification and management of symptoms

*Patients with history of mediastinal radiation and anthracycline use.
†With TBI-based conditioning.

should be started at 25 years or 8 years after mediastinal radiation therapy, whichever occurs later [86].

Late cardiovascular side effects

Cardiovascular disease is up to three times more frequent in ASCT recipients compared to their siblings and is seen in up to 43% of ASCT survivors [88,89]. Cardiac toxicity accounts for 2% of late deaths due to a higher incidence of ischemic heart disease, cardiomyopathy, stroke, vascular disease, and arrhythmias [86]. Compared to allogeneic transplant recipients, past ASCT recipients present the same incidence of cardiovascular risk factors except for hypertension, which seems more common after allogeneic transplantation [90]. Prior mediastinal radiation therapy and anthracyclines increase the risk of cardiomyopathy [86]. Known risk factors, such as smoking, metabolic syndrome, diabetes, smoking and hypertension, also increase the risk for cardiovascular events post transplant. Annual screening for cardiovascular risk factors and disease is recommended for patients surviving 1 year after transplantation.

Late pulmonary side effects

Bacterial and fungal infections can occur for several months after engraftment because of poor humoral and cell-mediated immunity. Patients not responding to empiric antibiotic therapy and manifesting pulmonary infiltrates need work-up for endemic fungal disease and uncommon infections like mycobacterial disease [92]. Restrictive and interstitial disease is common among ASCT recipients, especially with use of TBI and agents such as carmustine and busulfan [93–96].

Progression of lung disease is rare beyond 2 years after transplantation and these patients are often asymptomatic. Patients are recommended to avoid smoking and have annual surveillance. Patients with symptoms or signs of functional compromise must have follow-up evaluation with repeat pulmonary function tests and or imaging [86].

Endocrine side effects

Thyroid dysfunction and fertility issues are common among ASCT survivors. Hypothyroidism is seen in about 5–19% of patients and in nearly 50% of those receiving

TBI [83]. Thyroid neoplasms are also more common among children after ASCT. Thyroid function tests (TSH, free T_4 and T_3) should be checked regularly starting at 1 year from transplant [86,97,98].

Data on infertility after ASCT are sparse. It has been reported in 18% of male ASCT recipients and in 29% of female recipients. The degree of gonadal dysfunction depends on age, prior therapy, and preparative regimen used [99]. Given the high incidence of infertility, patients must be counseled about permanent infertility and offered specialist consultation.

Other side effects

Renal dysfunction is seen in up to 11% of ASCT recipients, especially those who have had abdominal radiation therapy or TBI-based therapy. Severe neuropathy occurs usually within 1 year of ASCT, but these patients continue to have a higher incidence until 20 years from transplant and symptoms could occur in about 14% of patients [98].

Conclusions

Patients receiving ASCT are at risk for early and late toxicities, which can occur several years after transplantation. It is important that patients and healthcare providers, especially nontransplant physicians, be educated about these side effects and the importance of screening for chronic conditions.

Conflict of interest

The authors have no conflicts of interest to declare relevant to the content of this chapter.

Further reading

Freifeld AG, Bow EJ, Sepkowitz KA *et al*. Clinical practice guideline for the use of antimicrobial agents in neutropenic patients with cancer: 2010 update by the Infectious Diseases Society of America. *Clin Infect Dis* 2011;**52**:e56–93.

Majhail NS, Rizzo JD, Lee SJ *et al*. Recommended screening and preventive practices for long-term survivors after hematopoietic cell transplantation. *Biol Blood Marrow Transplant* 2012;**18**:348–71.

Tomblyn M, Chiller T, Einsele H *et al*. Guidelines for preventing infectious complications among hematopoietic cell transplantation recipients: a global perspective. *Biol Blood Marrow Transplant* 2009;**15**:1143–238.

Wildes TM, Stirewalt DL, Medeiros B, Hurria A. Hematopoietic stem cell transplantation for hematologic malignancies in older adults: geriatric principles in the transplant clinic. *J Natl Compr Canc Netw* 2014;**12**:128–36.

References

1 Wildes TM, Stirewalt DL, Medeiros B, Hurria A. Hematopoietic stem cell transplantation for hematologic malignancies in older adults: geriatric principles in the transplant clinic. *J Natl Compr Canc Netw* 2014;**12**:128–36.

2 Hosing C, Saliba RM, Okoroji G-J *et al*. High-dose chemotherapy and autologous hematopoietic progenitor cell transplantation for non-Hodgkin's lymphoma in patients >65 years of age. *Ann Oncol* 2008;**19**:1166–71.

3 Wildes TM, Augustin KM, Sempek D *et al*. Comorbidities, not age, impact outcomes in autologous stem cell transplant for relapsed non-Hodgkin lymphoma. *Biol Blood Marrow Transplant* 2008;**14**:840–6.

4 Pasquini MC, Wang Z. Current use and outcome of hematopoietic stem cell transplantation: CIBMTR Summary Slides, 2013. Available at http://www.cibmtr.org

5 Hill BT, Rybicki L, Bolwell BJ *et al*. The non-relapse mortality rate for patients with diffuse large B-cell lymphoma is greater than relapse mortality 8 years after autologous stem cell transplantation and is significantly higher than mortality rates of population controls. *Br J Haematol* 2011;**152**:561–9.

6 Bhatia S, Robison LL, Francisco L *et al*. Late mortality in survivors of autologous hematopoietic-cell transplantation: report from the Bone Marrow Transplant Survivor Study. *Blood* 2005;**105**:4215–22.

7 Majhail NS, Bajorunaite R, Lazarus HM *et al*. Long-term survival and late relapse in 2-year survivors of autologous haematopoietic cell transplantation for Hodgkin and non-Hodgkin lymphoma. *Br J Haematol* 2009;**147**:129–39.

8 Majhail NS, Rizzo JD. Surviving the cure: long term followup of hematopoietic cell transplant recipients. *Bone Marrow Transplant* 2013;**48**:1145–51.

9 Majhail NS, Weisdorf DJ, Defor TE *et al*. Long-term results of autologous stem cell transplantation for primary refractory or relapsed Hodgkin's lymphoma. *Biol Blood Marrow Transplant* 2006;**12**:1065–72.

10 Sweetenham JW, Pearce R, Philip T *et al*. High-dose therapy and autologous bone marrow transplantation for intermediate and high grade non-Hodgkin's lymphoma in patients aged 55 years and over: results from the European Group for Bone Marrow Transplantation. *The EBMT Lymphoma Working Party. Bone Marrow Transplant* 1994;**14**:981–7.

11 Kusnierz-Glaz CR, Schlegel PG, Wong RM *et al*. Influence of age on the outcome of 500 autologous bone marrow

transplant procedures for hematologic malignancies. *J Clin Oncol* 1997;**15**:18–25.

12 Miller CB, Piantadosi S, Vogelsang GB *et al.* Impact of age on outcome of patients with cancer undergoing autologous bone marrow transplant. *J Clin Oncol* 1996;**14**:1327–32.

13 Jantunen E, Canals C, Rambaldi A *et al.* Autologous stem cell transplantation in elderly patients (≥60 years) with diffuse large B-cell lymphoma: an analysis based on data in the European Blood and Marrow Transplantation registry. *Haematologica* 2008;**93**:1837–42.

14 Lazarus HM, Carreras J, Boudreau C *et al.* Influence of age and histology on outcome in adult non-Hodgkin lymphoma patients undergoing autologous hematopoietic cell transplantation (HCT): a report from the Center for International Blood and Marrow Transplant Research (CIBMTR). *Biol Blood Marrow Transplant* 2008;**14**:1323–33.

15 Wadehra N, Farag S, Bolwell B *et al.* Long-term outcome of Hodgkin disease patients following high-dose busulfan, etoposide, cyclophosphamide, and autologous stem cell transplantation. *Biol Blood Marrow Transplant* 2006;**12**:1343–9.

16 Geisler CH, Kolstad A, Laurell A *et al.* Long-term progression-free survival of mantle cell lymphoma after intensive front-line immunochemotherapy with in vivo-purged stem cell rescue: a nonrandomized phase 2 multicenter study by the Nordic Lymphoma Group. *Blood* 2008;**112**:2687–93.

17 Villela L, Sureda A, Canals C *et al.* Low transplant related mortality in older patients with hematologic malignancies undergoing autologous stem cell transplantation. *Haematologica* 2003;**88**:300–5.

18 Auner HW, Sill H, Mulabecirovic A, Linkesch W, Krause R. Infectious complications after autologous hematopoietic stem cell transplantation: comparison of patients with acute myeloid leukemia, malignant lymphoma, and multiple myeloma. *Ann Hematol* 2002;**81**:374–7.

19 Gil L, Styczynski J, Komarnicki M. Infectious complication in 314 patients after high-dose therapy and autologous hematopoietic stem cell transplantation: risk factors analysis and outcome. *Infection* 2007;**35**:421–7.

20 Kuderer NM, Dale DC, Crawford J, Lyman GH. Impact of primary prophylaxis with granulocyte colony-stimulating factor on febrile neutropenia and mortality in adult cancer patients receiving chemotherapy: a systematic review. *J Clin Oncol* 2007;**25**:3158–67.

21 Jantunen E, Salonen J, Juvonen E *et al.* Invasive fungal infections in autologous stem cell transplant recipients: a nation-wide study of 1188 transplanted patients. *Eur J Haematol* 2004;**73**:174–8.

22 Freifeld AG, Bow EJ, Sepkowitz KA *et al.* Clinical practice guideline for the use of antimicrobial agents in neutropenic patients with cancer: 2010 update by the Infectious Diseases Society of America. *Clin Infect Dis* 2011;**52**:e56–93.

23 Rotstein C, Bow EJ, Laverdiere M, Ioannou S, Carr D, Moghaddam N. Randomized placebo-controlled trial of fluconazole prophylaxis for neutropenic cancer patients:

benefit based on purpose and intensity of cytotoxic therapy. *Clin Infect Dis* 1999;**28**:331–40.

24 Saral R, Burns WH, Laskin OL, Santos GW, Lietman PS. Acyclovir prophylaxis of herpes-simplex-virus infections. *N Engl J Med* 1981;**305**:63–7.

25 Williams KM, Agwu AG, Chen M *et al.* CIBMTR retrospective analysis reveals incidence, mortality, and timing of *Pneumocystis jiroveci* pneumonia (PCP) after hematopoietic stem cell transplantation (HSCT). *Biol Blood Marrow Transplant* 2014;**20**:S94.

26 Raser K, McNulty ML, Yanik G *et al.* Routine prophylaxis of *Pneumocystis jirovecii* pneumonia in recipients of autologous hematopoietic stem cell transplantation. *Biol Blood Marrow Transplant* 2014;**20**:S116–17.

27 Vagliano L, Feraut C, Gobetto G *et al.* Incidence and severity of oral mucositis in patients undergoing haematopoietic SCT: results of a multicentre study. *Bone Marrow Transplant* 2011;**46**:727–32.

28 Rubenstein EB, Peterson DE, Schubert M *et al.* Clinical practice guidelines for the prevention and treatment of cancer therapy-induced oral and gastrointestinal mucositis. *Cancer* 2004;**100**:2026–46.

29 Sonis ST, Oster G, Fuchs H *et al.* Oral mucositis and the clinical and economic outcomes of hematopoietic stem-cell transplantation. *J Clin Oncol* 2001;**19**:2201–5.

30 Sonis ST, Elting LS, Keefe D *et al.* Perspectives on cancer therapy-induced mucosal injury: pathogenesis, measurement, epidemiology, and consequences for patients. *Cancer* 2004;**100**:1995–2025.

31 Bolwell BJ, Kalaycio M, Sobecks R *et al.* A multivariable analysis of factors influencing mucositis after autologous progenitor cell transplantation. *Bone Marrow Transplant* 2002;**30**:587–91.

32 Spielberger R, Stiff P, Bensinger W *et al.* Palifermin for oral mucositis after intensive therapy for hematologic cancers. *N Engl J Med* 2004;**351**:2590–8.

33 Blijlevens N, de Chateau M, Krivan G *et al.* In a high-dose melphalan setting, palifermin compared with placebo had no effect on oral mucositis or related patien's burden. *Bone Marrow Transplant* 2013;**48**:966–71.

34 Nooka AK, Johnson HR, Kaufman JL *et al.* Pharmacoeconomic analysis of palifermin to prevent mucositis among patients undergoing autologous hematopoietic stem cell transplantation. *Biol Blood Marrow Transplant* 2014;**20**:852–7.

35 Crowther M, Avenell A, Culligan DJ. Systematic review and meta-analyses of studies of glutamine supplementation in haematopoietic stem cell transplantation. *Bone Marrow Transplant* 2009;**44**:413–25.

36 Papas AS, Clark RE, Martuscelli G, O'Loughlin KT, Johansen E, Miller KB. A prospective, randomized trial for the prevention of mucositis in patients undergoing hematopoietic stem cell transplantation. *Bone Marrow Transplant* 2003;**31**:705–12.

37 Figueiredo AL, Lins L, Cattony AC, Falcao AF. Laser therapy in the control of oral mucositis: a meta-analysis. *Rev Assoc Med Bras* 2013;**59**:467–74.

38 Bezinelli LM, de Paula Eduardo F, da Graca Lopes RM *et al.* Cost-effectiveness of the introduction of specialized oral care with laser therapy in hematopoietic stem cell transplantation. *Hematol Oncol* 2014;**32**:31–9.

39 Peterson DE, Bensadoun RJ, Roila F. Management of oral and gastrointestinal mucositis: ESMO Clinical Practice Guidelines. *Ann Oncol* 2011;**22**(Suppl 6):vi78–84.

40 Sirohi B, Powles R, Treleaven J *et al.* The role of autologous transplantation in patients with multiple myeloma aged 65 years and over. *Bone Marrow Transplant* 2000;**25**:533–9.

41 Mileshkin LR, Seymour JF, Wolf MM *et al.* Cardiovascular toxicity is increased, but manageable, during high-dose chemotherapy and autologous peripheral blood stem cell transplantation for patients aged 60 years and older. *Leukemia Lymphoma* 2005;**46**:1575–9.

42 Carreras E, Fernandez-Aviles F, Silva L *et al.* Engraftment syndrome after auto-SCT: analysis of diagnostic criteria and risk factors in a large series from a single center. *Bone Marrow Transplant* 2010;**45**:1417–22.

43 Maiolino A, Biasoli I, Lima J, Portugal AC, Pulcheri W, Nucci M. Engraftment syndrome following autologous hematopoietic stem cell transplantation: definition of diagnostic criteria. *Bone Marrow Transplant* 2003;**31**:393–7.

44 Spitzer TR. Engraftment syndrome following hematopoietic stem cell transplantation. *Bone Marrow Transplant* 2001;**27**:893–8.

45 Edenfield WJ, Moores LK, Goodwin G, Lee N. An engraftment syndrome in autologous stem cell transplantation related to mononuclear cell dose. *Bone Marrow Transplant* 2000;**25**:405–9.

46 Ravoet C, Feremans W, Husson B *et al.* Clinical evidence for an engraftment syndrome associated with early and steep neutrophil recovery after autologous blood stem cell transplantation. *Bone Marrow Transplant* 1996;**18**:943–7.

47 Afessa B, Abdulai RM, Kremers WK, Hogan WJ, Litzow MR, Peters SG. Risk factors and outcome of pulmonary complications after autologous hematopoietic stem cell transplant. *Chest* 2012;**141**:442–50.

48 Clark JG, Hansen JA, Hertz MI, Parkman R, Jensen L, Peavy HH. NHLBI workshop summary. Idiopathic pneumonia syndrome after bone marrow transplantation. *Am Rev Respir Dis* 1993;**147**:1601–6.

49 Kantrow SP, Hackman RC, Boeckh M, Myerson D, Crawford SW. Idiopathic pneumonia syndrome: changing spectrum of lung injury after marrow transplantation. *Transplantation* 1997;**63**:1079–86.

50 Rubio C, Hill ME, Milan S, O'Brien ME, Cunningham D. Idiopathic pneumonia syndrome after high-dose chemotherapy for relapsed Hodgkin's disease. *Br J Cancer* 1997;**75**:1044–8.

51 Bilgrami SF, Metersky ML, McNally D *et al.* Idiopathic pneumonia syndrome following myeloablative chemotherapy and autologous transplantation. *Ann Pharmacother* 2001;**35**:196–201.

52 Wingard JR, Sostrin MB, Vriesendorp HM *et al.* Interstitial pneumonitis following autologous bone marrow transplantation. *Transplantation* 1988;**46**:61–5.

53 Valteau D, Hartmann O, Benhamou E *et al.* Nonbacterial nonfungal interstitial pneumonitis following autologous bone marrow transplantation in children treated with high-dose chemotherapy without total-body irradiation. *Transplantation* 1988;**45**:737–40.

54 Wong R, Rondon G, Saliba RM *et al.* Idiopathic pneumonia syndrome after high-dose chemotherapy and autologous hematopoietic stem cell transplantation for high-risk breast cancer. *Bone Marrow Transplant* 2003;**31**:1157–63.

55 Robbins RA, Linder J, Stahl MG *et al.* Diffuse alveolar hemorrhage in autologous bone marrow transplant recipients. *Am J Med* 1989;**87**:511–18.

56 Afessa B, Tefferi A, Litzow MR, Peters SG. Outcome of diffuse alveolar hemorrhage in hematopoietic stem cell transplant recipients. *Am J Respir Crit Care Med* 2002;**166**:1364–8.

57 Jules-Elysee K, Stover DE, Yahalom J, White DA, Gulati SC. Pulmonary complications in lymphoma patients treated with high-dose therapy autologous bone marrow transplantation. *Am Rev Respir Dis* 1992;**146**:485–91.

58 Chao NJ, Duncan SR, Long GD, Horning SJ, Blume KG. Corticosteroid therapy for diffuse alveolar hemorrhage in autologous bone marrow transplant recipients. *Ann Intern Med* 1991;**114**:145–6.

59 Metcalf JP, Rennard SI, Reed EC *et al.* Corticosteroids as adjunctive therapy for diffuse alveolar hemorrhage associated with bone marrow transplantation. *University of Nebraska Medical Center Bone Marrow Transplant Group. Am J Med* 1994;**96**:327–34.

60 Schrier RW, Parikh CR. Comparison of renal injury in myeloablative autologous, myeloablative allogeneic and non-myeloablative allogeneic haematopoietic cell transplantation. *Nephrol Dial Transplant* 2005;**20**:678–83.

61 Kogon A, Hingorani S. Acute kidney injury in hematopoietic cell transplantation. *Semin Nephrol* 2010;**30**:615–26.

62 Sawinski D. The kidney effects of hematopoietic stem cell transplantation. *Adv Chronic Kidney Dis* 2014;**21**:96–105.

63 Merouani A, Shpall EJ, Jones RB, Archer PG, Schrier RW. Renal function in high dose chemotherapy and autologous hematopoietic cell support treatment for breast cancer. *Kidney Int* 1996;**50**:1026–31.

64 Lopes JA, Jorge S, Silva S *et al.* Acute renal failure following myeloablative autologous and allogeneic hematopoietic cell transplantation. *Bone Marrow Transplant* 2006;**38**:707.

65 Forbes GM, Davies JM, Herrmann RP, Collins BJ. Liver disease complicating bone marrow transplantation: a clinical audit. *J Gastroenterol Hepatol* 1995;**10**:1–7.

66 Kim BK, Chung KW, Sun HS *et al.* Liver disease during the first post-transplant year in bone marrow transplantation recipients: retrospective study. *Bone Marrow Transplant* 2000;**26**:193–7.

67 Ozdogan O, Ratip S, Ahdab YA *et al*. Causes and risk factors for liver injury following bone marrow transplantation. *J Clin Gastroenterol* 2003;**36**:421–6.

68 Shulman HM, Gooley T, Dudley MD *et al*. Utility of transvenous liver biopsies and wedged hepatic venous pressure measurements in sixty marrow transplant recipients. *Transplantation* 1995;**59**:1015–22.

69 Dulley FL, Kanfer EJ, Appelbaum FR *et al*. Venocclusive disease of the liver after chemoradiotherapy and autologous bone marrow transplantation. *Transplantation* 1987;**43**:870–3.

70 Lee SH, Yoo KH, Sung KW *et al*. Hepatic veno-occlusive disease in children after hematopoietic stem cell transplantation: incidence, risk factors, and outcome. *Bone Marrow Transplant* 2010;**45**:1287–93.

71 Kashyap A, Wingard J, Cagnoni P *et al*. Intravenous versus oral busulfan as part of a busulfan/cyclophosphamide preparative regimen for allogeneic hematopoietic stem cell transplantation: decreased incidence of hepatic venoocclusive disease (HVOD), HVOD-related mortality, and overall 100-day mortality. *Biol Blood Marrow Transplant* 2002;**8**:493–500.

72 Lee JH, Choi SJ, Lee JH *et al*. Decreased incidence of hepatic veno-occlusive disease and fewer hemostatic derangements associated with intravenous busulfan vs oral busulfan in adults conditioned with busulfan + cyclophosphamide for allogeneic bone marrow transplantation. *Ann Hematol* 2005;**84**:321–30.

73 de Lima M, Couriel D, Thall PF *et al*. Once-daily intravenous busulfan and fludarabine: clinical and pharmacokinetic results of a myeloablative, reduced-toxicity conditioning regimen for allogeneic stem cell transplantation in AML and MDS. *Blood* 2004;**104**:857–64.

74 McDonald GB, Hinds MS, Fisher LD *et al*. Veno-occlusive disease of the liver and multiorgan failure after bone marrow transplantation: a cohort study of 355 patients. *Ann Intern Med* 1993;**118**:255–67.

75 Richardson PG, Murakami C, Jin Z *et al*. Multi-institutional use of defibrotide in 88 patients after stem cell transplantation with severe veno-occlusive disease and multisystem organ failure: response without significant toxicity in a high-risk population and factors predictive of outcome. *Blood* 2002;**100**:4337–43.

76 Chopra R, Eaton JD, Grassi A *et al*. Defibrotide for the treatment of hepatic veno-occlusive disease: results of the European compassionate-use study. *Br J Haematol* 2000;**111**:1122–9.

77 Snider S, Bashir R, Bierman P. Neurologic complications after high-dose chemotherapy and autologous bone marrow transplantation for Hodgkin's disease. *Neurology* 1994;**44**:681–4.

78 Guerrero A, Perez-Simon JA, Gutierrez N *et al*. Neurological complications after autologous stem cell transplantation. *Eur Neurol* 1999;**41**:48–50.

79 Rosenfeld MR, Pruitt A. Neurologic complications of bone marrow, stem cell, and organ transplantation in patients with cancer. *Semin Oncol* 2006;**33**:352–61.

80 Vassal G, Deroussent A, Hartmann O *et al*. Dose-dependent neurotoxicity of high-dose busulfan in children: a clinical and pharmacological study. *Cancer Res* 1990;**50**:6203–7.

81 De La Camara R, Tomas JF, Figuera A, Berberana M, Fernandez-Ranada JM. High dose busulfan and seizures. *Bone Marrow Transplant* 1991;**7**:363–4.

82 Khera N, Storer B, Flowers ME *et al*. Nonmalignant late effects and compromised functional status in survivors of hematopoietic cell transplantation. *J Clin Oncol* 2012;**30**:71–7.

83 Majhail NS, Ness KK, Burns LJ *et al*. Late effects in survivors of Hodgkin and non-Hodgkin lymphoma treated with autologous hematopoietic cell transplantation: a report from the Bone Marrow Transplant Survivor Study. *Biol Blood Marrow Transplant* 2007;**13**:1153–9.

84 Vanderwalde AM, Sun CL, Laddaran L *et al*. Conditional survival and cause specific mortality after autologous hematopoietic cell transplantation for hematological malignancies. *Leukemia* 2013;**27**:1139–45.

85 Oddou S, Vey N, Viens P *et al*. Second neoplasms following high-dose chemotherapy and autologous stem cell transplantation for malignant lymphomas: a report of six cases in a cohort of 171 patients from a single institution. *Leukemia Lymphoma* 1998;**31**:187–94.

86 Majhail NS, Rizzo JD, Lee SJ *et al*. Recommended screening and preventive practices for long-term survivors after hematopoietic cell transplantation. *Biol Blood Marrow Transplant* 2012;**18**:348–71.

87 Metayer C, Curtis RE, Vose J *et al*. Myelodysplastic syndrome and acute myeloid leukemia after autotransplantation for lymphoma: a multicenter case-control study. *Blood* 2003;**101**:2015–23.

88 Chow EJ, Wong K, Lee SJ *et al*. Late cardiovascular complications after hematopoietic cell transplantation. *Biol Blood Marrow Transplant* 2014;**20**:794–800.

89 Sun CL, Francisco L, Kawashima T *et al*. Prevalence and predictors of chronic health conditions after hematopoietic cell transplantation: a report from the Bone Marrow Transplant Survivor Study. *Blood* 2010;**116**:3129–39; quiz 3377.

90 Chow EJ, Mueller BA, Baker KS *et al*. Cardiovascular hospitalizations and mortality among recipients of hematopoietic stem cell transplantation. *Ann Intern Med* 2011;**155**:21–32.

91 Palomo M, Diaz-Ricart M, Carbo C *et al*. Endothelial dysfunction after hematopoietic stem cell transplantation: role of the conditioning regimen and the type of transplantation. *Biol Blood Marrow Transplant* 2010;**16**:985–93.

92 Ip MS, Yuen KY, Chiu EK, Chan JC, Lam WK, Chan TK. Pulmonary infections in bone marrow transplantation: the Hong Kong experience. *Respiration* 1995;**62**:80–3.

93 Carlson K, Backlund L, Smedmyr B, Oberg G, Simonsson B. Pulmonary function and complications subsequent to autologous bone marrow transplantation. *Bone Marrow Transplant* 1994;**14**:805–11.

94 Badier M, Guillot C, Delpierre S, Vanuxem P, Blaise D, Maraninchi D. Pulmonary function changes 100 days and one year after bone marrow transplantation. *Bone Marrow Transplant* 1993;**12**:457–61.

95 Cerveri I, Zoia MC, Fulgoni P *et al*. Late pulmonary sequelae after childhood bone marrow transplantation. *Thorax* 1999;**54**:131–5.

96 Arvidson J, Bratteby LE, Carlson K *et al*. Pulmonary function after autologous bone marrow transplantation in children. *Bone Marrow Transplant* 1994;**14**:117–23.

97 Sanders JE, Hoffmeister PA, Woolfrey AE *et al*. Thyroid function following hematopoietic cell transplantation in children: 30 years' experience. *Blood* 2009;**113**:306–8.

98 Moser EC, Noordijk EM, Carde P *et al*. Late non-neoplastic events in patients with aggressive non-Hodgkin's lymphoma in four randomized European Organisation for Research and Treatment of Cancer trials. *Clin Lymphoma Myeloma* 2005;**6**:122–30.

99 Ranke MB, Schwarze CP, Dopfer R *et al*. Late effects after stem cell transplantation (SCT) in children: growth and hormones. *Bone Marrow Transplant* 2005;**35**(Suppl 1):S77–81.

100 Ruiz-Soto R, Sergent G, Gisselbrecht C *et al*. Estimating late adverse events using competing risks after autologous stem-cell transplantation in aggressive non-Hodgkin lymphoma patients. *Cancer* 2005;**104**:2735–42.

Long-term follow-up of lymphoma patients after allogeneic hematopoietic cell transplantation

Shylaja Mani and Navneet S. Majhail

Introduction

Allogeneic hematopoietic cell transplantation (HCT) is a treatment option for selected lymphoma patients with high-risk or relapsed disease. Approximately 1000 patients with lymphoma receive an allogeneic HCT in the United States annually [1]. Advances in transplantation technology and improvements in supportive care have led to improvements in early and late survival after allogeneic HCT in general [2]. Advances such as the introduction of reduced-intensity conditioning regimens and availability of alternative donor sources have directly impacted the utilization of allogeneic HCT for patients with lymphoma. As patients survive longer post transplantation, their risks of disease relapse progressively decrease over time. However, they continue to be at risk for morbidity and mortality from late complications. This chapter describes the general principles for long-term follow-up of lymphoma patients who have received an allogeneic HCT and reviews the application of guidelines for preventive practices and screening for late effects [3,4]. The review is primarily focused on follow-up of patients who have survived without disease progression for 1–2 years or more after transplantation. The general goal of long-term follow-up is to monitor for disease progression and late complications.

Long-term survival after allogeneic HCT for lymphoma

Several studies have described long-term survival in allogeneic HCT recipients who are alive and disease-free for 2–5 years after allogeneic transplantation [5–10]. Studies have generally described outcomes for all diagnoses and have not provided survival information specific to patients with lymphoma. An exception is a recent large study from the Center for International Blood and Marrow Transplant Research (CIBMTR) that included 10,632 survivors who were alive and disease-free for at least 2 years after allogeneic HCT using a myeloablative conditioning regimen [5]. Their analysis included 619 lymphoma patients. For these patients, median age at HCT was 34 years, HLA-identical sibling donor source was used for 80% of patients, and 83% of patients had received a total body irradiation (TBI)-based conditioning regimen. Chronic graft-versus-host disease (GVHD) had been reported in 50% of survivors. Probability of overall survival at 10 years after HCT for lymphoma patients was 84% and the 10-year cumulative incidences of relapse and nonrelapse mortality were 6% and 11%, respectively. In multivariate analysis, factors predictive of better long-term survival after allogeneic HCT for lymphoma included younger age at HCT (<25 years), use of an HLA-identical sibling donor, and no history of acute and chronic GVHD after transplantation. The relative mortality rate approached that expected in

Clinical Guide to Transplantation in Lymphoma, First Edition. Edited by Bipin N. Savani and Mohamad Mohty.
© 2015 John Wiley & Sons, Ltd. Published 2015 by John Wiley & Sons, Ltd.

general population controls of a comparable age and gender at approximately 10 years post transplantation. This was in contrast to survivors transplanted for acute leukemia and severe aplastic anemia, whose mortality rates remained higher than the general population until at least 15 years after HCT. These data provide a reference for long-term survival outcomes in lymphoma patients and highlight the relatively high rate of nonrelapse mortality seen in this population of 2-year disease-free survivors. However, the number of lymphoma patients in this analysis was small and studies that include a larger cohort of lymphoma patients are needed.

Follow-up schedule and duration

Long-term survivors need to be seen at periodic intervals to monitor for treatment complications and assess for lymphoma progression. The frequency and extent of these visits depends on the type of lymphoma and disease status at transplantation. For evaluation of disease progression, there are no prospective studies that can guide the optimal follow-up schedule or types of evaluation (e.g., comparing one imaging modality over another). In general, follow-up visits are scheduled every 3 months during the first year, then every 3–6 months thereafter up to 5 years since most lymphoma relapse occurs during this time. After 5 years of completion of therapy and in the absence of clinical findings to suggest lymphoma recurrence, patients can be evaluated once a year. At these visits, history and physical examination should be performed with complete blood count, chemistries, lactate dehydrogenase levels, and additional evaluations for late complications (see next section). The role of routine imaging for monitoring disease status in the longitudinal follow-up of asymptomatic patients is not clear and needs to be individualized to the needs of a specific patient. As described later in this chapter, patients need to be seen at least once a year for evaluation of late complications of transplantation and this follow-up should continue lifelong.

Risk factors for late complications

Allogeneic HCT involves unique exposures which are risk factors for late complications. In addition, pretransplant treatment exposures including chemotherapy and radiation

therapy contribute to late effects. Genetic and lifestyle factors can also increase the risks of late complications. Specific exposures are associated with particular complications (Table 11.1). For example, exposure to TBI and corticosteroids can lead to insulin resistance and increase risks of hypertension, diabetes and metabolic syndrome and ultimately cardiovascular complications [11–13]. Chronic GVHD is a strong risk factor for secondary cancers of the oropharyngeal mucosa and the skin, while TBI increases the risk of secondary breast cancer [14–16]. Pretransplant treatment exposures can contribute to increased risks of late complications post transplantation. For example, use of anthracyclines and radiation therapy to the chest

Table 11.1 Risk factors for late complications in allogeneic HCT recipients with lymphoma.

Exposure	Late complication
Pretransplant anthracycline chemotherapy	Cardiomyopathy
Pretransplant chest radiation	Coronary artery disease Cardiomyopathy
Conditioning chemotherapy	Secondary cancers Infertility
Total body irradiation	Xerophthalmia, cataracts Xerostosis Secondary cancers Cardiovascular complications Growth disturbance, hypothyroidism, hypogonadism Chronic kidney disease Infertility
Chronic GVHD	Prolonged immunodeficiency, late infections Xerophthalmia Xerostosis Bronchiolitis obliterans Secondary cancers Myopathy Complications associated with prolonged steroid exposure
Corticosteroids	Prolonged immunodeficiency, late infections Cataracts Cardiovascular complications Bone loss, avascular necrosis Myopathy
Red cell transfusions	Iron overload
Hepatitis B or C	Cirrhosis

region are well-known risk factors for cardiovascular complications in lymphoma survivors. Additional exposures at the time of transplantation that also contribute to cardiovascular late complications (e.g., TBI) may augment the risks of cardiac dysfunction and toxicity in patients who have already received anthracyclines or chest radiation prior to HCT.

Pertinent exposures that increase risks for late complications should be identified early post transplantation as they may influence the timing and frequency of long-term follow-up and the types of evaluations needed. For example, patients with chronic GVHD need more frequent follow-up compared to patients who do not have GVHD. Hence, the follow-up schedule and frequency has to be individualized for each patient based on time since transplantation, need for disease assessment and risk for lymphoma relapse, ongoing medical issues, and risk factors for late complications.

Guidelines for screening and prevention of late complications

Consensus guidelines for screening and preventive practices for HCT survivors were published in 2012 [3,4]. The recommendations were developed by an international group of experts and lay emphasis on specific transplant-related exposures such as age, gender, type of transplant, prolonged corticosteroid use, chronic GVHD, and use of TBI as part of the conditioning regimen. The guidelines identify late complications by organ system and recommend the minimum set of practices and evaluations that patients need to follow for their prevention and early detection and management. Follow-up for psychosocial issues, fertility, general health maintenance, and secondary cancers is also covered. Although this chapter focuses on allogeneic HCT survivors, the guidelines also apply to recipients of autologous HCT. The National Marrow Donor Program has developed physician and patient-friendly versions of the guidelines that are available online and as a smartphone app [available at www.BeTheMatchclinical.org (healthcare provider version) and www.BeTheMatch.

org/Patient (patient version)]. Table 11.2 lists recommendations for prevention of late complications for lymphoma survivors who have received allogeneic HCT. The table includes recommendations from published guidelines, as well as additional measures that are relevant to lymphoma survivors.

Delivery of care for lymphoma survivors

Lymphoma survivors who have received an allogeneic HCT have unique healthcare needs that are best addressed by a patient-centered multidisciplinary team. Depending on time since transplantation, and based on patient age, gender, and presence of transplant complications (e.g., GVHD), this team can include transplant providers, a hematologist-oncologist, primary care providers, as well as other specialists (e.g., ophthalmologist, dentist, and gynecologist). Studies that can guide the optimal mechanism for care delivery for lymphoma transplant survivors are lacking. However, it is likely that primary care providers will have a greater role to play in the care of patients who are further from transplant and do not have ongoing transplant-related complications such as GVHD. The transplant center or hematologist-oncologist has a greater role to play in patients with GVHD or other transplant complications and in patients who are at high risk for lymphoma progression. Irrespective of these factors, the optimal model for care delivery for lymphoma transplant survivors needs close partnership of several providers and the transplant center.

A treatment summary and survivorship care plan may facilitate the care of lymphoma survivors, especially as they transition from the transplant center back to their hematologist-oncologist or primary care provider. Although a template specific to HCT recipients is not available, this document usually contains a summary of a patient's pretransplant and transplant therapies and, based on his or her exposures, an outline of the preventive care and screening evaluations needed to prevent late complications or detect and treatment them early.

Table 11.2 Guidelines for screening and preventive practices for allogeneic HCT survivors with lymphoma.

Organ system	Late complications	Monitoring tests and preventive measures
Immune system	Infections	Immunizations post transplant according to published guidelines
		Antibiotics for endocarditis prophylaxis according to published guidelines
		Chronic GVHD: prophylaxis against encapsulated organisms and PCP and screening for cytomegalovirus reactivation
Ocular	Cataracts	Routine clinical evaluation at 6 months and 1 year and then at least yearly thereafter
	Sicca syndrome	Ophthalmologic examination with measurement of visual acuity and fundus examination at 1 year
	Microvascular retinopathy	and then at least yearly thereafter
		Chronic GVHD: patients may need clinical evaluation and ophthalmologic examination more frequently
Oral	Sicca syndrome	Clinical oral assessment at 6 months and 1 year and then at least yearly thereafter
	Caries	Dental examination at 1 year and then at least yearly thereafter
	Oropharyngeal cancer	*Chronic GVHD*: patients may need clinical and dental evaluation more frequently
Respiratory	Bronchiolitis obliterans	Routine clinical evaluation at 6 months and 1 year and at least yearly thereafter; PFTs and focused radiologic assessment for patients with symptoms or signs of lung compromise
	Cryptogenic organizing pneumonia	Assessment of tobacco use and counseling against smoking
	Sinopulmonary infections	*Chronic GVHD*: patients may need earlier and more frequent clinical evaluation
Cardiac and vascular	Cardiomyopathy	Routine clinical assessment of cardiovascular risk factors at 1 year and at least yearly thereafter
	Congestive heart failure	Education and counseling on "heart" healthy lifestyle (regular exercise, healthy weight, no smoking, dietary counseling)
	Arrhythmias	Early treatment of cardiovascular risk factors such as diabetes, hypertension, and dyslipidemia
	Coronary artery disease	*TBI and chest radiation recipients*: may need additional periodic work-up (e.g., echocardiogram) based on age and symptoms
	Cerebrovascular disease	*Anthracycline exposure*: patients with prior history of heart failure may need closer monitoring with echocardiogram and cardiology consultation
Liver	Hepatitis B	LFTs every 3–6 months in the first year and then at least yearly thereafter
	Hepatitis C	Monitor viral load by PCR for patients with known hepatitis B or C, with liver and infectious disease specialist consultation
	Iron overload	Consider liver biopsy at 8–10 years after HCT to assess cirrhosis in patients with chronic HCV infection
		Serum ferritin at 1 year after HCT in patients who have received red cell transfusions; consider liver biopsy or imaging study for abnormal results
Renal and genitourinary	Chronic kidney disease	Blood pressure assessment at every clinic visit (at least once a year), with aggressive hypertension management
	Bladder dysfunction	Assess renal function with BUN, creatinine and urine protein at 6 months, 1 year, and at least yearly thereafter
	Urinary tract infections	
Muscle and connective tissue	Myopathy	Follow general population guidelines for physical activity
	Fasciitis	Frequent clinical evaluation for myopathy in patients on corticosteroids
	Polymyositis	
Skeletal	Osteopenia/ osteoporosis	Dual-photon densitometry at 1 year; subsequent testing determined by defects or to assess response to therapy
	Avascular necrosis	Physical activity, vitamin D and calcium supplementation to prevent loss of bone density
		Chronic GVHD: patients with substantial corticosteroid exposure may need dual-photon densitometry earlier
		TBI and pelvic/spine radiation recipients: may need dual-photon densitometry earlier
Nervous system	Neuropsychological and cognitive deficits	Clinical evaluation for symptoms and signs of neurologic dysfunction at 1 year and yearly thereafter
	Peripheral neuropathy	

Table 11.2 *(Continued)*

Organ system	Late complications	Monitoring tests and preventive measures
Endocrine	Hypothyroidism	Thyroid function testing at least once yearly
	Hypoadrenalism	Clinical and endocrinologic gonadal assessment for postpubertal women at 1 year
	Hypogonadism	Gonadal function in men, including FSH, LH, and testosterone, as indicated based on clinical symptoms
	Growth retardation	
Mucocutaneous	Cutaneous sclerosis	Routine self-examination of skin
	Skin GVHD	Avoidance of excessive exposure to sunlight and use of sunscreen
	Genital GVHD	Annual gynecologic examination in women
	Skin cancer	
Second cancers	Solid tumors	Counsel patients about risks of secondary malignancies annually and encourage them to perform
	Hematologic	self examination (e.g., skin, testicles/genitalia)
	malignancies	Counsel patients to avoid high-risk behaviors (e.g., smoking)
	Post-transplant	Follow general population recommendations for colon cancer screening: annual fecal occult blood
	lymphoproliferative	testing, sigmoidoscopy every 5 years with fecal occult testing every 3 years, or colonoscopy every
	disorder	10 years starting at age 50 in the absence of family history
		Follow general population recommendations for breast cancer screening: screening mammograms every 1–2 years starting at age 40 (see below for patients with radiation exposure)
		Follow general population guidelines for cervical cancer screening: Pap smears every 1–3 years in women older than 21 years or within 3 years of initial sexual activity, whichever occurs earlier
		TBI and chest irradiation recipients: screening mammography in women starting at age 25 or 8 years after radiation exposure, whichever occurs later but no later than age 40
Psychosocial and sexual	Depression	Clinical assessment throughout recovery period, at 6 months, 1 year, and annually thereafter, with referral to a mental health professional for patients with recognized deficits
	Anxiety	Regularly assess level of spousal/caregiver psychological adjustment and family functioning
	Fatigue	
	Sexual dysfunction	Query adults about sexual function at 6 months, 1 year, and at least annually thereafter
Fertility	Infertility	Consider referral to appropriate specialists for patients who are contemplating on pregnancy or are having difficulty conceiving
		Counsel sexually active patients in the reproductive age group about birth control post HCT
General health		Screening for hypertension and hypercholesterolemia at least once a year
		Screening for type 2 diabetes at least once a year
		Screening for depression at least once a year
		Follow general population guidelines for physical activity: adults (age 18–64) should do 2½ hours a week of moderate-intensity, or 1¼ hours of vigorous-intensity aerobic physical activity or an equivalent combination of moderate- and vigorous-intensity aerobic exercise

BUN, blood urea nitrogen; FSH, follicle-stimulating hormone; HCT, hematopoietic cell transplantation; HCV, hepatitis C virus; LFT, liver function test; LH, luteinizing hormone; PCP, *Pneumocystis jirovecii* pneumonia; PCR, polymerase chain reaction; PFT, pulmonary function test.

References

1 Pasquini MC, Wang Z. Current use and outcome of hematopoietic stem cell transplantation: CIBMTR Summary Slides, 2013. Available at http://www.cibmtr.org

2 Majhail NS, Tao L, Bredeson C *et al.* Prevalence of hematopoietic cell transplant survivors in the United States. *Biol Blood Marrow Transplant* 2013;**19**:1498–501.

3 Majhail NS, Rizzo JD, Lee SJ *et al.* Recommended screening and preventive practices for long-term survivors after hematopoietic cell transplantation. *Biol Blood Marrow Transplant* 2012;**18**:348–71.

4 Majhail NS, Rizzo JD, Lee SJ *et al.* Recommended screening and preventive practices for long-term survivors after hematopoietic cell transplantation. *Bone Marrow Transplant* 2012;**47**:337–41.

5 Wingard JR, Majhail NS, Brazauskas R *et al.* Long-term survival and late deaths after allogeneic hematopoietic cell transplantation. *J Clin Oncol* 2011;**29**:2230–9.

6 Bhatia S, Francisco L, Carter A *et al.* Late mortality after allogeneic hematopoietic cell transplantation and functional status of long-term survivors: report from the Bone Marrow Transplant Survivor Study. *Blood* 2007;**110**:3784–92.

7 Goldman JM, Majhail NS, Klein JP *et al.* Relapse and late mortality in 5-year survivors of myeloablative allogeneic

hematopoietic cell transplantation for chronic myeloid leukemia in first chronic phase. *J Clin Oncol* 2010;**28**:1888–95.

8 Martin PJ, Counts GW Jr, Appelbaum FR *et al*. Life expectancy in patients surviving more than 5 years after hematopoietic cell transplantation. *J Clin Oncol* 2010;**28**:1011–16.

9 Nivison-Smith I, Simpson JM, Dodds AJ, Ma DD, Szer J, Bradstock KF. Relative survival of long-term hematopoietic cell transplant recipients approaches general population rates. *Biol Blood Marrow Transplant* 2009;**15**:1323–30.

10 Majhail NS, Rizzo JD. Surviving the cure: long term followup of hematopoietic cell transplant recipients. *Bone Marrow Transplant* 2013;**48**:1145–51.

11 Baker KS, Ness KK, Steinberger J *et al*. Diabetes, hypertension, and cardiovascular events in survivors of hematopoietic cell transplantation: a report from the Bone Marrow Transplantation Survivor Study. *Blood* 2007;**109**:1765–72.

12 Chow EJ, Mueller BA, Baker KS *et al*. Cardiovascular hospitalizations and mortality among recipients of hematopoietic stem cell transplantation. *Ann Intern Med* 2011;**155**:21–32.

13 Majhail NS, Flowers ME, Ness KK *et al*. High prevalence of metabolic syndrome after allogeneic hematopoietic cell transplantation. *Bone Marrow Transplant* 2009;**43**:49–54.

14 Majhail NS, Brazauskas R, Rizzo JD *et al*. Secondary solid cancers after allogeneic hematopoietic cell transplantation using busulfan-cyclophosphamide conditioning. *Blood* 2011;**117**:316–22.

15 Rizzo JD, Curtis RE, Socie G *et al*. Solid cancers after allogeneic hematopoietic cell transplantation. *Blood* 2009;**113**:1175–83.

16 Friedman DL, Rovo A, Leisenring W *et al*. Increased risk of breast cancer among survivors of allogeneic hematopoietic cell transplantation: a report from the FHCRC and EBMT Late Effect Working Party. *Blood* 2008;**111**:939–44.

CHAPTER 12

First 100 days of the autologous hematopoietic stem cell transplantation process in lymphoma

Angela Moreschi Woods

Introduction and orientation to transplant process

After arrival at the transplant center (before the transplant), each patient completes a thorough evaluation followed by stem cell collection. The term "transplant" is used, but the treatment is better summarized as high-dose chemotherapy (to treat the lymphoma) followed by autologous stem cell rescue, which is how the patient will recover from the toxic effects of the chemotherapy on the bone marrow. As individuals arrive at a transplant center, they are likely still learning what this process holds for them, even though they have been informed by their local or primary providers and by their family and friends, who have likely searched the internet. Now the patient is going to confirm what the future may hold. In 2010, non-Hodgkin lymphoma (NHL) was the second most common indication for autologous transplant for patients aged 50 years and older [1]. However, they will meet many other patients at their center, including those with other diseases such as multiple myeloma and leukemia and those who will receive stem cells from an allogeneic source (donor and recipient are not the same person). As this process unravels, they will realize there are some similarities with their friends in the waiting room, along with many differences. They will encounter various types of lymphoma and various types of transplant and chemotherapy, a variety of ages and physical conditions, and varying degrees of comorbidity (additional health conditions such as diabetes). For each patient all these aspects will likely have an effect on transplant outcome during the first 100 days.

The day of the stem cell infusion is considered day zero, when patients' previously frozen cells are returned. Before they were frozen, a preservative called dimethyl sulfoxide (DMSO) was added. The frozen bags are thawed, usually at the bedside with the patient's family and friends present, and the liquid/cells are injected intravenously into the patient. This liquid contains the stem cells that normally reside in the bone marrow and which mature into white blood cells, immune system cells, red blood cells, and platelets. There is a possibility of a reaction to DMSO, such as chills, flushing, headache, chest pressure, shortness of breath, nausea, vomiting, and a bad taste in the mouth. If these symptoms do occur, they commonly resolve quickly. Most patients receive premedication prior to the infusion to help prevent significant side effects from the DMSO. The 100-day time period begins as "day +1," which is the day after their pre-collected autologous stem cells are infused.

At many centers these days the patient is transplanted as an outpatient, walking, driving, or riding a shuttle to and from the clinic every day. Some centers still manage their transplant patients as inpatients, residing in a hospital ward for part of this time. This may be due to logistics such as transportation, lack of a 24-hour caregiver, inadequate clinic space or staff, or sometimes when a patient is considered more high risk for various reasons (Table 12.1).

Clinical Guide to Transplantation in Lymphoma, First Edition. Edited by Bipin N. Savani and Mohamad Mohty.
© 2015 John Wiley & Sons, Ltd. Published 2015 by John Wiley & Sons, Ltd.

Table 12.1 First 100 days of the autologous hematopoietic stem cell transplantation process in lymphoma.

Timeframe	General events	Side effects from chemotherapy (and radiation if given)	Fevers and infections
Days −13 to −1	Chemotherapy* administered	Side effects may begin, such as fatigue, decreased appetite, nausea, vomiting, diarrhea, constipation, mouth sores	Fevers may start and infections can occur
Day 0	Hematopoietic stem cell infusion		
Days 1–14	Awaiting engraftment of stem cells and blood count recovery. Supportive care	Most chemotherapy side effects (above) occur. Hair loss begins	Most patients are taking preventive antiviral, antibacterial, and antifungal medications. Most fevers and infections occur during this time
Days 10–14	Blood counts start to recover	Side effects start to improve as the body can heal itself with an increasing white blood cell count	
Days 15–30	White blood cell count is usually recovered	Patients start to feel better, similar to their baseline	Most original fevers/infections have resolved, but new episodes may begin
Days 31–100	Patient travels home if not already there. Less appointments with the transplant center, usually followed by their local hematologist	Energy level returns to normal if not already previously recovered	Immune system is slowly improving. Infectious precautions may prevent infections. Fever/infections still possible

*Chemotherapy is the conditioning/preparative regimen. In autologous transplantation, this is the cancer/disease treatment.

Impact of conditioning regimen

The treatment begins with chemotherapy and possible radiation therapy (also called the conditioning/preparative regimen), which starts and finishes prior to the stem cell infusion. As treatment starts, so does the risk of side effects, including nausea, vomiting, diarrhea, mouth sores, constipation, heartburn, indigestion, abdominal pain, decreased appetite, and fatigue. The risk of side effects usually remains until cell counts recover. An abundance of medications is usually available for nausea, vomiting, diarrhea, constipation, heartburn, indigestion, and pain. Although these medications help the side effects become tolerable, they are frequently unable to eradicate or resolve them completely. Depending on the chemotherapy, some patients are already pancytopenic (low blood counts) on day 0, while some patients still have normal blood counts. The blood counts at stem cell infusion do not affect the engraftment of stem cells (the process whereby stem cells return to the bone marrow, reproducing and making new blood cells, which is the beginning of rescue). The goal is for the chemotherapy medications to be excreted from the body prior to stem cell infusion. This is so the chemotherapy does not damage the previously collected and stored "new" stem cells. However, even when the chemotherapy medications are discontinued, their effects persist. This is why

the blood counts may continue to drop and unwanted effects may start or resume. Hair loss is delayed but almost always occurs. Each patient's hair loss may vary, especially with regard to facial and body hair.

Time to engraftment

The first 2 weeks are usually the most difficult for the majority of patients, as this is usually the period with the lowest blood counts and likely the most side effects. This means low white and red blood cells along with low platelets. Normal white blood cells fight infection and heal the body. Red blood cells carry oxygen, while platelets clot the blood, which stops bleeding. This is therefore the time when the majority of red blood cell and platelet transfusions occur. These transfusions can cause allergic reactions as the blood products are donated by people via the American Red Cross. Many centers use premedications such as acetaminophen and diphenhydramine to help prevent allergic reactions, although these drugs are not mandatory. Although the American Red Cross screens the blood products for diseases, there is a small chance of exposure to illnesses such as hepatitis and HIV. Despite the transfusions, the patients can still experience the symptoms and risks of anemia (low red blood cells) and thrombocytopenia (low platelets). Anemia places more pressure on the cardiac system, evidenced by possible symptoms of fatigue, breathlessness on exertion, shortness of breath, decreased stamina, chest pain, or cardiac/heart complications such as arrhythmias (atrial fibrillation is a common type) or myocardial infarction (heart attack). In addition, the patient may experience bruising and bleeding from low platelets. Bleeding can be spontaneous (i.e., unprovoked, versus provoked such as with shaving or falling), which can be mild and easily controlled, but severe bleeding is possible. Bleeding can occur anywhere in the body, but common locations include gums/ mouth sores, nose, in urine or stool, or even coughing or vomiting. Rarely bleeding can occur in the brain (e.g., stroke). Provoked bleeding is usually due to an injury; shaving is discouraged for this reason (until platelets recover), unless using an electric razor. The risk of falls causing bleeding is one reason why patients are usually required to have a decent performance status – a baseline ability to care for themselves and be able to walk to maintain strength. Whether inpatient or outpatient, patients are encouraged to maintain their activity and strength by walking, preferably twice daily. It is also good practice for patients to sit up in a chair most of the day, instead of lying in bed. Both these activities help maintain muscles, endurance, stamina, strength, and expansion of the lungs (which helps prevent pneumonia).

This period is also critical because of the low white blood cell count. There is a serious risk of infections, including pneumonias, when white cell counts are low and also for a period after the white cells normalize, as the entire immune system needs time to recover. Infections can be caused by bacteria, viruses, and/or fungi. Patients will therefore be taking medications such as antibacterials, antivirals, and antifungals, in order to prevent infections before they start. Many patients will also require extra medications, usually multiple antibacterials, because they still experience fevers and infections despite the attempt at prevention, and this combination of preventive and treatment medications leads to numerous pills to swallow or intravenous infusions. The causes of some of these fevers and infections are never found but resolve when the white blood cell count recovers. Sometimes patients even develop a phenomenon called "drug fever," when one of the medications, usually an antibiotic, causes a fever.

This is also the time when the patient's hair starts to fall out. As this hair may shed onto the pillow, many patients acknowledge this dreaded expectation and use electric clippers to "buzz" their head, which also helps decrease the itchiness from hair shedding. This must be done with an electric razor, as the platelet count is generally low.

Almost all patients have begun to recover their blood counts by day 14. Mouth sores, nausea, vomiting, diarrhea, and fatigue all start to resolve. With some patients this resolution happens quickly as blood counts recover, seemingly overnight. For others, more likely older patients, there is a slower healing process, and they may not feel that the fatigue or gastrointestinal symptoms resolve until days 21–30. The most common lingering symptoms include decreased taste and/or a metallic taste of food and drinks, fatigue, and nausea. For this reason, many patients lose weight. Their weight is not as important as maintaining their energy and strength in order to fight infections and being able to exercise, along with maintaining protein levels. A visible side effect of low protein levels is fluid accumulation, better known as swelling or edema, most commonly in the legs and feet.

First months after transplantation and back to home

The 30-day post-transplant period has likely been emotionally and physically draining for the patient and caregiver. Patients frequently say they do not remember certain periods, especially the time when they were sickest. At these times, patients receive support from nurses, physicians, social workers, chaplains, pharmacists, and many important support staff members and, significantly, are supported by the other patients, not in the physical or medical sense but with empathy and camaraderie. They compare "notes" and help each other out, possibly a simple ride to the grocery store, as some choose to bring their vehicles from home and others do not. Every transplant center is different, but it is important to provide information about, for example, the distance from the hospital to the lodging and grocery store, access to the laundry, and whether a fully equipped kitchen is available. Patients undergoing autologous transplantation are more adaptable as they are living at the transplant center for only 1–8 weeks, depending on the schedule for evaluation, collection, and transplant, whereas patients undergoing allogeneic transplantation may be away from home for 4 months solid.

Most centers require patients to stay locally, near the transplant center. For patients with autologous transplants, this period is usually about 28–30 days after stem cell infusion. Some centers will keep a patient longer if there are ongoing issues or side effects. Most patients are close to normal at the end of 30 days in regard to blood counts, eating, energy, and activity. Older patients are more likely to still have issues with these functions. Most patients are extremely excited to go home (around day 30), but some are hesitant and anxious about this transition. They worry about being away from their transplant team/staff, who know what they have been through and what to expect. They are anxious about what to do if they get sick and who will take care of them. They ask questions such as: Where should I go (primary care provider, home/local hematologist, emergency room provider), will these providers know what to do, and will I be able to contact the transplant center for questions or advice? The answer is yes to all these inquiries, and patients should carry the transplant center's phone number with them. Patients also worry about the risks of going home to family, friends, children, pets, neighbors, and church community, which are sometimes the same things they are most excited to have again. These cause anxiety as they now worry about infection more than ever. The transplant staff can provide cautious but realistic advice for going home. Delayed chemotherapy side effects (toxicities) and infections can still occur. Key points include always reporting worrisome symptoms quickly, for example infection/fever/chills, shortness of breath, chest pain, increased or new diarrhea, and bleeding. Avoiding sick people and large crowds, plus washing hands frequently, are very important ways to keep well. Avoiding most animals (other than dogs and cats that are up to date with vaccines) and any feces (*avoid* cat and bird feces), along with not touching or handling dirt, grass, flowers, wood, and chemicals (including any activity that would cause excessive inhalation of these dangers, such as mowing), will help prevent some infections. Because of these infectious risks and the likelihood that after an autologous stem cell transplant most people are not yet strong enough, patients should continue to rehabilitate for the first 100 days. Recommended activities include walking for exercise and light household duties such as cooking. Most patients do not usually return to work during this time as they are focusing on their health, strength, and stamina. However, occasional patients are able to achieve this because they have low-risk occupations or work from home. When in doubt, patients should check with their transplant center about safety. As these patients recover more immune function (usually by day 100), their lives become more normal again.

After they return home, the Center for International Blood and Marrow Transplant Research (CIBMTR) requires transplant centers to continue to monitor and report complications and disease status (if their disease/cancer remains or returns and how much is present). The patient's transplant center will likely perform disease-specific testing or make specific recommendations for follow-up at day 100, 6 months, 1 year, and annually. Disease-specific testing includes lactate dehydrogenase (LDH), computed tomography (CT) of neck, chest, abdomen and pelvis or positron emission tomography (PET)/CT depending on disease/patient, and may also include bone marrow biopsy with flow cytometry, karyotype/chromosome analysis, and possibly fluorescence *in situ* hybridization (FISH) and/or molecular testing.

Even though the risk of death is low, it is still possible in patients with autologous transplants as with any medical procedure. CIBMTR 2010 data show that 100-day mortality is highest for chemotherapy-resistant NHL compared to all other groups. These patients can die from infection or organ toxicity, likely due to these patients having the most treatments prior to transplant, which decreases their immune system and organ function. That being said, relapsed or progressive disease is still the most common cause of death after autologous transplant for any disease/cancer (CIBMTR data).

Reference

1 Pasquini MC, Wang Z. Current use and outcome of hematopoietic stem cell transplantation: CIBMTR Summary Slides, 2013. Available at http://www.cibmtr.org

CHAPTER 13

First 100 days of the allogeneic hematopoietic stem cell transplantation process in lymphoma

Angela Moreschi Woods

Introduction and orientation to transplant process

As individuals arrive at a transplant center, they are likely still learning what this process entails, even though they have been informed by their local or primary providers and by their family and friends, who have likely searched the internet. Now the patient is going to confirm what the future may hold. During 1998–2010, the highest numbers of reduced-intensity conditioning (RIC) allogeneic transplants were performed for types of lymphoma, including chronic lymphocytic leukemia, follicular lymphoma, mantle cell lymphoma, Hodgkin lymphoma, and diffuse large B-cell lymphoma (CIBMTR). However, they will meet many other patients at their center, including those with other diseases such as myelodysplastic syndrome and acute leukemia and those who will receive stem cells from an autologous source (recipient and donor are the same person). As this process unravels, they will realize there are some similarities with their friends in the waiting room, along with many differences. They will encounter various types of lymphoma and various types of transplant and chemotherapy, a variety of ages and physical conditions, and varying degrees of comorbidity (additional health conditions such as diabetes). For each patient all these aspects will likely have an effect on transplant outcome during the first 100 days.

The day of stem cell infusion is considered day zero. This usually occurs as an infusion, similar to a blood transfusion: a bag of liquid is infused intravenously, usually at the bedside, with the patient's family and friends and possibly the donor if it were to be a brother or sister. Because these cells are from a human other than the patient, there is a risk of reaction during this infusion, so the patient is monitored closely. This liquid contains the stem cells that normally reside in the bone marrow and which mature into white blood cells, immune system cells, red blood cells, and platelets. The 100-day time period begins as "day +1," which is the day after the donor's stem cells are infused. The myeloablative regimens (chemotherapy and possibly radiation) are more intense (compared with a reduced-intensity regimen), usually with more significant side effects (nausea, vomiting, diarrhea, mouth sores, need for intravenous nutrition, lung/liver/heart/kidney inflammation, bleeding) and higher risk for intensive care transfer. These regimens are usually used in the younger population. Older patients (or those with numerous previous treatments) usually receive the reduced-intensity or mini regimens, which are less intense with regard to expected side effects and thus enable older patients to tolerate treatment.

At many centers these days the patient is transplanted as an outpatient, walking, driving, or riding a shuttle to and from the clinic every day. Some centers still manage their transplant patients as inpatients, residing in a hospital ward for part of this time. This may be due to logistics such as transportation, lack of a 24-hour

Clinical Guide to Transplantation in Lymphoma, First Edition. Edited by Bipin N. Savani and Mohamad Mohty.

Table 13.1 First 100 days of the allogeneic hematopoietic stem cell transplantation process in lymphoma.

Timeframe	General events	Side effects from chemotherapy (and radiation if given)	Fevers and infections	GVHD
Days −13 to −1	Chemotherapy* administered	Side effects may begin, e.g., fatigue, decreased appetite, nausea, vomiting, diarrhea, constipation, mouth sores	Fevers may start and infections can occur	Not possible
Day 0	Hematopoietic stem cell infusion			
Days 1–14	Awaiting engraftment of stem cells and blood count recovery. Supportive care	Most chemotherapy side effects occur. Hair loss begins	Most patients are taking preventive antiviral, antibacterial, and antifungal medications. Many fevers and infections occur during this time	Uncommon forms of hyperacute GVHD can begin
Days 10–14	Blood counts start to recover	Side effects start to improve as the body can heal itself with an increasing white blood cell count		The risk of GVHD begins as donor cells start to engraft
Days 15–30	White blood cell count is usually recovered	Patients start to feel better, similar to their baseline	Most original fevers/ infections have resolved, but new episodes may begin	Most GVHD cases that occur during this timeframe are with myeloablative regimens
Days 31–100	Usually remain near their transplant center. Immune system is still low as most patients are still on medications to prevent GVHD, which prevent the immune system from returning to normal	Energy level is variable, as some patients recover similar to those undergoing autologous transplant but others experience infections and GVHD which cause new symptoms	The risk of fever and infection remains. Immune system recovery depends on preparative regimen/type of transplant along with GVHD activity. Infections include viral, bacterial, and fungal	Risk continues. GVHD depresses the immune system further, along with GVHD treatment, which also may increase infections. New symptoms arise, such as fatigue, fever, rash, nausea, vomiting, diarrhea, decreased appetite, weight loss, liver test abnormalities

*Chemotherapy is the conditioning/preparative regimen. With allogeneic transplant, it is partially a treatment for the cancer/disease and partially to prepare the recipient's body for the donor cells.

caregiver, inadequate clinic space or staff, or sometimes when a patient is considered more high risk for various reasons (e.g., myeloablative transplant) (Table 13.1).

Impact of conditioning regimen

In allogeneic transplantation, a conditioning/preparative regimen (chemotherapy and possible radiation) is used to prepare the recipient's body by treating any residual disease, making space for new cells by emptying the bone marrow, and inhibiting the immune system to prevent rejection of the donor cells. As the conditioning regimen commences (before day 0), so does the risk of side effects, including nausea, vomiting, diarrhea, mouth sores, constipation, heartburn, indigestion, abdominal pain, decreased appetite, and fatigue. The risk of side effects usually remains until cell counts recover. An abundance of medications is usually available for nausea, vomiting, diarrhea,

constipation, heartburn, indigestion, and pain. Although these medications help the side effects become tolerable, they are frequently unable to eradicate or resolve them completely. Depending on the conditioning/preparative regimen, some patients are already pancytopenic (low blood counts) on day 0, while some patients still have normal blood counts. The blood counts at stem cell infusion do not affect the engraftment of stem cells (the process whereby stem cells return to the bone marrow, reproducing and making new blood cells). The goal is for the chemotherapy medications to be excreted from the body prior to stem cell infusion. This is so the chemotherapy does not damage the donor stem cells. However, even when the chemotherapy medications are discontinued, their effects persist. This is why the blood counts may continue to drop and unwanted effects may start or resume. Hair loss is delayed but almost always occurs. Each patient's hair loss may vary, especially with regard to facial and body hair.

Time to engraftment

The first 2 weeks are usually the most difficult for the majority of patients, as this is usually the period with the lowest blood counts and likely the most side effects. This means low white and red blood cells along with low platelets. Normal white blood cells fight infection and heal the body. Red blood cells carry oxygen, while platelets clot the blood, which stops bleeding. This is therefore the time when the majority of red blood cell and platelet transfusions occur. These transfusions can cause allergic reactions as the blood products are donated by people via the American Red Cross. Many centers use premedications such as acetaminophen and diphenhydramine to help prevent allergic reactions, although these drugs are not mandatory. Although the American Red Cross screens the blood products for diseases, there is a small chance of exposure to illnesses such as hepatitis and HIV. Despite the transfusions, the patients can still experience the symptoms and risks of anemia (low red blood cells) and thrombocytopenia (low platelets). Anemia places more pressure on the cardiac system, evidenced by possible symptoms of fatigue, breathlessness on exertion, shortness of breath, decreased stamina, chest pain, or cardiac/heart complications such as arrhythmias (atrial fibrillation is a common type) or myocardial infarction (heart attack). In addition, the patient may experience bruising and bleeding from low platelets. Bleeding can be spontaneous (i.e., unprovoked, versus provoked such as with shaving or falling), which can be mild and easily controlled, but severe bleeding is possible. Bleeding can occur anywhere in the body, but common locations include gums/mouth sores, nose, in urine or stool, or even coughing or vomiting. Rarely bleeding can occur in the brain (e.g., stroke). Provoked bleeding is usually due to an injury; shaving is discouraged for this reason (until platelets recover), unless using an electric razor. The risk of falls causing bleeding is one reason why patients are usually required to have a decent performance status – a baseline ability to care for themselves and be able to walk to maintain strength. Whether inpatient or outpatient, patients are encouraged to maintain their activity and strength by walking, preferably twice daily. It is also good practice for patients to sit up in a chair most of the day, instead of lying in bed. Both these activities help maintain muscles, endurance, stamina, strength, and expansion of the lungs (which helps prevent pneumonia).

This period is also critical because of the low white blood cell count. There is a serious risk of infections, including pneumonias, when white cell counts are low and also for a period after the white cells normalize, as the entire immune system needs time to recover. Infections can be caused by bacteria, viruses, and/or fungi. Patients will therefore be taking medications such as antibacterials, antivirals, and antifungals, in order to prevent infections before they start. Many patients will also require extra medications, usually multiple antibacterials, because they still experience fevers and infections despite the attempt at prevention, and this combination of preventive and treatment medications leads to numerous pills to swallow or intravenous infusions. The causes of some of these fevers and infections are never found but resolve when the white blood cell count recovers. Sometimes patients even develop a phenomenon called "drug fever," when one of the medications, usually an antibiotic, causes a fever.

This is also the time when the patient's hair starts to fall out. As this hair may shed onto the pillow, many patients acknowledge this dreaded expectation and use electric clippers to "buzz" their head, which also helps decrease the itchiness from hair shedding. This must be done with an electric razor, as the platelet count is generally low.

First months after transplantation

Almost all patients receiving peripheral blood stem cells have started to recover their blood counts by day 14 (bone marrow recipients may take until day 21). "Engraftment" is the term used to describe this early recovery of blood counts, but it also describes the acceptance and incorporation of the donor cells. Mouth sores, nausea, vomiting, diarrhea, and fatigue all start to resolve. With some patients this resolution happens quickly as blood counts recover, seemingly overnight. For others, more likely older patients, there is a slower healing process, and they may not feel that the fatigue or gastrointestinal symptoms resolve until days 21–30. The most common lingering symptoms include decreased taste and/or a metallic taste of food and drinks, fatigue, and nausea. For this reason, many patients lose weight. Their weight is not as important as maintaining their energy and strength in order to fight infections and being able to exercise, along with maintaining protein levels. A visible side effect of low protein levels is fluid accumulation, better known as swelling or edema, most commonly in the legs and feet.

Patients receiving allogeneic transplants are also at risk for graft-versus-host disease (GVHD), which may start as early as a few days before the engraftment of the donor cells. Theoretically, the risk of GVHD can last forever, but usually persists for a few years. Unwanted immune reactions, such as rejection of the donor cells by the recipient's immune system, can occur and this is one of the reasons that patients receive chemotherapy (radiation sometimes) and immunosuppressive drugs such as cyclosporine or tacrolimus in addition to methotrexate or mycophenolate that help prevent rejection and ensure the recipient accepts the donor cells. GVHD is an immune reaction where the donor cells recognize the recipient as foreign, creating mild to severe side effects and complications. The occurrence of GVHD usually signifies that the recipient's body has accepted the donor cells and that the desired engraftment or "changeover" has begun. The goal is for the recipient to eventually possess the donor's bone marrow/blood cells (disease/cancer-free cells) plus the donor's immune system. Hopefully, developing the donor's immune system will ensure that the disease/cancer will not be able to grow again in the future, a phenomenon called the graft-versus-lymphoma effect. This positive immune reaction is the response that is desired. When GHVD occurs, which it does very often, the effects can be mild to severe, requiring few or sometimes major treatments. GVHD can be fatal, so it must be taken seriously. The presence of the GVHD immune response can inhibit other parts of the immune system, causing more infections to occur. In addition, GVHD treatment itself commonly depresses the immune system further, which also increases the risk of infections. Frequently, GVHD and infection occur simultaneously, evidenced as a new infection sometimes just days before the GVHD symptoms begin.

Beyond first months after transplantation and back to home

The 100-day post-transplant period has likely been emotionally and physically draining for the patient and caregiver. Patients frequently say they do not remember certain periods, especially the time when they were very unwell. At these times, patients receive support from nurses, physicians, social workers, chaplains, pharmacists, and many important support staff members and, significantly, are supported by the other patients, not in the physical or medical sense but with empathy and camaraderie. They compare "notes" and help each other out, possibly a simple ride to the grocery store, as some choose to bring their vehicles from home and others do not. Every transplant center is different, but it is important to provide information about, for example, the distance from the hospital to the lodging and grocery store, access to the laundry, and whether a fully equipped kitchen is available.

Most centers require patients to stay locally, near the transplant center. For patients with allogeneic transplants, this period is usually about 90–100 days after stem cell infusion. Some centers will keep a patient longer if there are ongoing issues or side effects, especially GVHD and infection. Most patients are close to normal at the end of 90 days in regard to blood counts, eating, energy, and activity. Most patients are extremely excited to go home around day 100, but some are hesitant and anxious about this transition. They worry about being away from their transplant team/staff, who know what they have been through and what to expect. They are anxious about what to do if they get sick and who will take care of them. They ask questions such as: Where should I go (primary care provider, home/local hematologist, emergency room provider), will these providers know what to do, and will I be able to contact the transplant center for questions or advice? The answer is yes to all these enquiries, and patients should carry the transplant center's phone number with them. Patients also worry about the risks of going home to family, friends, children, pets, neighbors, and church community, which are sometimes the same things they are most excited to have again. These cause anxiety as they now worry about infection more than ever. The transplant staff can provide cautious but realistic advice for going home. Delayed chemotherapy side effects (toxicities), GVHD, and infections can still occur. Key points include always reporting worrisome symptoms quickly, for example infection/fever/chills, shortness of breath, chest pain, nausea/vomiting/diarrhea, lack of appetite/weight loss, skin rash, and bleeding. Avoiding sick people and large crowds, plus washing hands frequently, are very important ways to keep well. Avoiding most animals (other than dogs and cats that are up to date with vaccines) and any feces (*avoid* cat and bird feces), along with not touching or handling dirt, grass, flowers, wood, and chemicals (including any activity that would cause excessive inhalation of these dangers, such as mowing), will help prevent some infections. Because of these infectious risks and the likelihood that after an allogeneic stem cell transplant most people are not yet strong enough, patients should continue to rehabilitate for the first 6 months. Recommended activities include walking for exercise and light household duties such as cooking. Most patients do not usually return to work during this time as they are focusing on their health, strength, and stamina. However, occasional patients are able to achieve this because they have low-risk occupations or work from home. When in doubt, patients should check with their transplant center about safety. As these patients recover more immune function (usually by 6 months unless there is active GVHD or ongoing treatment/prevention), their lives become more normal again.

After they return home, the Center for International Blood and Marrow Transplant Research (CIBMTR) requires transplant centers to continue to monitor and report complications and disease status (if their disease/cancer remains or returns and how much is present). The patient's transplant center will likely perform disease-specific testing or make specific recommendations for follow-up at 6 months, 1 year, and annually.

Disease-specific testing includes lactate dehydrogenase (LDH), computed tomography (CT) of neck, chest, abdomen and pelvis or positron emission tomography (PET)/CT depending on disease/patient, and likely includes bone marrow biopsy with flow cytometry, karyotype/chromosome analysis, and possibly fluorescence *in situ* hybridization (FISH) and/or molecular testing. The transplant center will likely perform transplant-specific testing for donor engraftment/status, such as sorted and unsorted chimerism or status of blood type conversion with Anti-A or Anti-B titers.

Even though the risk of death has become lower over the years, it is still possible. The percentage varies depending on, for example, age, disease, donor source, and conditioning regimen. CIBMTR 2010 data shows that 100-day mortality is highest for chemotherapy-resistant NHL compared to all other groups. These patients can die from infection or organ toxicity, likely due to these patients having the most treatments prior to transplant, which decreases their immune system and organ function.

Reference

1 Pasquini MC, Wang Z. Current use and outcome of hematopoietic stem cell transplantation: CIBMTR Summary Slides, 2013. Available at http://www.cibmtr.org

CHAPTER 14

Stem cell transplantation in follicular lymphoma

Satyajit Kosuri and Koen Van Besien

Introduction

Follicular lymphoma is the most common indolent non-Hodgkin lymphoma (NHL), with close to 30,000 new cases per year in the United States alone [1]. Although it is a chemosensitive disease, the majority of patients present in advanced stages and remain incurable with conventional strategies [2]. With the multitude of advancements in front-line and salvage settings, such as rituximab [3,4] and newer targeted agents [5], duration of responses and survival have improved. This progress and the somewhat sobering results of randomized studies of autologous transplant in first remission necessitate a reconsideration of the role of both autologous and allogeneic transplant in the management paradigm for follicular lymphoma.

Autologous transplant as consolidation for first remission

The linear log relationship between dose and tumor cytotoxicity [6] provides the theoretical basis for administering escalated doses of chemotherapy followed by stem cell rescue in an attempt to overcome disease resistance. Given the inevitability of tumor progression in many follicular lymphoma patients, autologous transplant was investigated as consolidation in first remission as an effort to improve survival. Three randomized studies were conducted in the pre-rituximab era which

found an improvement in progression-free survival (PFS), but due to transplant-associated toxicities no definitive overall survival advantage was established.

The German Low Grade Lymphoma Study Group (GLSG) randomized 240 patients with stage 3 or 4 follicular lymphoma with a partial or complete remission with induction therapy to either autologous transplant or interferon-alpha maintenance [7]. With a median follow-up of 4.2 years the study found a 2-year (79.1% vs. 52.7%) and estimated 5-year (64.7% vs. 33.3%) PFS favoring autologous transplant. Early mortality was 2.5% in both cohorts. However, the rate of secondary acute myeloid leukemia (AML)/myelodysplastic syndrome (MDS) was significantly higher with autologous transplant (3.5% vs. 0%). Two French study groups were able to comment on overall survival with mature data. The GELA group compared CHVP (cyclophosphamide, doxorubicin, vepeside, and prednisone) combined with interferon-alpha versus four cycles of CHOP (cyclophosphamide, doxorubicin, vincristine, and prednisone) followed by autologous transplant with cyclophosphamide, etoposide and total body irradiation (TBI) conditioning. After an extended 7.5-year median follow-up period, event-free survival (EFS) was 28% for the interferon arm and 38% for the transplant arm ($P = 0.11$) with no difference in overall survival between the groups (71 and 76%, $P = 0.53$) [8]. The GOELAMS study group investigated the use of an induction regimen of VCAP (vincristine, cyclophosphamide, doxorubicin, and prednisone) and IMVP-16 (ifosfamide,

Clinical Guide to Transplantation in Lymphoma, First Edition. Edited by Bipin N. Savani and Mohamad Mohty.
© 2015 John Wiley & Sons, Ltd. Published 2015 by John Wiley & Sons, Ltd.

methotrexate, etoposide) followed by autologous transplant against CHVP and interferon-alpha [9]. This initial study reported an EFS benefit with autologous transplant of 60% versus 48% ($P = 0.05$) at 5 years with no overall survival advantage. They too found increased incidences of secondary malignancies in the transplant arm (six MDS/AML, four solid tumors, with seven fatalities compared to no secondary malignancies in the interferon arm). The 5-year actuarial risk of secondary malignancy after transplant was 18.6%. After an extended follow-up period of 9 years the estimated PFS was 64% with autologous transplant and 39% for the chemotherapy group ($P = 0.004$) [10]. Since the inception of the study 12 secondary malignancies occurred after autologous transplant, half of which were MDS/AML compared to one secondary malignancy in the comparator arm. Interestingly, of 35 patients treated for relapse with chemotherapy, 15 underwent autologous transplant and all achieved a second complete remission, except one for whom the response was unknown.

As rituximab became a standard component in follicular lymphoma management, an Italian study group conducted a multicenter randomized Phase III trial comparing high-dose sequential therapy (R-HDS) with autologous transplant without TBI against R-CHOP in 136 stage III or IV follicular lymphoma patients under the age of 60 [11]. There was a statistically significant difference in EFS favoring transplant compared to chemotherapy only (61% vs. 28%, respectively). Even though there was a greater percentage of molecular remissions after autologous transplant, there was no difference in overall survival. This may be partly due to the fact that the cumulative incidence of secondary MDS/AML at 4 years was 6.6% for R-HDS compared with 1.7% for R-CHOP, with secondary solid tumors being equal. Also corroborating the long-term findings of the GOELAMS study group, a population of patients benefited from autologous transplant after having relapsed with standard chemotherapy. A recent meta-analysis including three randomized clinical trials totaling 701 patients confirmed the lack of overall survival benefit with autologous transplant as upfront consolidative therapy [12].

With maturation of earlier data, showing lack of overall survival benefit and increased occurrence of therapy-related MDS/AML, autologous transplant is not recommended as a consolidation strategy for follicular lymphoma patients in first remission. A recent consensus statement by the European Society for

Blood and Marrow Transplantation (EBMT) Lymphoma Working Party supports this notion [13].

Autologous transplant for relapsed follicular lymphoma

Most patients with follicular lymphoma will experience serial relapses and/or progression with the likelihood of inducing further remissions declining with each subsequent line of salvage therapy. Therefore, autologous transplant can play an important role in patients with recurrent follicular lymphoma, as it can induce durable remissions more often than other forms of salvage therapy with relatively limited toxicity.

The only Phase III randomized study which prospectively investigated the use of autologous transplant in the relapsed setting was the EBMT sponsored CUP (conventional chemotherapy, unpurged graft, purged graft) trial [14]. It compared salvage chemotherapy alone to chemotherapy followed by either an unpurged or purged TBI conditioned autologous transplant. Despite slow accrual resulting in early termination of the study, 89 patients less than age 65 who obtained at least a partial remission mostly after first relapse were randomized to one of the three arms. The purged and unpurged autologous transplant arms were combined due to the limited number of patients and demonstrated a notable difference in 2-year PFS and overall survival (55% and 71%, respectively) when compared to chemotherapy alone (26% and 46%, respectively). These survival benefits should be viewed in context of the fact that this study was conducted prior to the standard incorporation of rituximab in initial treatment strategies.

A large EBMT registry study retrospectively evaluated 693 follicular lymphoma patients treated from 1979 to 1995 with autologous transplant [15]. Almost all patients had chemosensitive disease, achieved a first or second remission, and most received TBI-based conditioning. The incidence of relapse at a median of 1.5 years post autologous transplant was 54%. This risk of relapse was related to disease status prior to transplant and was slightly higher in those receiving non-TBI-based conditioning. PFS was 31% and overall survival was 52% at 10 years for the entire cohort and 27% and 47%, respectively, at 15 years. Factors which contributed to a shorter overall survival on multivariate analysis included chemoresistant disease, age above 45 years, and TBI-based conditioning. The nonrelapse mortality was higher at 5 and 10 years for those receiving TBI compared to those who did not. This may be due in part to the higher incidence of, and death from, secondary neoplasms (13.5% vs. 3.5%), specifically MDS/AML (8.5% vs. 1.7%), among those receiving TBI versus chemotherapy only conditioning. This study confirmed the ability of autologous transplant to induce durable remissions and although conducted prior to rituximab it remains relevant because of its large cohort size and prolonged follow-up. A German retrospective analysis also included a large group of patients with median follow-up of 8 years [16]. Here, 241 follicular lymphoma patients underwent autologous transplant with TBI-based conditioning unless previously irradiated in which case they received BEAM (BCNU, etoposide, ara-C, melphalan) or Bu/Cy (busulfan/cyclophosphamide) conditioning. The 10-year relapse probability, PFS and overall survival were 47%, 49%, and 75%, respectively. Importantly the authors noted only a few relapses (3/103) occurring 6 years after autologous transplant and a plateau of the EFS curve at this time suggesting that approximately half of the patients were cured.

A joint English and American study retrospectively investigated the long-term outcomes of 121 follicular lymphoma patients who underwent autologous transplant compared to historical controls. All patients had been conditioned with cyclophosphamide and TBI and transplanted in second or subsequent remissions. With a minimum length of follow-up of 12 years, the authors reported that 48% of patients were free from disease progression, with 54% alive at 10 years. Importantly, those transplanted in second remission survived longer than those transplanted at a later time, lending credence to the concept that utilizing autologous transplant earlier in the disease course may offer a benefit compared to waiting for later responses [17].

More recent studies reflect the effects of rituximab use and of chemotherapy-based conditioning on transplant outcomes. A Canadian retrospective analysis conducted from 1993 to 2008 evaluated 100 follicular lymphoma patients under the age of 70 with good performance status who underwent autologous transplant after first or second relapse or for refractory disease [18]. TBI was administered to 59 patients. With a median follow-up of 65 months, 40 patients relapsed, the 5-year EFS was 56%, and overall survival was 70%, with projected 10-year rates of 54% and 63% respectively. The authors noted a significant prolongation in

EFS post autologous transplant compared to last line of therapy administered prior to transplant. Evaluation of the EFS curve revealed a plateau at 6 years. The authors noted that administration of rituximab within 6 months prior to autologous transplant improved EFS, especially in those with FLIPI (Follicular lymphoma International Prognostic Index) scores of 2–5 at the time of relapse prior to salvage therapy and autologous transplant. Importantly there was no difference in EFS between those who failed rituximab prior to autologous transplant versus those who did not. With a decreased rate of secondary malignancy compared to historical data [15,17], three of the four patients who developed secondary MDS/AML received TBI-based conditioning.

The largest single-center cohort analysis of BEAM conditioning in follicular lymphoma was undertaken by a British group [19]. They analyzed 70 patients aged less than 70 years with chemosensitive relapsed follicular lymphoma. Rituximab was administered in 66% of patients as part of front-line or salvage therapy prior to autologous transplant; 34% of patients were transplanted in first remission, 50% in second remission, and 16% in subsequent remissions. With a median follow-up of 6.8 years, the study demonstrated a 7-year PFS of 60% and overall survival of 76%. The authors noted a significant difference in overall survival for patients transplanted in first or second remission compared to those transplanted in subsequent remissions. Importantly, there was no significant difference in 7-year overall survival for those patients who received rituximab prior to autologous transplant compared to those who were rituximab naive (78% vs. 72%, respectively, $P = 0.51$). All three cases of secondary malignancy (two MDS/AML, one malignancy of the urogenital tract) occurred in patients transplanted in third remission. This study suggests that more lines of pretransplant chemotherapy may be a contributing factor to secondary malignancies. This concept is supported by data showing occult MDS in some patients prior to transplant [20]. The authors reported no overt relapses after 6.4 years with a plateau in the EFS curve in patients transplanted in first or second remission.

Collectively, these analyses (Table 14.1) establish four compelling findings. First, retrospective studies [15,16,18,19,21] consistently showed a plateau for EFS curves evident at approximately 6 years and beyond post autologous transplant. There exists a subgroup of approximately 50% of patients with chemotherapy-sensitive

Table 14.1 Autologous transplant performed for relapsed follicular lymphoma [17,19,25].

Study	No.	Median follow-up (years)	Conditioning	EFS/PFS (%)	Overall survival (%)	TRM (%)	Relapse rate (%)	Comments
Schouten et al. (2003) [14] prospective	89	5.75	TBI based	55	71	10	43	Only prospective trial comparing autologous transplant and chemotherapy only
Montoto et al. (2007) [15] retrospective	693	10.3	TBI based	31	52	9 (5-year)	54	13.5% secondary malignancies in TBI based vs. 3.5% in non-TBI conditioning
Rohatiner et al. (2007) [17] retrospective	121	13.5	TBI based	48	54	22	49.5	15 secondary AML/MDS, 4 other secondary malignancies
Kornacker et al. (2008) [16] retrospective	241	8	TBI based	49	75	6.2	47	Five secondary neoplasms; only 3/103 relapses occurred after 6 years
Peters et al. (2011) [18] retrospective	100	5.4	Variable, 40% TBI	56	70	7	40	Improved EFS if rituximab administered within 6 months of autologous transplant
Kothari et al. (2014) [19] retrospective	70	6.8	BEAM	60	76	12	NR	All secondary malignancies occurred in patients transplanted in later than second remission

EFS, event-free survival; PFS, progression-free survival; TRM, transplant-related mortality; TBI, total body irradiation; BEAM, BCNU/etoposide/Ara-C/melphalan.

recurrences in whom autologous transplant can be curative. Second, failure after prior rituximab exposure did not nullify the survival benefit seen with autologous transplant [18,19,22–24]. Third, TBI-based conditioning for autologous transplant in the relapsed setting was associated with higher rates of long-term nonrelapse mortality due to secondary malignancies, specifically MDS/AML [15,17,21] and therefore has largely been replaced with BEAM. Lastly, the ideal time to offer autologous transplant to chemosensitive follicular lymphoma patients may be in second remission as the benefits optimally outweigh the risks compared to first or later remissions [17,25].

Graft purging

As the relationship between autograft contamination by residual lymphoma cells and relapse risk was established in the early 1990s [26–28], the objective of eliminating these cells from the graft with various "purging" techniques became an important area of investigation. This concept was particularly pertinent to follicular and mantle cell lymphomas in which overt or occult bone marrow infiltration is a common feature [29]. These purging techniques have involved the use of monoclonal antibodies or chemotherapeutic drugs applied with both *ex vivo* and *in vivo* methods.

Numerous studies have been conducted, none of them conclusive. However, pooled data suggest a benefit to purging. This is best illustrated by a study from the Center for International Bone Marrow Transplant Registry (CIBMTR) which compared the outcomes of syngeneic, purged and unpurged autologous transplant with allogeneic stem-cell transplantation (allo-SCT) in NHL patients [30]. Recipients of purged autologous transplant had a lower risk of relapse ($P = 0.0009$), with increased disease-free survival (DFS) ($P = 0.003$) and overall survival ($P = 0.04$) compared to their unpurged counterparts. This study established an important proof of concept for the importance of a tumor-free graft. In their large assessment of autologous transplant versus allo-SCT specifically in follicular lymphoma, CIBMTR also compared purged and unpurged groups and reported a decrease in early and late disease recurrences as well as improved DFS and overall survival in the purged autologous transplant patients [31].

Despite these advantages, *ex vivo* purging methods were technically arduous as well as labor- and cost-intensive [29,31]. Therefore, *in vivo* purging with rituximab became the preferred field of inquiry. Based on preliminary data indicating concurrent administration of rituximab with high-dose Ara-C as a safe and efficient method for *in vivo* purging in follicular lymphoma and mantle cell lymphoma [32], an Italian group conducted a multicenter prospective trial investigating purging with rituximab and chemotherapy prior to autologous transplant in 64 patients with refractory or relapsed follicular lymphoma [33]. Following nested polymerase chain reaction (PCR) for *bcl-2* rearrangement as a marker of residual lymphoma, all 33 patients in whom this data was available obtained PCR-negative harvests and experienced favorable results compared to historical chemotherapy-only programs. Furthermore, *bcl-2* negativity in the blood, bone marrow, and leukapheresis product was associated with the persistence of clinical remission after autologous transplant.

However, a prospective randomized trial by the EBMT Lymphoma Working Party of 280 rituximab-naive patients with chemosensitive recurrence with a median follow-up period of 8.3 years failed to show a benefit for *in vivo* purging with rituximab [34]. They found no difference in PFS or overall survival between the purged and unpurged groups. The authors speculate that the lack of observed benefit may have been related to insufficient sample size – the trial was stopped for slow accrual – and also to the fact that rituximab was given as a single agent rather than with chemotherapy. In the same study, there was a second randomization to rituximab maintenance or not. Patients given four doses of maintenance chemotherapy had a significantly better PFS but not overall survival.

Allogeneic transplant for follicular lymphoma

With ideal timing autologous transplant is an effective part of the management paradigm for relapsed follicular lymphoma. However, a large percentage of patients will experience disease progression or relapse and are at risk of developing secondary AML/MDS. Many others will not qualify for autologous transplant because of insufficient response to salvage or because of inability to collect sufficient stem cells. As a result, the utilization of allo-SCT has been investigated as a potentially curative modality in select relapsed/refractory patients. Potential advantages for allo-SCT consist of the administration of a lymphoma-free graft that operates synergistically with a possible graft-versus-lymphoma (GVL) effect [35–38].

Other than patient selection, the issues which have surrounded the integration of allo-SCT into treatment strategies include the timing, intensity of conditioning regimens, and efforts to reduce transplant-related mortality (TRM) with methods such as graft manipulation and/or GVHD prophylaxis.

In an initial study CIBMTR [39] demonstrated the curative potential of allogeneic sibling transplant for indolent lymphoma. They identified 113 patients transplanted at 50 centers. The conditioning regimen included TBI in 82% of patients. Three-year probabilities of recurrence, survival, and DFS were 16%, 49%, and 49%, respectively. Higher survival was associated with pretransplant Karnofsky performance score of 90% or more, chemotherapy-sensitive disease, use of a TBI-containing conditioning regimen, and age less than 40 years. A subsequent CIBMTR analysis [31] studied 904 follicular lymphoma patients who underwent purged and unpurged autologous transplant (*N* = 728) and matched sibling donor allogeneic transplant (*N* = 176). All allogeneic patients received myeloablative conditioning, which was mostly TBI based (68%). The cumulative rate of relapse was reduced by 54% in the allo-SCT cohort. However, PFS and overall survival between the groups were similar. This was due to a striking increase in TRM with allo-SCT (30%) compared to autologous transplant (4.4 times higher on multivariate analysis). Importantly, in this analysis most relapses after allo-SCT occurred in the first year as opposed to autologous transplant, where relapses occurred over an extended period of time. Consistent with previous studies, all secondary malignancies during this follow-up period occurred after autologous transplant, even though there was a higher percentage of TBI usage in the allo-SCT group.

An EBMT registry report comparing autologous transplant and allo-SCT in early disease patients had similar outcomes [40]. In the low-grade NHL group, the authors similarly reported a lower relapse rate and comparable PFS but lower overall survival in the allo-SCT group, with a TRM at 4 years of 38%. As in the CIBMTR studies, allo-SCT patients tended to have more advanced and resistant disease prior to transplant and received TBI more often. Taken together these large registries demonstrated that allo-SCT with myeloablative conditioning may reduce relapse rates, but unfortunately the high TRM abrogated overall survival benefit. Significantly, CIBMTR studies repeatedly showed that survival and TRM were influenced by patient performance status and chemotherapy sensitivity. There were many subsequent efforts at developing strategies to maintain disease control while improving on the unacceptably high rates of TRM caused by allogeneic transplant.

By the late 1990s small retrospective cohorts found improved outcomes with reduced-intensity conditioning (RIC) compared to historical controls utilizing myeloablative conditioning [41]. To better define this comparison, the CIBMTR analyzed 208 follicular lymphoma patients who received conventional allo-SCT from matched sibling donors with either myeloablative conditioning or RIC from 1997 to 2002 [42]. A total of 120 patients received myeloablative conditioning with Cy-TBI or Bu-Cy; 95% ($N = 84$) of the patients in the RIC arm received a fludarabine-based regimen. Notably, prognostic features of disease sensitivity and performance score prior to transplant were well balanced between the two groups. The 3-year incidences of acute (a)GVHD and chronic (c)GVHD were higher in the RIC arm, and TRM was almost identical at 1 and 3 years post transplant. A significantly higher risk of progression/relapse with RIC did not translate to a difference in PFS or overall survival. Multivariate analysis reconfirmed that decreased performance score and chemotherapy-resistant disease were predictors of outcome, but not the type of conditioning regimen.

These investigations included young patients (40–50 years) and, as the authors from the CIBMTR noted, despite a therapeutic equivalence, the percentage of RIC allo-SCT increased exponentially from the late 1990s to the early 2000s, signifying a shift in practice (Table 14.2). RIC is generally considered a more widely inclusive and tolerable strategy even though the data do not directly establish superiority of one approach over another.

Expanding on the use of RIC, the group from the M.D. Anderson Cancer Center [43] published long-term outcomes of 47 young patients (median age 53 years) with good performance scores and chemosensitive relapsed follicular lymphoma. The cohort received RIC allo-SCT with mostly matched sibling donors ($N = 45$). The patients were administered fludarabine and cyclophosphamide with high-dose rituximab (375 mg/m² on day −13 and high doses of 1000 mg/m² on days −6, +1 and +8) for chemosensitization and as an effort to ameliorate rates of GVHD. All patients achieved complete remission with only two relapsing at a median of 19 months post transplant. PFS and overall survival with a median follow-up of 60 months were 83% and 85%, respectively. Rates of grade 2–4 aGVHD were 11% and extensive cGVHD was 36%. One-year TRM was 10%. In an update of this cohort with a median follow-up of 107 months the estimated PFS and overall survival were 72% and 78%, respectively. Only one further relapse occurred in addition to the two previously reported and occurred 6 years after allo-SCT. The reported incidence of greater than grade 2 aGVHD and extensive stage cGVHD remained virtually the same at 13% and 40%, respectively [44]. These mature data support the concept that RIC with fludarabine, cyclophosphamide and rituximab may be curative for certain relapsed follicular lymphoma patients. It is imperative to recognize that selection of young patients who have a good performance status and chemosensitive disease with matched sibling donors contributed to these outcomes in contrast to the heterogeneous populations and treatments studied together in the registry analyses. Also, the risk of developing cGVHD, one of the leading causes of late morbidity and TRM after allogeneic transplant [45], remains high after RIC. This adds justification for the pursuit of methods such as T-cell depletion to reduce the chance of developing this complication.

An English group investigated the use alemtuzumab for T-cell depletion in 88 patients with relapsed and refractory NHL. Cyclosporine was used as post-transplant GVHD prophylaxis. They noted only six cases of cGVHD and an overall TRM of only 8%. Three-year PFS was 65% for low-grade NHL but this included some patients who achieved remission after donor lymphocyte infusion (DLI) [46]. This was followed by a multicenter prospective study [38] evaluating 82 patients (median age 45 years) with chemosensitive disease who received allo-SCT from 1998 to 2009; 52% of patients received stem cells from an unrelated donor. With a 43-month median follow-up, median incidence of grade 2–3 aGVHD was 13% (8% in patients with

Table 14.2 Reduced-intensity conditioning allogeneic stem cell transplant for relapsed follicular lymphoma.

Study	No.	Median follow-up (years)	Conditioning	EFS/PFS (%)	Overall survival (%)	TRM (%)	Relapse rate (%)	Comments
Hari et al. (2008) [42]	RIC, 88	3	Follicular lymphoma based (RIC)	55	62	28	17	Day 100 grade 2–4 aGVHD, 44%; 3-year cGVHD, 62%
Khouri et al. (2008, 2012) [43,44]	47	8.9	FCR	72	78	15 (5-year)	6	Grade 2–3 aGVHD, 13%; 3-year cGHVD, 58%
Thomson et al. (2010) [38]	82	3.5	FMC	76	76	15	26	Grade 2–3 aGVHD, 13%; cGVHD, 30%
Delgado et al. (2011) [47]	164	4	Follicular lymphoma based (RIC) ± ATG/ alemtuzumab	52, T-cell depletion; 67, conventional	74, T-cell depletion; 74, conventional	18, T-cell depletion; 17, conventional	28, T-cell depletion; 14, conventional	Grade 2–4 aGVHD, 15% (T-cell depletion), 23% (conventional) cGVHD, 25% (T-cell depletion), 46% (conventional)

aGVHD, acute graft-versus-host disease; ATG, antithymocyte globulin; cGVHD, chronic graft-versus-host disease; EFS, event-free survival; FCR, fludarabine/cyclophosphamide/rituximab; FMC, fludarabine/melphalan/cyclophosphamide; PFS, progression-free survival; RIC, reduced-intensity conditioning; TRM, transplant-related mortality.

matched sibling donors and 18% in patients with unrelated donors). Incidence of extensive cGVHD was 11% for patients with matched sibling donors and 29% for patients with unrelated donors. TRM was 15%, with relapse or progression occurring in 23% of the complete cohort. A total of 13 patients required DLI for relapsed disease, 10 of whom then achieved complete remission. PFS and overall survival were 76% at 4 years. A European study compared outcomes of patients receiving a fludarabine and alkylator-based conditioning regimen with alemtuzumab or antithymocyte globulin (ATG) for T-cell depletion (N = 88) versus those without (N = 76) [47]. The incidence of grade 2 or greater aGVHD was lower in patients undergoing T-cell depletion than in those undergoing non-T-cell depletion (17% vs. 31%, P = 0.04). The incidence of cGVHD was considerably smaller (33% vs. 73%, P = 0.01). Despite a higher relapse rate after T-cell depletion, current PFS (which includes patients salvaged with DLI) was similar and overall survival was similar after T-cell depletion and non-T-cell depletion transplant. Disease status at transplantation was the best predictor of long-term outcome. With similar median term survival and concerns over late morbidity and mortality in patients with cGVHD, we continue to pursue T-cell depletion at our center.

Nonsibling donor allogeneic transplant in follicular lymphoma

Although most reports focus on matched sibling donors, in clinical practice most patients needing allo-SCT are without such a donor. For these patients, options include a matched unrelated donor (MUD), cord blood stem cells, or haploidentical donors.

An EBMT registry analysis evaluated 131 patients who received a MUD transplant from 2000 to 2005. The majority of these patients received RIC and 47% had failed previous autologous transplant. With a median follow-up of 36 months, PFS was 47% and overall survival was 51%, with 37% and 48% of patients developing stage 2–4 aGVHD and cGVHD respectively [48].

Another EBMT registry study evaluated unrelated single or double umbilical cord transplants in patients with lymphoid malignancies [49]. A single cord was transplanted in 75% of the cases, with 64% of the patients receiving RIC. The authors reported nonrelapse mortality, PFS, and overall survival rates of 20%, 60%, and 68%, respectively at 1 year in those with indolent lymphoma. Overall, they concluded that umbilical cord transplant is a viable alternative for patients without an HLA-matched donor in chemosensitive lymphoid malignancies. Haploidentical stem cells are also under investigation

(NCT01597778) in hematologic malignancies including follicular lymphoma with encouraging results [50,51].

RIC allogeneic versus autologous transplant

Choosing which transplant procedure would more highly benefit certain patients in the primary relapsed setting can be challenging. A recent EBMT registry study evaluated follicular lymphoma patients who relapsed after a first remission and underwent either autologous transplant ($N = 726$) or RIC allo-SCT ($N = 149$) [52]. Patient characteristics were similar between the groups, but there were a higher percentage with chemoresistant disease in the allo-SCT arm (20% vs. 7%). Patients received a fludarabine-based RIC regimen. The 3-year cumulative incidence of nonrelapse mortality was 5% with autologous transplant compared to 22% with allo-SCT. A higher proportion of relapses occurred in the autologous transplant arm, with close to half of patients relapsing at a median time of 5.4 months post transplant. The allogeneic transplant patients fared much better, with a 20% incidence of relapse occurring at a median of 13 months post transplant. With a median follow-up of 5 years, PFS was similar in the first year after transplant but afterwards favored those patients who underwent allo-SCT (48% vs. 57%). However, there was no difference in overall survival in the two arms. A plateau was present in the PFS curves in the allo-SCT group. In another recent retrospective NCCN analysis of follicular lymphoma in first relapse [24], nonrelapse mortality was much higher in the allo-SCT group which conferred an overall survival advantage for the autologous transplant arm. It must be noted that the allo-SCT group was much smaller ($N = 49$) and combined both related and unrelated donors administered "mostly" RIC. A previous attempt to prospectively investigate autologous transplant and RIC allo-SCT in a biologic assignment study by the Bone Marrow Transplant Clinical Trials Network [53] was closed early due to slow accrual (eight patients in the allo-SCT arm).

Transformed follicular lymphoma

With an annual reported risk of 3–5%, transformation to a more aggressive histology will occur in a percentage of follicular lymphoma patients [54,55]. Outcomes of patients with disease transformation have been poor, with median survival ranging from 1 to 2 years after transformation [15,54]. In the largest early study the EBMT group analyzed autologous transplant consolidation in 50 transformed lymphoma patients with chemosensitive disease and reported 5-year PFS and overall survival rates of 30% and 51%, respectively [56]. Smaller studies showed similar 5-year PFS and overall survival [56–61].

A recent Canadian study addressed the role of transplant in the rituximab era [62]. The authors compared three groups of patients with transformed lymphoma: those undergoing autologous transplant ($N = 22$), allo-SCT ($N = 97$), and only rituximab-containing chemotherapy ($N = 53$). The approximate time from diagnosis to transformation for the entire cohort was 4 years. The authors reported 5-year overall survival of 65% with autologous transplant, 46% with allo-SCT, and 61% with the rituximab chemotherapy group ($P = 0.24$). On multivariate analysis no significant differences in survival were noted between the transplant groups, although an improvement in overall survival was noted between autologous transplant and the rituximab cohort. Even though allo-SCT may have the benefit of a GVL effect, the higher TRM may have contributed to lower survivals. On further adjustment the authors concluded that autologous transplant offers a modest benefit for physically fit patients with chemosensitive nonbulky follicular lymphoma. Another CIBMTR study compared autologous transplant ($N = 108$) and allo-SCT ($N = 33$) in transformed lymphoma. Among allo-SCT, those patients undergoing RIC experienced better survival than myeloablative conditioning because of decreased TRM. Regardless of age, histological transformation, or previous rituximab use, the authors noted that autologous transplant provided durable survival in a group of patients [63].

The optimal approach for the management of transformed lymphoma remains under investigation and should be tailored to each individual case. Certain clinical and patient characteristics, such as disease stage and burden, response to salvage chemotherapy, performance status, and comorbid conditions, must be accounted for when formulating a management strategy, not unlike the nontransformed disease setting. Based on these concepts there is a role for both autologous transplant and RIC allo-SCT in select individuals with follicular lymphoma.

Chemorefractory follicular lymphoma

There is a group of patients in whom standard chemo-therapeutic regimens fail to induce a substantive complete or partial response. Although autologous transplant is not recommended in this setting, these patients may derive benefit from undergoing allo-SCT. A recent large analysis by the CIBMTR evaluated patients with chemorefractory NHL undergoing allo-SCT with both myeloablative and RIC regimens [64]. A total of 80 patients were diagnosed with grade 3 refractory follicular lymphoma. One-quarter of refractory patients, both diffuse large B-cell lymphoma (DLBCL) and follicular lymphoma, experienced remission up to 3 years post transplant. Among this group, those patients with refractory follicular lymphoma demonstrated better outcomes than those diagnosed with refractory DLBCL. Therefore, this large registry study supports previous analyses [65–67] that allo-SCT can benefit a subset of patients with chemorefractory low-grade lymphoma and follicular lymphoma. However, identifying those most likely to benefit remains a challenge. Our data and those of others suggest that serum lactate dehydrogenase may be a better predictor of outcome than positron emission tomography [67,68].

Post-transplant relapse

Choices for relapsed follicular lymphoma after autologous transplant range from localized radiation to rituximab to allo-SCT. Consideration must be given to the previous type of transplant, whether there is localized or wide-spread relapse, chemosensitivity, duration of remission, and patient characteristics. With the advent of targeted therapies, recent data offer promise for treatment extending to follicular lymphoma in this particular setting [5].

Relapse after allogeneic transplant also has features of interest. Management options in this setting include manipulation of immune suppression or DLI [69] or, if possible, a second allo-SCT. Follicular lymphoma has high rates of response to immunological therapies. For example, in one series 28 patients who underwent allo-SCT and received DLI in NHL included 19 follicular lymphoma patients, five of whom had transformed lymphoma. With 17 patients receiving DLI for progressive disease, 13 achieved a complete response with a median time to response of 12 months. Importantly, the authors noted a 5-year PFS and overall survival of 76% and 88% in this group [37]. In our own series, relapse more than 6 months after transplant was associated with a median survival of 16.3 months. Of 15 such patients, nine remained alive, mostly in remission, and only two deaths were attributed to lymphoma [67].

Minimal residual disease detection

Data from the Dana Farber group [26–28] helped to establish that detection of minimal residual disease (MRD) can act as an important prognostic tool in follicular lymphoma. Long-term analysis from this group [70] revealed that MRD negativity by PCR in follicular lymphoma grafts translated to a significant difference in PFS compared to patients who received MRD-positive grafts (67% vs. 26%). Two Italian studies confirmed the relevance of this concept in the rituximab era. A previously mentioned Italian prospective trial investigating purging strategies prior to autologous transplant in relapsed follicular lymphoma followed nested PCR for *bcl-2* and revealed how loss of molecular response was invariably followed by clinical relapse [33]. These findings were recently reconfirmed by another Italian study [71]. Although these data provide some insight and justification for following MRD in follicular lymphoma, considerable work is left to achieve a standardized approach. Questions pertaining to the best method to utilize, what constitutes a positive test, what level of positivity correlates with impending pending relapse, and when should clinical intervention be considered continue to linger. Detecting MRD at the level of bone marrow and peripheral blood can be used as part of a combination which includes imaging to gauge response to treatment or to detect relapsing disease once prospectively validated. It may offer valuable information in the future for guiding follicular lymphoma management in the post-transplant period.

Conclusion

The variable clinical course of follicular lymphoma makes it difficult to predict individual prognosis at the time of diagnosis. Unlike certain myeloid malignancies, current biologic and genetic determinations to assess disease risk are not yet sufficient to predict outcome in follicular lymphoma [13], necessitating assessment of

Table 14.3 Consensus recommendations on role of transplant in follicular lymphoma.

Autologous transplant

Not appropriate for first remission consolidation

Appropriate for chemosensitive second remission

Appropriate for chemosensitive transformed follicular lymphoma

Allogeneic stem cell transplant

Not appropriate for first remission consolidation

Myeloablative conditioning: appropriate for good performance score/healthy patients with refractory disease

Reduced-intensity conditioning: appropriate for carefully selected patients

Consider in autologous transplant failures

Appropriate for refractory or post autologous transplant relapsed transformed follicular lymphoma

---

Source: adapted from Montoto *et al.* [13].

disease course to contemplate optimal timing for transplantation. The question of which patients benefit from autologous transplant or allo-SCT requires the clinician to individualize management options based on both patient and disease characteristics. These include chemosensitivity, duration and depth of remission, physiologic age and performance score, availability of an HLA-matched donor, comorbid conditions and, often overlooked, social and psychological hurdles.

Novel approaches incorporating new agents such as immunomodulators, BTK and PI3K inhibitors further complicate the therapeutic landscape and will in the near future once again require repositioning of the role of transplant. Currently, for patients with chemosensitive disease and good performance score in later than first remission, the data support offering autologous transplant, which can result in long-term DFS and possibly cure [13,25]. For patients with refractory disease and HLA-matched donors, or for post autologous transplant relapse, allo-SCT is an attractive approach (Table 14.3). The transplant community continues to investigate innovative methods to further improve rates of disease control and ameliorate toxicities by limiting effects of GVHD without reducing the potential GVL effect [72].

References

1 Howlader N, Noone AM, Krapcho M *et al.* (eds) *SEER Cancer Statistics Review, 1975–2011*. Bethesda, MD: National Cancer Institute, 2014.

2 Salles GA. Clinical features, prognosis and treatment of follicular lymphoma. *Hematology Am Soc Hematol Educ Program* 2007;**216–25**.

3 Salles G, Seymour JF, Offner F *et al.* Rituximab maintenance for 2 years in patients with high tumour burden follicular lymphoma responding to rituximab plus chemotherapy (PRIMA): a phase 3, randomised controlled trial. *Lancet* 2011;**377**:42–51.

4 Hiddemann W, Kneba M, Dreyling M *et al.* Frontline therapy with rituximab added to the combination of cyclophosphamide, doxorubicin, vincristine, and prednisone (CHOP) significantly improves the outcome for patients with advanced-stage follicular lymphoma compared with therapy with CHOP alone: results of a prospective randomized trial of the German Low-Grade Lymphoma Study Group. *Blood* 2005;**106**:3725–32.

5 Gopal AK, Kahl BS, de Vos S *et al.* PI3Kδ inhibition by idelalisib in patients with relapsed indolent lymphoma. *N Engl J Med* 2014;**370**:1008–18.

6 Frei E, Teicher BA, Holden SA *et al.* Preclinical studies and clinical correlation of the effect of alkylating dose. *Cancer Res* 1988;**48**:6417–23.

7 Lenz G, Dreyling M, Schiegnitz E *et al.* Myeloablative radiochemotherapy followed by autologous stem cell transplantation in first remission prolongs progression-free survival in follicular lymphoma: results of a prospective randomized trial of the German Low-Grade Lymphoma Study Group. *Blood* 2004;**104**:2667–74.

8 Sebban C, Mounier N, Brousse N *et al.* Standard chemotherapy with interferon compared with CHOP followed by high-dose therapy with autologous stem cell transplantation in untreated patients with advanced follicular lymphoma: the GELF-94 randomized study from the Groupe d'Etude des Lymphomes de l'Adulte (GELA). *Blood* 2006;**108**:2540–4.

9 Deconinck E, Foussard C, Milpied N *et al.* High-dose therapy followed by autologous purged stem-cell transplantation and doxorubicin-based chemotherapy in patients with advanced follicular lymphoma: a randomized multicenter study by GOELAMS. *Blood* 2005;**105**:3817–23.

10 Gyan E, Foussard C, Bertrand P *et al.* High-dose therapy followed by autologous purged stem cell transplantation and doxorubicin-based chemotherapy in patients with advanced follicular lymphoma: a randomized multicenter study by the GOELAMS with final results after a median follow-up of 9 years. *Blood* 2009;**113**:995–1001.

11 Ladetto M, De Marco F, Benedetti F *et al.* Prospective, multicenter randomized GITMO/IIL trial comparing intensive (R-HDS) versus conventional (CHOP-R) chemoimmunotherapy in high-risk follicular lymphoma at diagnosis: the superior disease control of R-HDS does not translate into an overall surviva. *Blood* 2008;**111**:4004–13.

12 Al Khabori, de Almeida JR, Guyatt GH, Kuruvilla J, Crump M. Autologous stem cell transplantation in follicular lymphoma: a systematic review and meta-analysis. *J Natl Cancer Inst* 2012;**104**:18–28.

13 Montoto S, Corradini P, Dreyling M *et al.* Indications for hematopoietic stem cell transplantation in patients with follicular lymphoma: a consensus project of the EBMT-Lymphoma Working Party. *Haematologica* 2013;**98**:1014–21.

14 Schouten HC, Qian W, Kvaloy S *et al.* High-dose therapy improves progression-free survival and survival in relapsed follicular non-Hodgkin's lymphoma: results from the randomized European CUP trial. *J Clin Oncol* 2003;**21**:3918–27.

15 Montoto S, Canals C, Rohatiner AZ *et al.* Long-term follow-up of high-dose treatment with autologous haematopoietic progenitor cell support in 693 patients with follicular lymphoma: an EBMT registry study. *Leukemia* 2007;**21**:2324–31.

16 Kornacker M, Stumm J, Pott C *et al.* Characteristics of relapse after autologous stem cell transplantation for follicular lymphoma: a long-term follow-up. *Ann Oncol* 2009;**20**:722–8.

17 Rohatiner AZS, Nadler L, Davies AJ *et al.* Myeloablative therapy with autologous bone marrow transplantation for follicular lymphoma at the time of second or subsequent remission: long-term follow-up. *J Clin Oncol* 2007;**25**:2554–9.

18 Peters AC, Duan Q, Russell JA, Duggan P, Owen C, Stewart DA. Durable event-free survival following autologous stem cell transplant for relapsed or refractory follicular lymphoma: positive impact of recent rituximab exposure and low-risk Follicular lymphoma International Prognostic Index score. *Leukemia Lymphoma* 2011;**52**:2124–9.

19 Kothari J, Peggs KS, Bird A *et al.* Autologous stem cell transplantation for follicular lymphoma is of most benefit early in the disease course and can result in durable remissions, irrespective of prior rituximab exposure. *Br J Haematol* 2014;**165**:334–40.

20 Abruzzese BE, Radford JE, Miller JS *et al.* Detection of abnormal pretransplant clones in progenitor cells of patients who developed myelodysplasia after autologous transplantation. *Blood* 1999;**94**:1814–19.

21 Metzner B, Pott C, Müller TH *et al.* Long-term clinical and molecular remissions in patients with follicular lymphoma following high-dose therapy and autologous stem cell transplantation. *Ann Oncol* 2013;**24**:1609–15.

22 Kang TY, Rybicki LA, Bolwell BJ *et al.* Effect of prior rituximab on high-dose therapy and autologous stem cell transplantation in follicular lymphoma. *Bone Marrow Transplant* 2007;**40**:973–8.

23 Le Gouill S, De Guibert S, Planche L *et al.* Impact of the use of autologous stem cell transplantation at first relapse both in naive and previously rituximab exposed follicular lymphoma patients treated in the GELA/GOELAMS follicular lymphoma 2000 study. *Haematologica* 2011;**96**:1128–35.

24 Evens AM, Vanderplas A, LaCasce AS *et al.* Stem cell transplantation for follicular lymphoma relapsed/refractory after prior rituximab: a comprehensive analysis from the NCCN lymphoma outcomes project. *Cancer* 2013;**119**:3662–71.

25 Montoto S, Matthews J, Greaves P *et al.* Myeloablative chemotherapy for chemo-sensitive recurrent follicular lymphoma: potential benefit in second relapse. *Haematologica* 2013;**98**:620–5.

26 Gribben JG, Freedman AS, Neuberg D *et al.* Immunologic purging of marrow assessed by PCR before autologous bone marrow transplantation for B-cell lymphoma. *N Engl J Med* 1991;**325**:1525–33.

27 Gribben BJG, Saporito L, Barber M *et al.* Bone marrows of non-Hodgkin's lymphoma patients with a bcl-2 translocation can be purged of polymerase chain reaction-detectable lymphoma cells using monoclonal antibodies and immunomagnetic bead depletion. *Blood* 1992;**80**:1083–9.

28 Gribben JG, Neuberg D, Freedman AS *et al.* Detection by polymerase chain reaction of residual cells with the bcl-2 translocation is associated with increased risk of relapse after autologous bone marrow transplantation for B-cell lymphoma. *Blood* 1993;**81**.3449–57.

29 Belhadj K, Delfau-Larue MH, Elgnaoui T *et al.* Efficiency of in vivo purging with rituximab prior to autologous peripheral blood progenitor cell transplantation in B-cell non-Hodgkin's lymphoma: a single institution study. *Ann Oncol* 2004;**15**:504–10.

30 Bierman PJ, Sweetenham JW, Loberiza FR *et al.* Syngeneic hematopoietic stem-cell transplantation for non-Hodgkin's lymphoma: a comparison with allogeneic and autologous transplantation. The Lymphoma Working Committee of the International Bone Marrow Transplant Registry and the European Group for Blood. *J Clin Oncol* 2003;**21**:3744–53.

31 Van Besien K, Loberiza FR Jr, Bajorunaite R *et al.* Comparison of autologous and allogeneic hematopoietic stem cell transplantation for follicular lymphoma. *Blood* 2003;**102**:3521–9.

32 Arcaini L, Orlandi E, Alessandrino EP *et al.* A model of in vivo purging with rituximab and high-dose AraC in follicular and mantle cell lymphoma. *Bone Marrow Transplant* 2004;**34**:175–9.

33 Arcaini L, Montanari F, Alessandrino EP *et al.* Immunochemotherapy with in vivo purging and autotransplant induces long clinical and molecular remission in advanced relapsed and refractory follicular lymphoma. *Ann Oncol* 2008;**19**:1331–5.

34 Pettengell R, Schmitz N, Gisselbrecht C *et al.* Rituximab purging and/or maintenance in patients undergoing autologous transplantation for relapsed follicular lymphoma: a prospective randomized trial from the Lymphoma Working Party of the European Group for Blood and Marrow Transplantation. *J Clin Oncol* 2013;**31**:1624–30.

35 Jones RJ, Ambinder RF, Piantadosi S, Santos GW. Evidence of a graft-versus-lymphoma effect associated with allogeneic bone marrow transplantation. *Blood* 1991;**77**:649–53.

36 Mandigers CM, Verdonck LF, Meijerink JP, Dekker AW, Schattenberg AV, Raemaekers JM. Graft-versus-lymphoma effect of donor lymphocyte infusion in indolent lymphomas relapsed after allogeneic stem cell transplantation. *Bone Marrow Transplant* 2003;**32**:1159–63.

37 Bloor AJC, Thomson K, Chowdhry N *et al.* High response rate to donor lymphocyte infusion after allogeneic stem cell transplantation for indolent non-Hodgkin lymphoma. *Biol Blood Marrow Transplant* 2008;**14**:50–8.

38 Thomson KJ, Morris EC, Milligan D *et al*. T-cell-depleted reduced-intensity transplantation followed by donor leukocyte infusions to promote graft-versus-lymphoma activity results in excellent long-term survival in patients with multiply relapsed follicular lymphoma. *J Clin Oncol* 2010;**28**:3695–700.

39 Van Besien K, Sobocinski KA, Rowlings PA *et al*. Allogeneic bone marrow transplantation for low-grade lymphoma. *Blood* 1998;**92**:1832–6.

40 Peniket AJ, Ruiz de Elvira MC, Taghipour G *et al*. An EBMT registry matched study of allogeneic stem cell transplants for lymphoma: allogeneic transplantation is associated with a lower relapse rate but a higher procedure-related mortality rate than autologous transplantation. *Bone Marrow Transplant* 2003;**31**:667–78.

41 Corradini P, Dodero A, Farina L *et al*. Allogeneic stem cell transplantation following reduced-intensity conditioning can induce durable clinical and molecular remissions in relapsed lymphomas: pre-transplant disease status and histotype heavily influence outcome. *Leukemia* 2007;**21**:2316–23.

42 Hari P, Carreras J, Zhang M-J *et al*. Allogeneic transplants in follicular lymphoma: higher risk of disease progression after reduced-intensity compared to myeloablative conditioning. *Biol Blood Marrow Transplant* 2008;**14**:236–45.

43 Khouri IF, McLaughlin P, Saliba RM *et al*. Eight-year experience with allogeneic stem cell transplantation for relapsed follicular lymphoma after nonmyeloablative conditioning with fludarabine, cyclophosphamide, and rituximab. *Blood* 2008;**111**:5530–6.

44 Khouri IF, Saliba RM, Erwin WD *et al*. Nonmyeloablative allogeneic transplantation with or without 90 yttrium ibritumomab tiuxetan is potentially curative for relapsed follicular lymphoma : 12-year results. *Blood* 2012;**119**:6373–8.

45 Bhatia S, Francisco L, Carter A *et al*. Late mortality after allogeneic hematopoietic cell transplantation and functional status of long-term survivors: report from the Bone Marrow Transplant Survivor Study. *Blood* 2007;**110**:3784–92.

46 Morris E, Thomson K, Craddock C *et al*. Outcomes after alemtuzumab-containing reduced-intensity allogeneic transplantation regimen for relapsed and refractory non-Hodgkin lymphoma. *Blood* 2004;**104**:3865–71.

47 Delgado J, Canals C, Attal M *et al*. The role of in vivo T-cell depletion on reduced-intensity conditioning allogeneic stem cell transplantation from HLA-identical siblings in patients with follicular lymphoma. *Leukemia* 2011;**25**:551–5.

48 Avivi I, Montoto S, Canals C *et al*. Matched unrelated donor stem cell transplant in 131 patients with follicular lymphoma: an analysis from the Lymphoma Working Party of the European Group for Blood and Marrow Transplantation. *Br J Haematol* 2009;**147**:719–28.

49 Rodrigues CA, Sanz G, Brunstein CG *et al*. Analysis of risk factors for outcomes after unrelated cord blood transplantation in adults with lymphoid malignancies: a study by the Eurocord-Netcord and lymphoma working party of the European Group for Blood and Marrow Transplantation. *J Clin Oncol* 2009;**27**:256–63.

50 Luznik L, O'Donnell PV, Symons HJ *et al*. HLA-haploidentical bone marrow transplantation for hematologic malignancies using nonmyeloablative conditioning and high-dose, post-transplantation cyclophosphamide. *Biol Blood Marrow Transplant* 2008;**14**:641–50.

51 Bashey A, Zhang X, Sizemore CA *et al*. T-cell-replete HLA-haploidentical hematopoietic transplantation for hematologic malignancies using post-transplantation cyclophosphamide results in outcomes equivalent to those of contemporaneous HLA-matched related and unrelated donor transplantation. *J Clin Oncol* 2013;**31**:1310–16.

52 Robinson SP, Canals C, Luang JJ *et al*. The outcome of reduced intensity allogeneic stem cell transplantation and autologous stem cell transplantation when performed as a first transplant strategy in relapsed follicular lymphoma: an analysis from the Lymphoma Working Party of the EBMT. *Bone Marrow Transplant* 2013;**48**:1409–14.

53 Tomblyn MR, Ewell M, Bredeson C *et al*. Autologous versus reduced-intensity allogeneic hematopoietic cell transplantation for patients with chemosensitive follicular non-Hodgkin lymphoma beyond first complete response or first partial response. *Biol Blood Marrow Transplant* 2011;**17**:1051–7.

54 Al-Tourah AJ, Gill KK, Chhanabhai M *et al*. Population-based analysis of incidence and outcome of transformed non-Hodgkin's lymphoma. *J Clin Oncol* 2008;**26**:5165–9.

55 Villa D, Crump M, Keating A, Panzarella T, Feng B, Kuruvilla J. Outcome of patients with transformed indolent non-Hodgkin lymphoma referred for autologous stem-cell transplantation. *Ann Oncol* 2013;**24**:1603–9.

56 Williams CD, Harrison CN, Lister TA *et al*. High-dose therapy and autologous stem-cell support for chemosensitive transformed low-grade follicular non-Hodgkin's lymphoma: a case-matched study from the European Bone Marrow Transplant Registry. *J Clin Oncol* 2001;**19**:727–35.

57 Friedberg JW, Neuberg D, Gribben JG *et al*. Autologous bone marrow transplantation after histologic transformation of indolent B cell malignancies. *Biol Blood Marrow Transplant* 1999;**5**:262–8.

58 Chen CI, Crump M, Tsang R, Stewart AK, Keating A. Autotransplants for histologically transformed follicular non-Hodgkin's lymphoma. *Br J Haematol* 2001;**113**:202–8.

59 Hamadani M, Benson DM, Lin TS, Porcu P, Blum KA, Devine SM. High-dose therapy and autologous stem cell transplantation for follicular lymphoma undergoing transformation to diffuse large B-cell lymphoma. *Eur J Haematol* 2008;**81**:425–31.

60 Hamadani M, Awan FT, Elder P *et al*. Feasibility of allogeneic hematopoietic stem cell transplantation for follicular lymphoma undergoing transformation to diffuse large B-cell lymphoma. *Leukemia Lymphoma* 2008;**49**:1893–8.

61 Eide MB, Lauritzsen GF, Kvalheim G *et al*. High dose chemotherapy with autologous stem cell support for patients with histologically transformed B-cell non-Hodgkin lymphomas. A Norwegian multi centre phase II study. *Br J Haematol* 2011;**152**:600–10.

62 Villa D, Crump M, Panzarella T *et al.* Autologous and allogeneic stem-cell transplantation for transformed follicular lymphoma: a report of the Canadian Blood and Marrow Transplant Group. *J Clin Oncol* 2013;**31**:1164–71.

63 Wirk B, Fenske TS, Hamadani M *et al.* Outcomes of hematopoietic cell transplantation for diffuse large B cell lymphoma transformed from follicular lymphoma. *Biol Blood Marrow Transplant* 2014;**20**:951–9.

64 Hamadani M, Saber W, Ahn KW *et al.* Impact of pretransplantation conditioning regimens on outcomes of allogeneic transplantation for chemotherapy-unresponsive diffuse large B cell lymphoma and grade III follicular lymphoma. *Biol Blood Marrow Transplant* 2013;**19**:746–53.

65 Van Besien KW, Khouri IF, Giralt SA *et al.* Allogeneic bone marrow transplantation for refractory and recurrent low-grade lymphoma: the case for aggressive management. *J Clin Oncol* 1995;**13**:1096–102.

66 Van Besien K, Champlin IK, McCarthy P. Allogeneic transplantation for low-grade lymphoma: long-term follow-up. *J Clin Oncol* 2000;**18**:702–3.

67 Kenkre VP, Horowitz S, Artz AS *et al.* T-cell-depleted allogeneic transplant without donor leukocyte infusions results in excellent long-term survival in patients with multiply relapsed lymphoma. Predictors for survival after transplant relapse. *Leukemia Lymphoma* 2011;**52**:214–22.

68 Armand P, Kim HT, Ho VT *et al.* Allogeneic transplantation with reduced-intensity conditioning for Hodgkin and non-Hodgkin lymphoma: importance of histology for outcome. *Biol Blood Marrow Transplant* 2008;**14**:418–25.

69 Van Besien KW, de Lima M, Giralt SA *et al.* Management of lymphoma recurrence after allogeneic transplantation: the relevance of graft-versus-lymphoma effect. *Bone Marrow Transplant* 1997;**19**:977–82.

70 Brown JR, Feng Y, Gribben JG *et al.* Long-term survival after autologous bone marrow transplantation for follicular lymphoma in first remission. *Biol Blood Marrow Transplant* 2007,**13**.1057–65.

71 Ladetto M, Lobetti-Bodoni C, Mantoan B *et al.* Persistence of minimal residual disease in bone marrow predicts outcome in follicular lymphomas treated with a rituximab-intensive program. *Blood* 2013;**122**:3759–66.

72 Cohen S, Kiss T, Lachance S *et al.* Tandem autologous–allogeneic nonmyeloablative sibling transplantation in relapsed follicular lymphoma leads to impressive progression-free survival with minimal toxicity. *Biol Blood Marrow Transplant* 2012;**18**:951–7.

CHAPTER 15

Chronic lymphocytic leukemia/small lymphocytic lymphoma

Salyka Sengsayadeth and Wichai Chinratanalab

Introduction

In Western countries, chronic lymphocytic leukemia (CLL)/small lymphocytic lymphoma (SLL) is the most common leukemia diagnosed, with more than 14,500 newly diagnosed cases each year [1]. The clinical course of CLL is very heterogeneous, with some patients having a very indolent course requiring no therapeutic interventions while some have very rapidly progressive courses requiring urgent and aggressive treatment. As most patients are typically diagnosed in the sixth or seventh decade of life, consideration of therapy should be focused on treating symptoms and ultimately preserving quality of life, as many of these patients will not be eligible for curative treatment [2]. Currently, two accepted clinical staging classification schemes are used to determine risk and median survival, and can help guide clinicians regarding timing of treatment [3,4]. Additionally, guidelines from the International Workshop on Chronic Lymphocytic Leukemia published by the National Cancer Institute Working Group are helpful in determining when to initiate treatment and the recommended treatments for patients with active disease; typically this includes patients who have symptomatic disease, bulky progressive lymphadenopathy, or evidence of marrow failure [5].

For patients with good performance status requiring treatment for symptomatic or rapidly progressive disease, preferred regimens include fludarabine-based therapy in combination with cyclophosphamide and rituximab (FCR). This regimen has been shown to be most effective in producing a complete response (CR) in both previously untreated and treated patients [6–8]. Alemtuzumab is an anti-CD52 monoclonal antibody that is approved for patients with previously untreated CLL as well as for those with fludarabine refractory disease. It has also been shown to be efficacious for patients with 17p deletions or p53 mutations [9]. Recently, there has been a significant increase in development of targeted therapies for the treatment of CLL, which have improved response rates and tolerability. Their role in upfront treatment of CLL remains to be defined.

Indication for transplantation in CLL/SLL

For the majority of patients diagnosed with CLL/SLL, hematopoietic stem cell transplant is not a viable treatment option as most are elderly with many medical comorbidities. Additionally, many often do not need treatment for an oftentimes indolent disease. Determining which patients may benefit from hematopoietic stem cell transplant remains a challenge.

Allogeneic stem cell transplantation (allo-SCT) is now considered the mainstay of transplant treatment for patients with high-risk or refractory CLL, employing reduced-intensity conditioning (RIC) or nonmyeloablative (NMA) conditioning allo-SCT and either related or unrelated donors. In regards to who should be referred for consideration of allo-SCT, the European Society for Blood and Marrow Transplantation (EBMT) guidelines outline in which patients allo-SCT should be considered. Allo-SCT is an efficacious and reasonable treatment

Clinical Guide to Transplantation in Lymphoma, First Edition. Edited by Bipin N. Savani and Mohamad Mohty.
© 2015 John Wiley & Sons, Ltd. Published 2015 by John Wiley & Sons, Ltd.

option in younger patients with (i) purine analog refractoriness, defined as no response or early relapse within 12 months; (ii) relapse within 2 years after purine analog combination therapy; and (iii) patients with del 17p/p53 mutation in whom treatment is required [10]. In particular, in patients who harbor the p53 abnormality, allo-SCT should be considered in first complete remission (CR1) as their prognoses are very poor. It is recommended that these patients be referred to transplant centers early for discussion of transplantation and identification of potential donors [2]. It should be noted that the EBMT consensus states that no chemotherapeutic regimen, including those with high-dose chemotherapy followed by autologous transplant, is curative whereas allo-SCT is the only curative treatment modality.

Timing and preparation of patients for transplantation in CLL/SLL

Allo-SCT was first reported in 1988 [11] and over the years has struggled with high transplant-related mortality (TRM) in patients who underwent myeloablative conditioning (MAC). With the advent of RIC and NMA conditioning, interest in this treatment modality has resurfaced and outcomes have been improved, with less morbidity and mortality. Although there is no definitive evidence to suggest otherwise, it is thought that the success of allo-SCT decreases as more cytotoxic therapies are used prior to transplant [10]. This suggests that consideration of allo-SCT should be done early in patients who may be able to derive benefit, such as younger patients with poor-risk disease.

The underlying mechanism of the therapeutic efficacy of allo-SCT in CLL is based on the principle of the graft-versus-leukemia (GVL) effect; thus, a reduced-intensity regimen has been shown to reduce TRM without impacting the efficacy of the GVL effect [10]. This is particularly important in older patients who may have comorbid illnesses but who have good disease control. For younger patients with poor disease control, it may be reasonable to consider a more ablative regimen [12]. In general, the evidence suggests that RIC allo-SCT is an effective treatment for patients with poor-risk CLL, although there is not sufficient evidence to specifically identify a superior conditioning regimen [10].

In preparing patients for consideration of allo-SCT, referring physicians must not only consider their age,

but other factors as well. Most transplant centers will consider patients up to the age of 70 with sufficient organ function to undergo RIC allo-SCT. These patients must have acceptable cardiac, pulmonary, hepatic, and renal function along with good performance status, typically with a Karnofsky performance status (KPS) of at least 80%. Additionally, the patient's disease should be chemosensitive with optimal tumor cytoreduction prior to transplant to optimize outcomes, as predictors of outcome after NMA or RIC allo-SCT are often dependent on pretransplant disease status, with patients who had higher disease burdens or high bone marrow involvement before transplant being at higher risk of post-transplant relapse.

If patients have siblings of adequate age and donor eligibility, these patients and their siblings should be considered for human leukocyte antigen (HLA) typing. There are no data to suggest that related or unrelated donors are better than one another, and a retrospective analysis from the National Marrow Donor Program (NMDP) demonstrated that allo-SCT with unrelated donors is feasible and effective [13]. Thus recommendations regarding donor source would simply be based on donor availability and degree of HLA match [10]. The degree of matching may impact outcomes, as described by Michallet *et al.* [14] in a retrospective analysis of the EBMT registry which showed no difference in overall survival (OS) between HLA-identical siblings and well-matched unrelated donors but conversely showed that patients with mismatched donors had statistically worse outcomes with regard to OS due to excess in TRM. There are no firm data on the superiority of bone marrow versus peripheral blood stem cell grafts, and either is considered suitable for transplantation. Alternative sources, including umbilical cord grafts and haploidentical donor transplants, are less commonly performed. However, recent data suggest that umbilical cord transplants are feasible and have demonstrated encouraging results with no difference in outcomes when compared with matched unrelated donors [15,16].

Transplant outcome in CLL/SLL

Autologous stem cell transplantation
The stem cell transplant landscape has changed for CLL over the past decade, with a shift from autologous stem cell transplantation (auto-SCT) to primarily allo-SCT.

Initial data in the 1990s and early 2000s suggested that there was a possible survival benefit to auto-SCT for high-risk patients [17,18]. Michallet *et al.* [19] published results of a Phase III prospective randomized trial that investigated autografting versus observation alone for patients who had responded to first- or second-line treatment. Most patient received fludarabine-based therapy but only 4% received a combination of purine analog and rituximab-based treatment. Autografts received a cyclophosphamide/total body irradiation (Cy/TBI) or carmustine, etoposide, cytarabine, and melphalan (BEAM) preparative regimen. The study showed that event-free survival (EFS) was prolonged in the auto-SCT group (51.2 months vs. 24.4 months in the observation group), but 5-year OS was similar in both groups (85.5% vs. 84.3% for autografting and observation, respectively; $P = 0.77$).

Another prospective randomized trial by Brion *et al.* [20] reported on the impact of high-dose chemotherapy followed by auto-SCT in CLL in the Groupe Ouest Est d'Etude des Leucemies Aigues et Maladies due Sang LLC 98 trial (GOELAMS LLC 98). This study compared conventional chemotherapy with 6-monthly courses of CHOP (cyclophosphamide, hydroxydaunorubicin, vincristine, prednisone) followed by six CHOP courses every 3 months in those achieving CR or partial response (PR) with patients who received high-dose therapy using a Cy/TBI preparative regimen followed by auto-SCT after three courses of CHOP. The study demonstrated that the auto-SCT group had a better progression-free survival (PFS) of 53 months compared to 22 months in the conventional chemotherapy group. However, no difference in OS was noted in this study that was notably accrued in the pre-rituximab era.

Similarly, Sutton *et al.* [21] reported results from a prospective, randomized, multicenter European trial that compared auto-SCT with observation in patients with advanced CLL. Patients received two courses of mini-CHOP followed by three courses of fludarabine. Those who achieved a CR were then randomized to auto-SCT versus observation, while those who did not achieve a CR were randomized to a dexamethasone, high-dose aracytin, cisplatin (DHAP) salvage regimen followed by auto-SCT or three courses of fludarabine/cyclophosphamide (FC). EFS was superior in those that had a CR compared to the observation group (79.8% vs. 35.5%, adjusted hazard ratio 0.3, 95% CI 0.1–0.7; $P = 0.003$). No difference in survival was observed

however. No difference was seen in the auto-SCT and FC groups that required DHAP salvage.

It should be noted that as these important clinical trials were accruing, the era of rituximab therapy in treatment of CLL was only beginning to emerge. Hallek *et al.* [22] would publish a large randomized trial of fludarabine, cyclophosphamide, and rituximab (FCR) versus fludarabine and cyclophosphamide alone (FR) and showed that in previously untreated patients the addition of rituximab would add a statistically significant survival benefit.

In one of the few studies to compare auto-SCT with allo-SCT, Gribben *et al.* [23] reported that there was no difference in OS, cumulative incidence of disease recurrence, or deaths between the two groups, with decreased TRM in the RIC allograft group. In their long-term follow-up study, which included 162 patients with high-risk CLL who underwent transplantation at their center from 1989 to 1999, they showed that PFS was significant longer following auto-SCT than allo-SCT but no difference in OS was detected. They also reported a good response to therapy with donor lymphocyte infusion (DLI) for relapse after transplant, indicating a robust GVL effect, which had also been previously described [24].

Thus, based on the fact that the auto-SCT trials were done in the pre-rituximab era and that no OS benefit was shown, the general consensus is that there is no superiority of auto-SCT compared to conventional chemotherapy in the rituximab era. Additionally, the negative impact of biomarkers that typically lead to chemotherapy resistance (e.g., *TP53* mutations) cannot be overcome by autografting, whereas data have shown that such high-risk genetic aberrations can be overcome by allografts. There is currently no role for auto-SCT in the treatment of advanced CLL and it should not be recommended outside of a clinical trial [25].

Allogeneic stem cell transplantation

With the advent of RIC or NMA conditioning in stem cell transplantation, interest in studying allo-SCT as a potentially curative treatment modality in older patients has again resurfaced. These types of transplant reduced the previously seen high morbidity and mortality associated with the myeloablative transplants [26–28].

Michallet *et al.* [29] published a retrospective cohort study looking at patients with CLL who were younger than 60 years old and had an HLA-identical sibling donor that was reported to the EBMT or the International Bone Marrow Transplant registry from 1984 to 1992, with most patients receiving a myeloablative regimen of Cy/TBI followed by a bone marrow graft. Their results showed that 70% of their 54 evaluable patients achieved hematologic remission with a median OS of 27 months. Their study showed that allo-SCT was feasible and can result in long-term survival.

Because of the high TRM associated with myeloablative transplants, investigators began looking at nonmyeloablative or reduced-intensity conditioning strategies for CLL. Khouri et al. [26] described an NMA fludarabine-based conditioning regimen in 15 patients with advanced refractory CLL or lymphoma followed by HLA-identical sibling transplant and showed that this type of transplant was feasible with regard to successful engraftment and durable GVL effect. They also further demonstrated direct evidence of GVL by the use of DLI in patients with post-transplant relapse.

Later studies would be done which showed again the feasibility of nonablative transplant along with the evidence that allo-SCT could overcome poor prognostic genomic factors. For example, it is now known that patients with overexpression of the zeta-chain-associated protein (ZAP)-70 and presence of 17p mutations can be overcome by a potent GVL effect with allo-SCT. Khouri et al. [30] demonstrated in patients who were treated with fludarabine, cyclophosphamide and rituximab-based nonablative regimens had an OS of 48% and PFS of 44% at 4 years, with multivariate analysis indicating that chemorefractory disease and mixed T-cell chimerism, not ZAP-70 expression, were associated with risk of disease progression after allo-SCT. Similarly, Schetelig et al. [31] published data from the EBMT database of 44 patients with 17p deletion CLL who underwent a matched sibling or alternative donor transplant, with the majority receiving RIC (89%) and showed that 3-year OS and PFS were 44% and 37%, respectively. No relapses occurred in their cohort of patients who had longer than 4-year follow-up. Their conclusion was that allo-SCT has the potential to induce long-term disease-free survival in patients with 17p deletion CLL.

Dreger et al. [32] published a landmark prospective multicenter Phase II trial which investigated the long-term outcome of RIC allo-SCT in patients with poor-risk CLL with fludarabine and cyclophosphamide-based conditioning. A total of 90 evaluable patients were

reported, with 4-year OS of 65%, EFS of 42%, and nonrelapse mortality (NRM) of 23%. Their EFS was similar for all genetic subsets, including patients with 17p deletion. The authors were able to study a subset of patients with minimal residual disease (MRD) using flow cytometry or real-time quantitative polymerase chain reaction and showed that these patients had a superior EFS of 89%. Multivariate analysis showed that uncontrolled disease and in vivo T-cell depletion with alemtuzumab, but not 17p deletion, were adverse predictors of outcome. They concluded that up to half of patients with poor disease could have a good long-term outcome that was independent of the underlying genomic risk profile, with those who were able to achieve MRD negativity post transplant having superior outcomes. Other studies of patients who underwent allo-SCT with NMA conditioning for relapsed/refractory disease showed that other variables which potentially impact outcomes, including below-normal serum IgG levels and CD4 count less than $100/mm^3$, were associated with reduced OS [33].

Delgado et al. [34] studied 41 patients treated with fludarabine, melphalan, and alemtuzumab conditioning followed by HLA-matched sibling, unrelated and mismatched donor transplant, demonstrating a 2-year OS of 51% and NRM of 26%. Their conclusion was that an alemtuzumab-based regimen was feasible and effective, with a low rate of graft-versus-host disease (GVHD) but a relatively high TRM due to excess viral and fungal infections.

The conclusion from the allo-SCT with RIC/NMA conditioning strategies is that they are feasible and have evidence to show that a reasonable number of patients with high-risk or refractory CLL can achieve long-term disease-free survival without excess TRM. Thus, for patients who are physically fit and harbor high-risk disease, early allo-SCT should be considered.

Management of relapses after transplantation for CLL/SLL

Although it is the only curative therapy for patients with CLL, relapse after allo-SCT remains a major cause of treatment failure. Three-year risk of relapse has been estimated to be 10–20% and even up to 50% [32,34–38], or more in a subset of patients [39,40]. Thus, optimization of post-transplant outcomes must take into account this relapse risk, and effective management strategies are needed.

As previously discussed, the efficacy of allo-SCT in the treatment of CLL is based on the GVL effect, which has been demonstrated in studies showing a median survival of 5 years after nonmyeloablative transplant [35,39]. Additionally, rapid complete donor chimerism conversion is indicative of a GVL effect and is suggested to be important in early control of CLL [41]. Patients who have longer duration of mixed chimerisms have been shown to have reduced PFS [36,37] as have patients who have undergone T cell depleted grafts [39,42].

Currently, there are no established predictors of relapse, although one study has shown that MRD quantification using primers and high-throughput immunoglobulin heavy chain sequencing was predictive of post allo-SCT relapse in CLL [43].

Early versus late relapses

Treatment of relapsed disease after allo-SCT for CLL remains difficult but durable responses have been reported with a variety of approaches. Often very early relapses are indicative of inadequate tumor control after pretransplant chemotherapy and/or the conditioning regimen. In other words, a mature and robust GVL effect has not yet been established to control disease sufficiently. For patients who achieve a remission but relapse shortly after, an inadequate sustained GVL may be responsible [44]. Evidence of GVL deficiency has been demonstrated in cases of T-cell-depleted transplants [39] in which decreased PFS is seen as well as in patients who have prolonged duration of mixed donor chimerism [42]. In these cases, immune modulation via withdrawal of immune suppression (WIS) and DLI are potentially efficacious in augmenting the GVL effect [44].

Late relapses, on the other hand, can be seen many months or years after transplant in CLL, and they can occur for several reasons. First, there may be loss of the GVL effect, either through clonal evolution of the previous CLL clone or "immune escape," in which the immune system no longer detects the CLL cells as malignant, thus leading to proliferation of disease. Another consideration is development of *de novo* CLL that originates from the stem cell donor. This should be a consideration in patients who may have been recipients of stem cells from older matched siblings or unrelated donors [44]. Donor-derived CLL presenting as late relapse has been described in patients who received

transplants from donors with the precursor-state monoclonal B-cell lymphocytosis (MBCL) [45,46]. This condition has been detected in up to 18% of unaffected members of CLL families and more than 5% of the general population [47–51]. Thus, it is important to keep these possibilities in mind in patients who may have received a matched sibling transplant from a donor with a lineage of CLL or an unrelated donor who was noted to have the MBCL precursor state. Identification of MBCL among prospective sibling transplant donors will become an ever more common occurrence in transplant practice as transplantation is increasingly offered to older individuals with CLL.

Recommended treatment approaches for relapsed CLL after allogeneic stem cell transplant

There are no large randomized controlled studies which help guide in the optimal management of relapsed CLL after allo-SCT. In 2010, the National Cancer Institute convened its first international workshop to focus on the biology, prevention, and treatment of relapse after allo-SCT. Its committee published treatment guidelines for management of relapses for hematologic diseases including CLL. As with most approaches to post-transplant relapse, considerations of the degree of donor engraftment, level of current immune suppression, and status of GVHD must be taken into account for each individual patient. In CLL, it is also important to consider the timing of the relapse for management of disease [44].

For patients with early relapses, an inadequate GVL effect is likely contributing to relapse, particularly in cases of mixed chimerisms. On suspicion of relapsed disease, complete disease restaging including assessment of the bone marrow as well as peripheral blood chimerisms are necessary. Once relapse had been confirmed, treatment approaches should target tumor control and boosting the GVL effect. In the absence of ongoing acute GVHD, immune manipulation to accomplish the aforementioned may include WIS with or without DLI. The results of DLI in management of post-transplant relapse vary widely with disparate results that reflect the heterogeneity of factors such as disease status, donor chimerisms, treatment indications, and the actual DLI products themselves [36,52,53]. Thus it is difficult to draw firm conclusions based on the available data but some patients have been able to achieve a durable CR after DLI. For patients who have achieved full donor chimerism without overt progression of disease, watchful waiting, WIS, and/or DLI are all felt to be reasonable considerations. The altered immune system in CLL patients may contribute to the GVL failure of the transplanted immune system, including imbalances in T-cell subsets, suppressed T-cell signaling response, and natural killer (NK) cell function.

For patients with active GVHD, consideration of non-immunomodulatory treatment strategies are required. Patients with indolent progression may be considered for monoclonal antibody therapy with agents such as rituximab. In early relapses, a novel chemotherapy regimen or targeted agent is likely required given the expected short interval between last treatment and post-transplant relapse [44]. For patients who have disease progression after treatment of GVHD, a reduced GVL effect should be suspected. Unfortunately, management of these patients is very difficult given the tenuous balance of GVHD and disease control. Reasonable considerations included local radiation, rituximab, and/or single-agent chemotherapy. The safety and efficacy of intensive chemotherapy regimens in this setting is unclear.

Similarly to early relapses, evaluation of possible late transplant relapse should include complete disease restaging including bone marrow evaluation and peripheral blood chimerism studies. In addition, due to the possibility of transformation, post-transplant lymphoproliferative disease, or donor-derived CLL, biopsy of active nodal disease should be considered. Late relapses often are related to waning GVL potency with immune escape or development of new post-transplant clones. Treatments should look to establish disease sensitivity and restoring GVL potency. For indolent late relapses, strategies such as WIS followed by DLI and/or rituximab are reasonable treatment strategies. For patients who have more aggressive late relapses, salvage chemotherapy with or without DLI may be required to control disease and also subsequently may lead to restoration of the GVL effect through the lymphoid depletion from cytotoxic therapy. If there has been a significant amount of time between the last chemotherapy treatment regimen and post-transplant relapse, it would be reasonable to consider the last effective chemotherapeutic regimen. It is likely that late relapses are less responsive to immune manipulations such as WIS and DLI. Interestingly, a patient with late

relapsed disease may be more sensitive to cytotoxic or new targeted therapies if a new clone or transformed clone is present [44].

Very late recurrences, particularly in the bone marrow, should lead to consideration of possible donor-derived CLL, particularly in patients who receive grafts from sibling donors with family history of lymphoid malignancies. Additionally, consideration of donor-derived CLL should be considered in patients with older donors, particularly those over 50 years old where the prevalence of MBCL is higher. If donor-derived CLL is felt to be contributing to post-transplant CLL, then management should be according to CLL guidelines for *de novo* CLL. There would be no role for immune manipulation such as WIS or DLI [44].

In summary, there is no standard of care on optimal management of disease relapse for transplant for CLL. Because of the heterogeneity of patients and their individual post-transplant disease and GVHD status, treatments should be individualized to each patient to account for these factors. The possible therapeutic options range from watchful waiting to intensive chemotherapy, and thus each patient's clinical status must be weighed carefully. Clinical trials are needed to ascertain safety and efficacy of standard treatment options as well as the multiple new agents that have recently been approved for management of CLL.

Standard chemotherapy post transplant

The data regarding the use of standard chemotherapy post transplant are limited. Often patients who have CLL that meet the indication for transplant are refractory to fludarabine-based chemotherapy regimens, and this likely predicts a poor response to post-transplant cytotoxic chemotherapy. However, there are some case series that report varying responses to cytotoxic chemotherapy with or without monoclonal antibodies, and these may be reasonable to consider in some patients [24,34,35]. It is important to consider the possible effects of cytotoxic agents on engraftment, GVL effect, and GVHD when considering various therapeutic regimens. For example, fludarabine and cyclophosphamide are active drugs in refractory disease but may be rather myelosuppressive, particularly with regard to lymphocyte depletion and, if used, may ultimately require donor stem cell support. Bendamustine and pentostatin are other drugs that may be considered in the post-transplant relapse setting [44].

With regard to monoclonal antibodies, several options are available for consideration. Alemtuzumab, while effective in relapsed disease, has not been shown to lead to durable responses post transplant [34]. Data regarding the use of rituximab are also limited but in theory it may have synergistic effects in treating both relapsed CLL and potentially reducing the risk of GVHD, thereby allowing reduction of immune suppression therapy [54]. Another anti-CD20 monoclonal antibody, ofatumumab, which targets a different CD20 epitope than rituximab, has been shown to have good single-agent activity for relapsed CLL [55], but similarly to its monoclonal antibody counterparts lacks data in the post-transplant setting.

Novel therapies and their integration in transplantation for CLL/SLL

Recently, several new drugs have been developed and this has ushered in a new era of targeted therapy for treatment of CLL. This has resulted in the approval by the Food and Drug Administration (FDA) of several new drugs that are now available in the CLL therapeutic arsenal. This has been due in large part to the elucidation of the critical importance of the B-cell receptor (BCR) and its signal transduction pathway in controlling the survival and proliferation of B cells in CLL. This has led to the development of several small-molecule inhibitors that have demonstrated both improved disease control with PFS and OS benefit along with preservation of quality of life without the major toxic effects of traditional chemotherapy.

While the new drug developments have spurred excitement in the treatment of patients with CLL, it is not known what their utility and role is in the realm of allo-SCT at this time, either in the pretransplant conditioning regimen or in the post-transplant maintenance setting. One consideration is that as these new drugs becoming increasingly used in the upfront or relapsed setting, it is likely that many patients who have undergone an allo-SCT will have been exposed to them at some point in their treatment. Thus, these drugs may not be useful in the post-transplant relapsed setting. As in many hematologic diseases in the post-transplant setting, maintenance therapy is an attractive option that may prolong PFS and OS. In CLL, there are no data to support post-transplant maintenance therapy at this

time. These novel agents are discussed briefly in the following sections but their role in the peritransplant period remains unclear.

Ibrutinib

Ibrutinib is a new oral Bruton's tyrosine kinase inhibitor that has recently been approved by the FDA for treatment of relapsed CLL. It has previously shown impressive preclinical activity in targeting the Bruton's tyrosine kinase [56–58], which plays an essential role in BCR signaling, mediation of interactions with the tumor microenvironment, and promotion of survival and proliferation of CLL cells. In relapsed disease, ibrutinib has been shown in a Phase Ib-2 multicenter trial to have an overall response rate (ORR) of 71% that was independent of disease stage, number of prior therapies, and the 17p deletion, with PFS and OS of 75% and 83% at 26 months. It is overall well tolerated and conveniently administered as a pill once daily [59]. In treatment-naive older patients, it has been shown to have a projected 24-month PFS in 95% of patients [60]. It has been noted to cause a prolonged lymphocytosis lasting from several months to greater than 1 year in some patients that is not reflective of disease progression [61], but which may make progression of disease assessment post transplant more difficult. There are several ongoing clinical trials investigating the role of ibrutinib in combination with other drugs in treatment of CLL as well as other B-cell non-Hodgkin lymphomas (clinicaltrials.gov).

Idelalisib

Idelalisib is a new first in class small-molecule oral inhibitor of the delta isoform of phosphatidylinositol 3-kinase (PI3K), which mediates the BCR signaling pathway, a key pathway in the pathogenesis of CLL. The PI3Kδ is highly expressed in lymphoid cells and is the most critical isoform in the malignant phenotype of CLL [62]. Moreover, it has been shown to be effective in patients with relapsed CLL with significant medical comorbidities when used in combination with rituximab compared with rituximab alone [63]. These authors conducted a Phase III, randomized, double-blind, placebo-controlled trial of combination therapy with idelalisib and rituximab in older patients (78% were older than 65 years) with significant medical comorbidities (renal dysfunction, poor marrow function, and cumulative illness rating scale, CIRS, of >6) and showed an ORR of 81% and OS at 12 months of 92% with a PFS not yet reached. Improvement in PFS was observed not only in the overall study population but also in all subgroups examined, including patients with poor prognostic features, such as 17p deletion or *TP53* mutations and unmutated *IGHV*. Overall the drug was well tolerated. There are several ongoing studies of this novel agent in combination with other drugs for treatment of patients with CLL and other non-Hodgkin lymphomas.

Obinutuzumab

CD20 is an effective target in CLL therapy, as demonstrated by efficacy with drugs such as rituximab and ofatumumab. Recently, obinutuzumab, a new anti-CD20 monoclonal antibody, has been demonstrated to be effective in older patients with significant coexisting medical conditions, which is the largest population of patients afflicted by CLL. Obinutuzumab differs from prior anti-CD20 monoclonal antibodies in that it harbors a glycoengineered Fc region and type 2 CD20 binding. The increased binding affinity of the Fc portion of obinutuzumab to the Fcγ receptor III on innate immune effector cells leads to antibody-dependent cell-mediated cytotoxicity and antibody-dependent cellular phagocytosis [64,65]. Goede *et al.* [66] reported data from a three-arm Phase II study that showed obinutuzumab (formerly Ga101) plus chlorambucil was superior to rituximab plus chlorambucil and chlorambucil alone in previously untreated patients. This study is important for the primary reason that it addresses the unmet need of a viable treatment option for elderly patients with multiple coexisting medical conditions that may make them ineligible for treatment with chemotherapy. The median age in this study was 73 years, with a CIRS score of 8 at baseline. The authors demonstrated that the combination of obinutuzumab and chlorambucil prolonged OS [hazard ratio (HR) for death 0.41, 95% CI 0.23–0.74; $P = 0.002$] compared to chlorambucil alone. A PFS prolongation was also seen in the obinuzutumab/chlorambucil treatment group compared to the rituximab/chlorambucil group (HR 0.39, 95% CI 0.31–0.49; $P < 0.001$) along with higher rates of CR (20.7% vs. 7.0%) and molecular response. Overall treatment was well tolerated. As a result of this trial, obinutuzumab has already been approved for first-line therapy in the United States for CLL. There are several ongoing studies evaluating the impact of obinutuzumab with other drugs in CLL and other non-Hodgkin lymphomas (clinicaltrials.gov).

Chimeric antigen receptors

Chimeric antigen receptor-modified T cells has also received a large amount of attention and interest as it relates to treatment for CLL. Porter *et al.* [67] first described this treatment modality in a case report of a patient with advanced p53-deficient (17p deletion) CLL who had been refractory to previous treatments, in which the use of autologous T cells expressing an anti-CD19 chimeric antigen receptor (CAR19) in combination with chemotherapy achieved a complete remission. Autologous T cells were collected by leukapheresis and subsequently transduced with a lentivirus to express a CD19-specific chimeric antigen receptor. The investigators additionally incorporated a CD137 (4-1BB) signaling domain as preclinical models had demonstrated that there was increased antitumor activity and increased persistence of the chimeric antigen receptor with the addition of this domain [68]. Their protocol included pre-infusion chemotherapy in the form of pentostatin 40 mg/m^2 plus cyclophosphamide 600 mg/m^2. Four days after chemotherapy the patient received a dose of 1.42×10^7 transduced cells (1.4×10^5 cells/kg) split into three consecutive daily intravenous doses. No infusion reaction was observed but approximately 22 days after the infusion tumor lysis syndrome was diagnosed. Repeat disease assessment at day 28 showed no further palpable lymphadenopathy, no morphologic evidence of CLL in the bone marrow, with cytogenetics showing normal karyotype and fluorescence *in situ* hybridization negative for 17p deletion consistent with complete remission. At the time of publication, the authors reported that the patient had sustained remission of approximately 10 months. A Phase I study has also been published looking at the role of donor-derived CD19-redirected virus-specific T cells for relapsed B-cell malignancies after allogeneic stem cell transplant which showed objective antitumor activity in a small number of patients [9]. This area of study for B-cell malignancies will continue to grow and it is likely that more data will emerge regarding the role of this novel treatment modality for patients in CLL.

Flavopiridol

Flavopiridol is a cyclin-dependent kinase inhibitor that had previously shown promising preclinical activity in the treatment of CLL and other diseases. However, clinical trials have been disappointing. Byrd *et al.* [70] have shown significant clinical activity in patients with refractory, bulky, and high-risk disease, with some patients achieving durable responses in a Phase I clinical trial. It has also been shown to have activity in combination with cyclophosphamide and rituximab with durable responses in a small number of patients [71]. Its role in the transplant setting is not known.

Summary

Patients with high-risk CLL should be referred for consideration of allo-SCT. Data have shown that patients can have long-term disease-free survival and acceptable transplantation-related risk. Allo-SCT is not only curative but has the potential to overcome the poor prognosis associated with high-risk disease. Young fit patients with high-risk or refractory disease should be referred to transplant centers early for consideration of this potentially curative treatment modality.

Case study

A 50-year-old female with a past medical history significant for hypertension and hyperlipidemia presented to her primary care physician with new symptoms of night sweats and unintentional weight loss in the preceding 2 months. She denied any palpable lymphadenopathy. Her primary care physician performed further work-up, and her complete blood count (CBC) was notable for leukocytosis of 63,000/μL with a lymphocyte predominance of 80%, hemoglobin of 10.5 g/dL, and platelet count of 50,000/μL. Her family history was negative for hematologic malignancies, and she has four fully related otherwise healthy siblings. She went on to have peripheral blood flow cytometry performed which was consistent with the diagnosis of chronic lymphocytic leukemia (CLL). Because of her cytopenias, a bone marrow biopsy was ordered and again confirmed the diagnosis of CLL, with 60–70% marrow involvement. Cytogenetics and fluorescence *in situ* hybridization (FISH) were notable for 17p deletion. Because of her symptoms, she was started on chemotherapy with fludarabine, cyclophosphamide, and rituximab (FCR). What is the next appropriate step in management of this patient?

A Continue treatment with four cycles of FCR and proceed with maintenance therapy after she achieves a complete remission (CR).

B Begin with HLA typing of the patient and referral for consideration of a myeloablative allogeneic stem cell transplant from an unrelated donor.

C Refer to a transplant center for consideration of autologous stem cell transplant for consolidation.

D Begin HLA typing of the patient and her siblings and, if match identified, proceed with reduced-intensity allogeneic transplant from a sibling donor

E Continue with FCR treatment until progression of disease.

Correct answer: D

The patient is young and otherwise healthy but has a diagnosis of high-risk CLL as defined by the 17p deletion in her cytogenetic and FISH analyses. This genetic aberration is associated with very high risk disease and poor outcomes. The standard recommendation for these patients is early referral for reduced-intensity allogeneic stem cell transplant either from a sibling or a matched unrelated donor (if a sibling donor is not available). Answer A is incorrect as there is no defined role for maintenance therapy for CLL. Answer B is incorrect because myeloablation is generally not recommended for patients undergoing allogeneic transplants as previous studies have shown excessive TRM without improvement in transplant outcome. Answer C is incorrect as there is evidence that there is no survival benefit in patients undergoing autologous stem cell transplant, and there is no role for it in the standard treatment of CLL outside of a clinical trial. Answer E is incorrect as early transplant referral, not continued chemotherapy, would be the standard recommendation for young fit patients with high-risk CLL.

References

1 Jemal A, Siegel R, Xu J, Ward E. Cancer statistics, 2010. *CA: Cancer J Clin* 2010;60:277–300.

2 Gribben JG. How I treat CLL up front. *Blood* 2010;115: 187–97.

3 Rai KR, Sawitsky A, Cronkite EP, Chanana AD, Levy RN, Pasternack BS. Clinical staging of chronic lymphocytic leukemia. *Blood* 1975;46:219–34.

4 Binet JL, Auquier A, Dighiero G *et al.* A new prognostic classification of chronic lymphocytic leukemia derived from a multivariate survival analysis. *Cancer* 1981;48:198–206.

5 Hallek M, Cheson BD, Catovsky D *et al.* Guidelines for the diagnosis and treatment of chronic lymphocytic leukemia: a report from the International Workshop on Chronic Lymphocytic Leukemia updating the National Cancer Institute-Working Group 1996 guidelines. *Blood* 2008;111: 5446–56.

6 Tam CS, O'Brien S, Wierda W *et al.* Long-term results of the fludarabine, cyclophosphamide, and rituximab regimen as initial therapy of chronic lymphocytic leukemia. *Blood* 2008;112:975–80.

7 Keating MJ, O'Brien S, Albitar M *et al.* Early results of a chemoimmunotherapy regimen of fludarabine, cyclophosphamide, and rituximab as initial therapy for chronic lymphocytic leukemia. *J Clin Oncol* 2005;23:4079–88.

8 Wierda W, O'Brien S, Wen S *et al.* Chemoimmunotherapy with fludarabine, cyclophosphamide, and rituximab for relapsed and refractory chronic lymphocytic leukemia. *J Clin Oncol* 2005;23:4070–8.

9 Stilgenbauer S, Dohner H. Campath-1H-induced complete remission of chronic lymphocytic leukemia despite p53 gene mutation and resistance to chemotherapy. *N Engl J Med* 2002;347:452–3.

10 Dreger P, Corradini P, Kimby E *et al.* Indications for allogeneic stem cell transplantation in chronic lymphocytic leukemia: the EBMT transplant consensus. *Leukemia* 2007;21:12–17.

11 Bandini G, Michallet M, Rosti G, Tura S. Bone marrow transplantation for chronic lymphocytic leukemia. *Bone Marrow Transplant* 1991;7:251–3.

12 Montserrat E, Moreno C, Esteve J, Urbano-Ispizua A, Gine E, Bosch F. How I treat refractory CLL. *Blood* 2006; 107:1276–83.

13 Pavletic SZ, Khouri IF, Haagenson M *et al.* Unrelated donor marrow transplantation for B-cell chronic lymphocytic leukemia after using myeloablative conditioning: results from the Center for International Blood and Marrow Transplant Research. *J Clin Oncol* 2005;23:5788–94.

14 Michallet M, Sobh M, Milligan D *et al.* The impact of HLA matching on long-term transplant outcome after allogeneic hematopoietic stem cell transplantation for CLL: a retrospective study from the EBMT registry. *Leukemia* 2010;24: 1725–31.

15 Rodrigues CA, Rocha V, Dreger P *et al.* Alternative donor hematopoietic stem cell transplantation for mature lymphoid malignances after reduced-intensity conditioning regimen: similar outcomes with umbilical cord blood and unrelated donor peripheral blood. *Haematologica* 2014;99:370–7.

16 McClune BL, Defor T, Brunstein C *et al.* Reduced intensity allogeneic haematopoietic cell transplantation for chronic lymphocytic leukaemia: related donor and umbilical cord allografting. *Br J Haematol* 2012;156:273–5.

17 Rabinowe SN, Soiffer RJ, Gribben JG *et al.* Autologous and allogeneic bone marrow transplantation for poor prognosis patients with B-cell chronic lymphocytic leukemia. *Blood* 1993;82:1366–76.

18 Dreger P, Stilgenbauer S, Benner A *et al.* The prognostic impact of autologous stem cell transplantation in patients with chronic lymphocytic leukemia: a risk-matched analysis based on the VH gene mutational status. *Blood* 2004;103:2850–8.

19 Michallet M, Dreger P, Sutton L *et al.* Autologous hematopoietic stem cell transplantation in chronic lymphocytic leukemia: results of European intergroup randomized trial comparing autografting versus observation. *Blood* 2011;117:1516–21.

20 Brion A, Mahe B, Kolb B *et al.* Autologous transplantation in CLL patients with B and C Binet stages: final results of the prospective randomized GOELAMS LLC 98 trial. *Bone Marrow Transplant* 2012;47:542–8.

21 Sutton L, Chevret S, Tournilhac O *et al.* Autologous stem cell transplantation as a first-line treatment strategy for chronic lymphocytic leukemia: a multicenter, randomized, controlled trial from the SFGM-TC and GFLLC. *Blood* 2011;117:6109–19.

22 Hallek M, Fischer K, Fingerle-Rowson G *et al.* Addition of rituximab to fludarabine and cyclophosphamide in patients with chronic lymphocytic leukaemia: a randomised, open-label, phase 3 trial. *Lancet* 2010;376:1164–74.

23 Gribben JG, Zahrieh D, Stephans K *et al.* Autologous and allogeneic stem cell transplantations for poor-risk chronic lymphocytic leukemia. *Blood* 2005;106:4389–96.

24 Sorror ML, Maris MB, Sandmaier BM *et al.* Hematopoietic cell transplantation after nonmyeloablative conditioning for advanced chronic lymphocytic leukemia. *J Clin Oncol* 2005;23:3819–29.

25 Montserrat E, Gribben JG. Autografting CLL: the game is over! *Blood* 2011;117:6057–8.

26 Khouri IF, Keating M, Korbling M *et al.* Transplant-lite: induction of graft-versus-malignancy using fludarabine-based nonablative chemotherapy and allogeneic blood progenitor-cell transplantation as treatment for lymphoid malignancies. *J Clin Oncol* 1998;16:2817–24.

27 Maloney DG, Sandmaier BM, Mackinnon S, Shizuru JA. Non-myeloablative transplantation. *Hematology Am Soc Hematol Educ Program* 2002;392–421.

28 Sorror M, Storer B, Sandmaier BM *et al.* Hematopoietic cell transplantation-comorbidity index and Karnofsky performance status are independent predictors of morbidity

and mortality after allogeneic nonmyeloablative hemato-poietic cell transplantation. *Cancer* 2008;112:1992–2001.

29 Michallet M, Archimbaud E, Bandini G *et al.* HLA-identical sibling bone marrow transplantation in younger patients with chronic lymphocytic leukemia. European Group for Blood and Marrow Transplantation and the International Bone Marrow Transplant Registry. *Ann Intern Med* 1996; 124:311–15.

30 Khouri IF, Saliba RM, Admirand J *et al.* Graft-versus-leu-kaemia effect after non-myeloablative haematopoietic transplantation can overcome the unfavourable expression of ZAP-70 in refractory chronic lymphocytic leukaemia. *Br J Haematol* 2007;137:355–63.

31 Schetelig J, van Biezen A, Brand R *et al.* Allogeneic hemato-poietic stem-cell transplantation for chronic lymphocytic leukemia with 17p deletion: a retrospective European Group for Blood and Marrow Transplantation analysis. *J Clin Oncol* 2008;26:5094–100.

32 Dreger P, Dohner H, Ritgen M *et al.* Allogeneic stem cell transplantation provides durable disease control in poor-risk chronic lymphocytic leukemia: long-term clinical and MRD results of the German CLL Study Group CLL3X trial. *Blood* 2010;116:2438–47.

33 Khouri IF, Bassett R, Poindexter N *et al.* Nonmyeloablative allogeneic stem cell transplantation in relapsed/refractory chronic lymphocytic leukemia: long-term follow-up, prog-nostic factors, and effect of human leukocyte histo-compatibility antigen subtype on outcome. *Cancer* 2011;117: 4679–88.

34 Delgado J, Thomson K, Russell N *et al.* Results of alemtu-zumab-based reduced-intensity allogeneic transplantation for chronic lymphocytic leukemia: a British Society of Blood and Marrow Transplantation Study. *Blood* 2006;107:1724–30.

35 Sorror ML, Storer BE, Sandmaier BM *et al.* Five-year follow-up of patients with advanced chronic lymphocytic leukemia treated with allogeneic hematopoietic cell transplantation after nonmyeloablative conditioning. *J Clin Oncol* 2008;26: 4912–20.

36 Khouri IF, Lee MS, Saliba RM *et al.* Nonablative allogeneic stem cell transplantation for chronic lymphocytic leukemia: impact of rituximab on immunomodulation and survival. *Exp Hematol* 2004;32:28–35.

37 Brown JR, Kim HT, Li S *et al.* Predictors of improved pro-gression-free survival after nonmyeloablative allogeneic stem cell transplantation for advanced chronic lymphocytic leukemia. *Biol Blood Marrow Transplant* 2006;12:1056–64.

38 Schmitz N, Dreger P, Glass B, Sureda A. Allogeneic trans-plantation in lymphoma: current status. *Haematologica* 2007;92:1533–48.

39 Schetelig J, Thiede C, Bornhauser M *et al.* Evidence of a graft-versus-leukemia effect in chronic lymphocytic leu-kemia after reduced-intensity conditioning and allogeneic stem-cell transplantation: the Cooperative German Transplant Study Group. *J Clin Oncol* 2003;21:2747–53.

40 Delgado J, Pillai S, Benjamin R *et al.* The effect of in vivo T cell depletion with alemtuzumab on reduced-intensity allogeneic hematopoietic cell transplantation for chronic lymphocytic leukemia. *Biol Blood Marrow Transplant* 2008; 14:1288–97.

41 Shaffer BC, Modric M, Stetler-Stevenson M *et al.* Rapid complete donor lymphoid chimerism and graft-versus-leu-kemia effect are important in early control of chronic lymphocytic leukemia. *Exp Hematol* 2013;41:772–8.

42 Hoogendoorn M, Jedema I, Barge RM *et al.* Characterization of graft-versus-leukemia responses in patients treated for advanced chronic lymphocytic leukemia with donor lym-phocyte infusions after in vitro T-cell depleted allogeneic stem cell transplantation following reduced-intensity condi-tioning. *Leukemia* 2007;21:2569–74.

43 Logan AC, Zhang B, Narasimhan B *et al.* Minimal residual disease quantification using consensus primers and high-throughput IGH sequencing predicts post-transplant relapse in chronic lymphocytic leukemia. *Leukemia* 2013;27:1659–65.

44 Porter DL, Alyea EP, Antin JH *et al.* NCI First International Workshop on the Biology, Prevention, and Treatment of Relapse after Allogeneic Hematopoietic Stem Cell Transplantation: Report from the Committee on Treatment of Relapse after Allogeneic Hematopoietic Stem Cell Transplantation. *Biol Blood Marrow Transplant* 2010;16: 1467–503.

45 Pavletic SZ, Zhou G, Sobocinski K *et al.* Genetically identical twin transplantation for chronic lymphocytic leukemia. *Leukemia* 2007;21:2452–5.

46 Hardy NM, Grady C, Pentz R *et al.* Bioethical considerations of monoclonal B-cell lymphocytosis: donor transfer after haematopoietic stem cell transplantation. *Br J Haematol* 2007;139:824–31.

47 Caporaso N, Marti GE, Goldin L. Perspectives on familial chronic lymphocytic leukemia: genes and the environment. *Semin Hematol* 2004;41:201–6.

48 Rawstron AC, Green MJ, Kuzmicki A *et al.* Monoclonal B lymphocytes with the characteristics of "indolent" chronic lymphocytic leukemia are present in 3.5% of adults with normal blood counts. *Blood* 2002;100:635–9.

49 Marti GE, Rawstron AC, Ghia P *et al.* Diagnostic criteria for monoclonal B-cell lymphocytosis. *Br J Haematol* 2005; 130:325–32.

50 Marti GE, Carter P, Abbasi F *et al.* B-cell monoclonal lym-phocytosis and B-cell abnormalities in the setting of familial B-cell chronic lymphocytic leukemia. *Cytometry Part B* 2003;52:1–12.

51 Rawstron AC, Yuille MR, Fuller J *et al.* Inherited predisposition to CLL is detectable as subclinical monoclonal B-lymphocyte expansion. *Blood* 2002;100:2289–90.

52 Dreger P, Brand R, Hansz J *et al.* Treatment-related mortality and graft-versus-leukemia activity after allogeneic stem cell transplantation for chronic lymphocytic leukemia using intensity-reduced conditioning. *Leukemia* 2003;17:841–8.

53 Rondon G, Giralt S, Huh Y *et al.* Graft-versus-leukemia effect after allogeneic bone marrow transplantation for chronic lymphocytic leukemia. *Bone Marrow Transplant* 1996;18:669–72.

54 Alousi AM, Uberti J, Ratanatharathorn V. The role of B cell depleting therapy in graft versus host disease after allogeneic hematopoietic cell transplant. *Leukemia Lymphoma* 2010;51:376–89.

55 Coiffier B, Lepretre S, Pedersen LM *et al.* Safety and efficacy of ofatumumab, a fully human monoclonal anti-CD20 antibody, in patients with relapsed or refractory B-cell chronic lymphocytic leukemia: a phase 1–2 study. *Blood* 2008;111: 1094–100.

56 Herman SE, Gordon AL, Hertlein E *et al.* Bruton tyrosine kinase represents a promising therapeutic target for treatment of chronic lymphocytic leukemia and is effectively targeted by PCI-32765. *Blood* 2011;117:6287–96.

57 Ponader S, Chen SS, Buggy JJ *et al.* The Bruton tyrosine kinase inhibitor PCI-32765 thwarts chronic lymphocytic leukemia cell survival and tissue homing in vitro and in vivo. *Blood* 2012;119:1182–9.

58 de Rooij MF, Kuil A, Geest CR *et al.* The clinically active BTK inhibitor PCI-32765 targets B-cell receptor- and chemokine-controlled adhesion and migration in chronic lymphocytic leukemia. *Blood* 2012;119:2590–4.

59 Byrd JC, Furman RR, Coutre SE *et al.* Targeting BTK with ibrutinib in relapsed chronic lymphocytic leukemia. *N Engl J Med* 2013;369:32–42.

60 O'Brien S, Furman RR, Coutre SE *et al.* Ibrutinib as initial therapy for elderly patients with chronic lymphocytic leukaemia or small lymphocytic lymphoma: an open-label, multicentre, phase 1b/2 trial. *Lancet Oncol* 2014;15:48–58.

61 Woyach JA, Smucker K, Smith LL *et al.* Prolonged lymphocytosis during ibrutinib therapy is associated with distinct molecular characteristics and does not indicate a suboptimal response to therapy. *Blood* 2014;123:1810–17.

62 Herman SE, Gordon AL, Wagner AJ *et al.* Phosphatidylinositol 3-kinase-delta inhibitor CAL-101 shows promising preclinical activity in chronic lymphocytic leukemia by antagonizing intrinsic and extrinsic cellular survival signals. *Blood* 2010; 116:2078–88.

63 Furman RR, Sharman JP, Coutre SE *et al.* Idelalisib and rituximab in relapsed chronic lymphocytic leukemia. *N Engl J Med* 2014;370:997–1007.

64 Mossner E, Brunker P, Moser S *et al.* Increasing the efficacy of CD20 antibody therapy through the engineering of a new type II anti-CD20 antibody with enhanced direct and immune effector cell-mediated B-cell cytotoxicity. *Blood* 2010;115:4393–402.

65 Honeychurch J, Alduaij W, Azizyan M *et al.* Antibody-induced nonapoptotic cell death in human lymphoma and leukemia cells is mediated through a novel reactive oxygen species-dependent pathway. *Blood* 2012;119: 3523–33.

66 Goede V, Fischer K, Busch R *et al.* Obinutuzumab plus chlorambucil in patients with CLL and coexisting conditions. *N Engl J Med* 2014;370:1101–10.

67 Porter DL, Levine BL, Kalos M, Bagg A, June CH. Chimeric antigen receptor-modified T cells in chronic lymphoid leukemia. *N Engl J Med* 2011;365:725–33.

68 Carpentino C, Milone MC, Hassan R *et al.* Control of large established tumor xenografts with genetically retargeted human T cells containing CD28 and CD137 domains. *Proc Natl Acad Sci USA* 2009;106:3360–5.

69 Cruz CR, Micklethwaite KP, Savoldo B *et al.* Infusion of donor-derived CD19-redirected virus-specific T cells for B-cell malignancies relapsed after allogeneic stem cell transplant: a phase 1 study. *Blood* 2013;122:2965–73.

70 Byrd JC, Lin TS, Dalton JT *et al.* Flavopiridol administered using a pharmacologically derived schedule is associated with marked clinical efficacy in refractory, genetically high-risk chronic lymphocytic leukemia. *Blood* 2007;109: 399–404.

71 Stephens DM, Ruppert AS, Maddocks K *et al.* Cyclophosphamide, alvocidib (flavopiridol), and rituximab, a novel feasible chemoimmunotherapy regimen for patients with high-risk chronic lymphocytic leukemia. *Leukemia Res* 2013;37:1195–9.

CHAPTER 16

Diffuse large B-cell lymphoma

Lauren Veltri, Bipin N. Savani, Mohamed A. Kharfan-Dabaja,
Mehdi Hamadani and Abraham S. Kanate

Introduction

Diffuse large B-cell lymphoma (DLBCL) is the most common subtype of non-Hodgkin lymphoma (NHL), comprising approximately 30% of all cases [1]. While conventional cytotoxic chemotherapy provides around 50% complete remission (CR) rates [2], the addition of rituximab to chemotherapy (chemoimmunotherapy) has dramatically improved response rates, progression-free survival (PFS), and overall survival (OS) and is considered the standard of care in the initial treatment of DLBCL [3,4]. Risk stratification based on the original International Prognostic Index (IPI), the new National Comprehensive Cancer Network (NCCN)-IPI, gene expression profiling, chromosomal aberrations (e.g., *myc* rearrangement), and interim functional imaging with positron emission tomography (PET) has prognostic value but is not currently utilized to tailor therapy in individual patients [5–10]. Even with optimal upfront therapy, disease progression/relapse remains a significant concern [11], warranting additional therapy including hematopoietic cell transplantation (HCT) in a subset of patients.

Indications for transplantation in DLBCL

The successful use of HCT in the management of hematologic malignancies was one of the great scientific achievements of the twentieth century. In-depth details pertaining to the historical perspectives and therapeutic rationale of HCT is discussed elsewhere in this book. The premise of autologous (auto)-HCT is the use of high-dose therapy (HDT) with cytotoxic agents with nonoverlapping toxicities, in order to maximize the steep dose–response curve followed by rescue of the patient's hematopoietic system with autologous progenitor cells. Chemosensitive/radiosensitive diseases such as DLBCL are especially amenable to this therapeutic strategy [12]. Auto-HCT is well tolerated, with non-relapse mortality (NRM) rates below 5% in most centers, but continued risk of disease relapse after auto-HCT remains a significant problem and usually portends poor outcomes. In contrast, allogeneic (allo)-HCT not only relies on cytoreductive effects of the conditioning regimen, but also provides therapeutic benefit via potent graft-versus-lymphoma (GVL) reactions; however, it is associated with higher NRM. In the context of DLBCL, HDT and auto-HCT is considered the standard second-line approach for patients with relapsed disease that is sensitive to salvage therapy. Upfront utilization of auto-grafting as a consolidative strategy in first CR (especially for high-risk disease) is more controversial. For chemo-refractory DLBCL and for progressive disease after auto-graft, alternative therapy including allo-HCT is warranted and can provide long-term disease-free survival (DFS).

Timing and preparation of patients for transplantation in DLBCL

Selecting the appropriate patient and timing for HCT is of paramount importance in balancing the toxicity and benefit of the proposed treatment approach and is

Clinical Guide to Transplantation in Lymphoma, First Edition. Edited by Bipin N. Savani and Mohamad Mohty.

contingent on patient- and disease-specific factors [13]. Previously, older patients were excluded from transplantation owing to higher toxicity and NRM. The European Group for Blood and Marrow Transplantation (EMBT) registry reviewed the impact of age on outcomes with HDT and auto-HCT in DLBCL in older (≥60, N = 2612) versus younger (<60, N = 2149) patients. While older age was associated with higher 1-year NRM (8.7% vs. 4.7%, P = 0.002) as well as inferior 3-year PFS (51% vs. 62%, P < 0.001) and OS (60% vs. 70%, P < 0.001), more than 50% of older individuals were disease-free and alive 3 years post HCT [14]. Several other studies have demonstrated that comorbidities and performance status (PS) play a more important role in determining HCT outcomes than simply patient's chronological age. A retrospective study specific to DLBCL reviewed 152 patients who received BEAM (carmustine, etoposide, cytarabine, melphalan) conditioning, with 59 patients being over 60 years of age. Charlson Comorbidity Index Score, but not chronological patient age, predicted NRM (P = 0.03) [15]. While older patients are more likely to have more comorbidities and poorer PS, chronological age alone can no longer be considered an exclusion criterion for auto-HCT and reduced-intensity conditioning (RIC) allo-HCT. The decision to proceed with transplantation should be an individualized decision.

With the excellent responses and long-term disease control noted in most patients with modern chemoimmunotherapies, HCT is routinely not considered in first remission. If relapse/progression or refractory disease is suspected, repeat tissue biopsy and re-imaging studies are essential to confirm active lymphoma and extent of involvement. In DLBCL, transplantation is considered an integral part of patient management in relapsed disease and transplant eligibility of the patient must be factored at the outset. Salvage therapy with chemoimmunotherapy with or without radiotherapy is essential to demonstrate chemoresponsiveness of DLBCL prior to proceeding to HCT. The secondary age-adjusted IPI (aa-IPI) [comprising three factors: PS, lactate dehydrogenase (LDH) and stage] calculated at disease relapse is predictive of OS and PFS following second-line therapy, and can also predict auto-HCT outcomes in chemosensitive disease [16]. Response to salvage therapy is probably the most important disease-specific parameter in predicting the utility and response to autografting. Pretransplant negative PET (i.e., chemosensitive disease) is highly predictive of post-autograft PFS and OS [17,18].

Autograft should be considered for relapsed/refractory DLBCL patients achieving only a partial remission (without attaining a CR) as shown in studies by the Grupo Español de Linfomas/Trasplante Autólogo de Médula Ósea (GELTAMO) [19,20]. Pretransplant positive PET and, more importantly, chemoresistant disease portend poor outcomes with HDT and auto-HCT [21] and alternative therapeutic strategies including allo-HCT, novel therapies, and clinical trials should be considered.

The optimal salvage chemotherapy has not been established but is usually center-specific. The two most commonly used regimens include DHAP (dexamethasone, cytarabine, cisplatin) and ICE (ifosfamide, carboplatin, etoposide) with rituximab (R). The international randomized Collaborative Trial in Relapsed Aggressive Lymphoma (CORAL) study compared salvage regimens R-DHAP and R-ICE (N = 477) in relapsed/refractory DLBCL and demonstrated similar response rates (63%). All chemosensitive patients underwent HDT and auto-HCT and the choice of salvage regimen had no impact on 3-year event-free survival (EFS) and OS [22]. Similarly, the choice of HDT (conditioning regimen) aimed at eradicating the lymphoma clone is arbitrary and center-specific. Commonly used regimens include BEAM, CBV (cyclophosphamide, etoposide, cytarabine), BEAC (carmustine, etoposide, cytarabine, cyclophosphamide), and total body irradiation (TBI)-containing regimens. Acknowledging the lack of randomized studies in this field, the use of TBI-based regimens may be associated with higher NRM, risk of secondary malignancies, and inferior PFS and OS [23]. Several investigators have attempted to augment HDT with radioimmunotherapeutic agents. However, a Phase III trial (N = 224) which randomized patients to receive BEAM conditioning with either rituximab or ^{131}I-labeled tositumomab followed by auto-HCT reported similar 2-year PFS and OS with either approach [24]. While the incorporation of monoclonal antibodies and radioimmunotherapy to conditioning regimens is feasible, it is mostly limited to institutional preference and not widely practiced.

There is a continued risk of relapse after auto-HCT owing possibly to either tumor contamination of the graft or persistence of lymphoma clone in the patient following HDT. For relapsing patients and those with chemoresistant DLBCL (thus not eligible for HDT and auto-HCT), adoptive immunotherapy by allo-HCT is potentially a curative option [25]. However, allo-HCT is

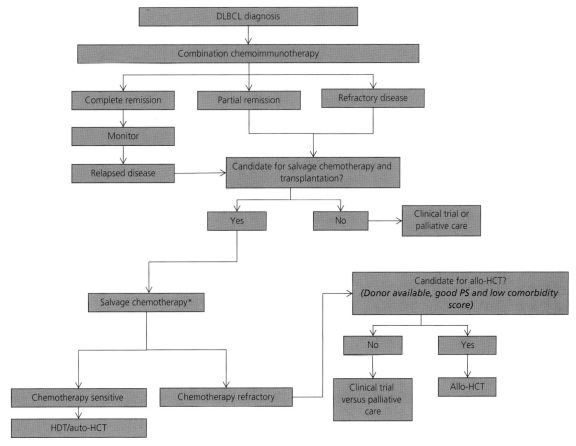

Figure 16.1 Suggested treatment algorithm for diffuse large B-cell lymphoma (DLBCL). Auto-HCT, autologous hematopoietic cell transplantation; aaIPI, age-adjusted International Prognostic Index; allo-HCT, allogeneic hematopoietic cell transplantation; HDT, high-dose therapy; PS, performance status. Asterisk indicates that autograft may be considered if chemotherapy sensitivity is demonstrable with salvage therapy. Adapted from Klyuchnikov *et al.* [54].

complicated by significant and sometimes prohibitive therapy-related morbidity and mortality and selection of the appropriate patient, donor, and conditioning regimen is extremely important. Figure 16.1 represents a suggested algorithm incorporating transplantation in DLBCL.

Autologous hematopoietic cell transplantation for DLBCL

In the previous sections we broadly discussed the role, timing, salvage, and conditioning regimens of auto-HCT. Here we will explore the pertinent data of HDT and auto-HCT in DLBCL.

Autologous hematopoietic cell transplantation consolidation in first remission
Pre-rituximab era
The use of auto-HCT earlier in the disease course as a consolidative strategy following first-line therapies for aggressive lymphomas has been evaluated. Based on promising results of small pilot studies, many randomized controlled trials in the pre-rituximab era explored the role of HDT and auto-HCT consolidation following front-line chemotherapies in patients with aggressive NHL (predominantly DLBCL). Although inconsistent, a majority of the trials did not show a PFS and/or OS benefit with upfront auto-HCT consolidation [26–30]. A few trials, including the subset analysis

of a large prospective study, did show improvement in PFS and OS, especially for patients with intermediate–high and high-risk IPI [31–33]. Interestingly, one study evaluating ACVBP (doxorubicin, cyclophosphamide, vincristine, bleomycin, prednisone) versus early HDT and auto-HCT found inferior OS and EFS with auto-grafting [34]. A systematic review and meta-analysis of 15 prospective studies with 2728 patients found no evidence of improved OS or EFS with early HDT and auto-HCT. In those with good risk aa-IPI, worse OS [hazard ratio (HR) 1.46, CI 1.02–2.09] was noted with autografting [35].

Rituximab era

Studies evaluating the role of upfront consolidation with HDT and auto-HCT in patients with high-risk DLBCL treated with rituximab-based chemoimmunotherapy have also produced conflicting results. Two randomized studies showed no PFS or OS benefit with auto-HCT consolidation, with one of them ($N = 262$) showing inferior OS in intermediate/high-risk aa-IPI patients receiving HDT [36,37]. Contrastingly, two studies have demonstrated superior PFS with upfront auto-HCT [38,39]. In the SWOG (South-West Oncology Group) study ($N = 253$), exploratory analysis showed an OS benefit in the high-risk aa-IPI group with early auto-grafting; however, this study included a large number of patients who did not receive rituximab-based front-line therapy that questions the relevance of these data in the rituximab era [39].

Considering the cumulative data from the pre-rituximab and rituximab eras and the excellent survival with current chemoimmunotherapy regimens (50–90% based on IPI), there does not appear to be a clear role for upfront auto-HCT and this modality cannot be recommended for routine practice.

Autologous hematopoietic cell transplantation in relapsed/refractory DLBCL

Relapsed (chemosensitive) DLBCL

Unlike in the upfront setting, HDT and auto-HCT is considered the standard of care in chemosensitive relapsed DLBCL. The PARMA trial conducted in the pre-rituximab era ($N = 215$) established the role of auto-HCT in relapsed DLBCL. Patients who demonstrated response to salvage chemotherapy with DHAP were randomized to receive additional DHAP plus radiation

therapy versus BEAC/TBI conditioning followed by auto-HCT. The respective 5-year EFS and OS were 46% and 12% ($P = 0.0001$) and 53% and 32% ($P = 0.038$), in the transplant and nontransplant cohorts, respectively [40]. Several retrospective registry studies have evaluated the role of HDT and auto-HCT in relapsed chemosensitive DLBCL with or without prior rituximab exposure [41–43]. The European Society for Blood and Marrow Transplantation (EBMT) study ($N = 470$), in which 25% of patients had prior rituximab use, showed 5-year OS and PFS of 63% and 48%, respectively [41]. Similarly, a Center for International Blood and Marrow Transplant Research (CIBMTR) study ($N = 994$) also found excellent outcomes with auto-HCT in DLBCL patients, who received rituximab-based therapies prior to auto-HCT [43].

Although auto-HCT is beneficial in relapsed chemosensitive DLBCL in the rituximab era, it may be noted that the relapse after initial therapy with rituximab-based therapy may be associated with less favorable outcomes [44,45]. An exploratory analysis of the CORAL study found DLBCL relapse within 12 months of initial diagnosis, prior rituximab use, and high second-line aa-IPI score to be associated with inferior EFS [22]. While the CORAL study does not dispute the utility of HDT and auto-HCT (3-year PFS, 51%), it identified a cohort with early relapse and prior rituximab exposure in whom the 3-year PFS was only 23% [22]. Unlike the CORAL results, a recent CIBMTR analysis reported 3-year OS and PFS of about 45% in DLBCL patients who experience early rituximab failure, but were subsequently able to undergo auto-HCT, after demonstrating evidence of chemosensitive disease with salvage therapies [46].

Refractory disease

Disease refractoriness in lymphoma, defined as less than 50% reduction in tumor size with therapy or disease progression while on therapy, is associated with poor prognosis. Even with optimal front-line chemoimmunotherapies, approximately 10–20% of patients have suboptimal responses [3]. In the relapsed setting, about 30% of patients do not respond to salvage therapy [22]. In relapsed DLBCL several studies have confirmed chemoresistance to salvage therapy as a predictor of poor outcome with subsequent HDT and auto-HCT [12,47–49].

An interesting retrospective study of 100 patients with relapsed/refractory intermediate- or high-grade

NHL who underwent auto-HCT divided the patient cohort into primary refractory, resistant relapse, and sensitive relapse based on responses to chemotherapy and noted 3-year post-autograft DFS of 0%, 14%, and 36%, respectively [50]. The Autologous Blood and Marrow Transplant Registry (ABMTR) reviewed 184 patients with aggressive NHL (mostly DLBCL) who underwent HDT and auto-HCT without ever achieving CR. Post-transplantation CR/CRu was 44%, with a 3-year OS of 37%. In multivariate analysis chemotherapy resistance, poor PS, age over 55, more than three lines of prior chemotherapy, and not receiving pre- or post-transplant involved-field radiation therapy predicted inferior survival [51]. Similarly, the GELTAMO reported 114 patients with DLBCL not in CR with induction treatment and found that one-third of these attained a CR with autograft, but confirmed the futility of HDT in chemoresistant disease [19,20]. The role of auto-HCT in DLBCL not attaining CR has been noted in other studies as well [52,53].

To summarize, HDT and auto-HCT has a clear role in relapsed chemosensitive DLBCL and should be considered the standard of care. Patients with chemoresistant disease following salvage attempts are best managed on clinical trials. Failure to attain a CR with primary therapy should not be considered a contraindication for HDT if chemosensitivity is demonstrable with subsequent therapies.

Allogeneic hematopoietic cell transplantation for DLBCL

The addition of chemoimmunotherapy and autologous transplantation to the therapeutic arsenal has improved the overall outcomes in relapsed DLBCL, but about 30–40% of patients will experience therapy failure [54]. The two subsets of DLBCL patients with particularly inferior outcomes include those relapsing after an autograft and those with chemoresistant disease. GVL effects are well recognized in several lymphoid malignancies but are potentially less robust in DLBCL owing to its inferior antigen-presenting ability [55,56]. However, clinically relevant GVL has been demonstrated in DLBCL [57,58]. In one report, 15 patients not in remission at day +100 were managed with withdrawal of immunosuppression or donor lymphocyte infusion (DLI) with or without chemotherapy, resulting in nine

responses including eight CRs [57]. Despite the presumed benefits, the use of allo-HCT in DLBCL has been limited secondary to higher rate of NRM, as well as the lack of randomized trials.

Allogeneic transplantation after autograft failure

Disease progression after auto-HCT portends poor prognosis, with a median survival of 3 months and 1-year OS of 10% or less [59]. Registry data have suggested feasibility and possible benefit with second auto-HCT in lymphoma patients (not specific to DLBCL), but may be limited to those with longer time to relapse from the first auto-HCT [60,61]. It may be noted that in the CIBMTR report, 62% of patients after a second auto-HCT had disease progression and relapse was the major cause of death [60]. While a second auto-HCT is a consideration for patients with no other options including allo-HCT, the data are limited and thus specific recommendations cannot be made.

The lack of tumor contamination of graft, potential GVL effects, and the possibility of cure makes allo-HCT a reasonable consideration. Several recent reports evaluating the role of allo-HCT in DLBCL have included those with prior autograft failure [58,62–64]. An EBMT study limited to allo-HCT in disease relapse after auto-HCT ($N = 101$) included both myeloablative conditioning (MAC) and RIC regimens and showed a 3-year PFS of 42% and OS of 54% [63]. Longer remission status after auto-HCT predicted better outcomes with allo-HCT. Similarly, retrospective data reviewing 165 DLBCL patients (all had prior auto-HCT) showed median PFS and OS of 52% and 39%, respectively [64]. These studies report NRM rates of 25–45% and relapse rates of 25–40% [58,62–64]. Careful patient selection and conditioning regimen is extremely important to balance the risk of toxicity and relapse (as discussed in subsequent sections). In eligible patients with available donors and chemosensitive disease, consideration for allo-HCT after failure of a prior auto-HCT is reasonable.

Allogeneic transplantation in refractory DLBCL

In clinical practice, the majority of patients who relapse after an auto-HCT will not proceed to allo-HCT due to inability to tolerate further therapy or due to resistant/progressive disease. According to the Gruppo Italiano Trapianto di Midollo Osseo (GITMO) database, of 884 patients who relapsed after an auto-HCT, only 165 (19%) proceeded to a subsequent allo-HCT [64].

Studies appraising the role of allo-HCT in DLBCL generally report 3- to 5-year PFS and OS of 35–48% and 41–47%, respectively [58,62,65]. The reports suggest very poor outcomes in patients with chemoresitant and progressive disease. Hamadani *et al.* [66] evaluated the outcomes of chemorefractory aggressive NHL (*N* = 46) including 18 patients with DLBCL who underwent allo-HCT. The 5-year OS, PFS, and NRM were 38%, 34%, and 35%, respectively. The OS and PFS were 46% and 46%, respectively, for those with stable disease at the time of transplant compared to 21% and 7%, respectively, for those with progressive disease. Based on the evidence provided, albeit limited, allo-HCT should be considered for chemotherapy-refractory DLBCL, but very careful patient selection is warranted weighing the risks and benefits.

Role of conditioning regimen in allogeneic transplantation

MAC regimens, while conferring additive cytoreduction to GVL effects, is associated with high NRM especially in patients who undergo prior auto-HCT, thus limiting its use [63,67–69]. RIC regimens have broadened the applicability of allo-HCT, especially in patients who are older and those with comorbid conditions. The EBMT reported significantly higher 3-year NRM offset by reduced (not statistically significant) relapse risk leading to comparable PFS with MAC compared to RIC in a cohort of 101 patients who underwent allo-HCT after autograft [63]. A CIBMTR registry study analyzed 396 patients with DLBCL who received an HLA-matched related to unrelated allo-HCT following MAC, RIC, or nonmyeloablative (NMA) conditioning. The 1-year NRM for the MAC group (47%) was significantly higher than that for the RIC/NMA group (31% and 29%, *P* = 0.004). The 1-year relapse rate was lower with MAC (26%) compared to 32% and 37%, respectively, with RIC and NMA (*P* = 0.04). However, no difference was noted in the 5-year PFS and OS between the groups [69]. Another CIBMTR study evaluating the role of conditioning regimen on allo-HCT outcomes in chemotherapy-unresponsive DLBCL and grade III follicular lymphoma found that MAC was associated with a higher 3-year NRM compared with RIC (53% vs. 42%, *P* = 0.03) and a reduced risk for

progression (relative risk 0.66). At 3 years the conditioning regimen did not impact the PFS, but the OS with MAC and RIC was 19% and 28%, respectively (*P* = 0.02).

Table 16.1 shows selected recent studies evaluating allo-HCT in DLBCL. Acknowledging the lack of prospective studies, the available data do not suggest that more intense conditioning in DLBCL patients undergoing allo-HCT is associated with improved outcomes, but may be associated with higher rates of NRM.

Post-transplantation disease monitoring for DLBCL

Disease monitoring after transplantation serves two purposes: (i) to detect early relapse for those undergoing HCT in CR and (ii) to monitor response to therapy if not in CR at the time of transplant. The optimal follow-up schedule after HCT is controversial. Re-imaging with computed tomography (CT) or PET/CT at day 90–100 post transplantation to document end-of-therapy disease status is reasonable and widely practiced by transplant centers. For those with documented bone marrow involvement before HCT, a repeat marrow aspiration and biopsy is appropriate to document remission. PET is often associated with high false-positive results in this setting and there are few data to recommend its routine use [70,71]. Patients should be followed clinically for disease relapse every 3 months for the first year, every 4–6 months for 3 years, every 6–12 months for up to 5 years, and annually thereafter. Many centers perform re-imaging at regular intervals following HCT, although the utility of this approach is questionable [72]. Those patients with active disease may need more frequent monitoring (every 3–6 months) to document response to therapy and to institute additional therapy when warranted. A strategy that is guided by patient symptoms and physical examination (good clinical evaluation) may be more useful than routine surveillance scans [73]. Besides monitoring for disease relapse, allo-HCT recipients should be followed closely for assessment of their graft function. In our practice we assess chimerism by DNA genotyping of polymorphic markers of simple sequence length that encode short tandem repeats until full donor chimerism is documented at 3–6 monthly intervals.

Table 16.1 Selected recent studies of transplant outcomes in patients with DLBCL.

Study	No. of patients (DLBCL)	Median age, years (range)	Disease status at transplant	Prior auto (%)	Donor type	Conditioning	Percent NRM (years)	Percent relapse (years)	Percent OS (years)	Percent PFS (years)
Rodriguez et al. (2006) [100]	88 (16 DLBCL)	MAC: 44 (13–54) RIC: 51 (20–67)	CS: 63%	24	MUD: 28%	MA: N = 48 (55%) RIC: N = 40 (45%)	33 (1) 28 (1)	13 28	52 (2) 53 (2)	46 (2) 40 (2)
Rezvani et al. (2008) [62]	32	52 (18–67)	CR: 44% RD: 72%	75	MRD: 66% URD: 34%	NMAC: N = 32 (100%)	25 (3)	41 (3)	45 (3)	35 (3)
Thomson et al. (2009) [58]	48	46 (23–64)	RD: 17%	71	MRD: 62% URD: 38%	RIC: N = 48 (100%)	32 (4)	33 (4)	47 (4)	48 (4)
Hamadani et al. (2009) [66]	46 (18 DLBCL)	46 (22–63)	CR: 0% RD: 100%	0	MRD: 85% URD: 15%	MAC: N = 43 (93%) RIC: N = 3 (7%)	34 (5)	35 (5)	38 (5)	34 (5)
Sirvent et al. (2010) [101]	68	48 (17–66)	CR: 47% RD: 19%	79 (1 prior allo)	MRD: 82% URD: 18%	RIC: N = 50 (74%) NMAC: N = 17 (24%)	23 (1)	41 (2)	49 (2)	44 (2)
Lazarus et al. (2010) [42]	79	46 (21–59)	CR: 30% RD: 42%	0	MRD: 100%	MAC: N = 65 (82%) Other: 18%	45 (5)	33 (5)	22 (5)	22 (5)
van Kampen et al. (2011) [63]	101	46 (18–66)	CR: 36% RD: 26%	100	MRD: 71% URD: 29%	MAC: N = 37 (37%) RIC: N = 64 (63%)	41 (3) 20 (3)	30 (3)	52 (3)	42 (3)
Rigacci et al. (2012) [64]	165	43 (16–65)	CR: 55% RD: 33%	100	MRD: 65% URD: 35%	MAC: N = 49 (30%) RIC: N = 116 (70%)	56 (5)	26 (5)	18	18 (5)
Bacher et al. (2012) [69]	396	48 (18–69)	CR2: 21% RD: 36%	32	MRD: 33% URD: 67%	MAC: N = 165 RIC: N = 143 NMAC: N = 88	56 (5) 47 (5) 36 (5)	26 (5) 38 (5) 36 (5)	18 (5) 20 (5) 26 (5)	18 (5) 15 (5) 25 (5)
Hamadani et al. (2013) [74]	533 (453 DLBCL)	MAC: 46 (9–66) RIC: 53 (20–70)	RD: 100%	25	MRD: 48% URD: 52%	MAC: N = 307 (58%)* RIC/NST: N = 226 (42%)	53 (3) 42 (3)	28 (3) 35 (3)	19 (3) 28 (3)	19 (3) 23 (3)
Kim et al. (2014) [102]	30	39 (22–59)	RD: 43.3%	100	MRD: 63% URD: 37%	MAC: N = 7 (23%) RIC: N = 23 (77%)	16.7	35 (5)	38 (5)	43 (5)

CR, complete remission; CS, chemosensitive; DLBCL, diffuse large B-cell lymphoma; MAC, myeloablative conditioning; MAC, myeloablative conditioning; MRD, matched related donor; MUD, matched unrelated donor; NMAC, nonmyeloablative conditioning; RD, resistant disease; RIC, reduced-intensity conditioning; URD, unrelated donor.

Management of relapses after transplantation for DLBCL

Identifying risk factors that impact post-transplant outcomes including disease progression is essential to identify high-risk patients, thus enabling practitioners to consider closer monitoring as well as strategies to minimize the risk of relapse. Patient- and disease-related risk factors associated with higher risk of relapse include disease status, chemorefractory disease, PS, duration of initial response, and high second-line aa-IPI [22,40,50,59,63,74]. It is theoretically possible that implementation of post-HCT maintenance and/or consolidation strategies would improve responses and decrease relapse risk. Rituximab maintenance was studied in a large randomized controlled trial after auto-HCT in DLBCL but showed no impact on survival and is thus not recommended [75]. The use of planned pre- or post-autograft radiation therapy may be another technique to improve local disease control and relapse risk [51,76]. The incorporation of novel agents into salvage regimens, conditioning regimens and as maintenance therapy holds promise and is under evaluation.

A practical approach to the management of DLBCL progressing after an autograft is presented in Figure 16.2. The main consideration in this context is to assess the ability of the patient to proceed to an allo-HCT. For those eligible, additional salvage therapy is often considered for cytoreduction and enable donor search. No salvage therapy has been found to be superior over the other and common regimens, including DHAP (dexamethasone, cisplatin, cytarabine), ESHAP (methylprednisolone, etoposide, cytarabine, cisplatin), GemOX (gemcitabine, oxaliplatin), GDP (gemcitabine, dexamethasone, cisplatin), and ICE (ifosfamide, carboplatin, etoposide). The allo-HCT conditioning should be carefully chosen taking into account patient's age, PS, and comorbidities. Evaluation of novel agents and their combinations for salvage and conditioning regimens in the context of clinical trials is recommended for allograft candidates. Patients who are not allograft candidates should ideally be always treated on appropriate clinical trials, when available. Recently, bendamustine (120 mg/m²) with rituximab was evaluated in transplant-ineligible patients and is a reasonable option [77]. Proteasome inhibitors, lenalidomide, and Bruton's tyrosine kinase (Btk) inhibitors also hold promise for relapsed DLBCL of the activated B-cell phenotype.

Patients who experience relapse post allo-HCT have poor outcomes [58,63,69]. Apart from having exhausted most of the available treatment options, a significant fraction of these patients is unable to tolerate further therapy due to poor PS, end-organ damage, concomitant graft-versus-host disease (GVHD), infectious disease complications, and rapidly progressive disease. The treatment decision in this setting is highly individualized, noting that palliation/best supportive care may be the optimal option for some patients (Figure 16.2). When appropriate the immediate goals of therapy include cytoreduction to reduce disease bulk and strategies to augment the GVL effects. No specific recommendations regarding the choice of therapy for cytoreduction can be made based on available data. It has been noted that true evidence of GVL effects is characterized by tumor regression after withdrawal of immunosuppression and/or administration of DLI [55]. In the absence of active and severe GVHD, discontinuation of immunosuppression (if ongoing) is usually considered with or without cytoreductive therapy. In patients who are not on immunosuppression, DLIs are often considered. The available data evaluating the role of withdrawal of immunosuppression and DLI are limited [25,78–80]. One prospective study evaluating RIC with alemtuzumab ($N = 88$, aggressive NHL = 37) used DLI for conversion of mixed chimerism ($N = 15$) and disease progression ($N = 21$) and reported a 3-year PFS of 34% for high-grade NHL [79]. Wudhikarn et al. [80] evaluated outcomes in 72 patients (DLBCL, $N = 15$) with disease progression after allo-HCT who were treated with withdrawal of immunosuppression ($N = 58$), DLI ($N = 7$), and other strategies and noted objective responses in 38 including CR in 30 patients. Although 79% died from disease progression, factors predicting survival post HCT included good PS (0–2), normal LDH, early-stage disease (stage I–III), isolated extranodal organ involvement, and late relapse (>100 days) post HCT [80]. A study specific to DLBCL not in remission at day +100 after allo-HCT ($N = 15$) managed these patients with withdrawal of immunosuppression ($N = 10$) and DLI ($N = 5$) and reported eight patients in CR with six alive at 42–83 months [25]. Acknowledging the lack of large prospective trials and based on the limited data available, withdrawal of immunosuppression and DLI with or without cytoreductive therapy is reasonable in carefully selected individuals. The

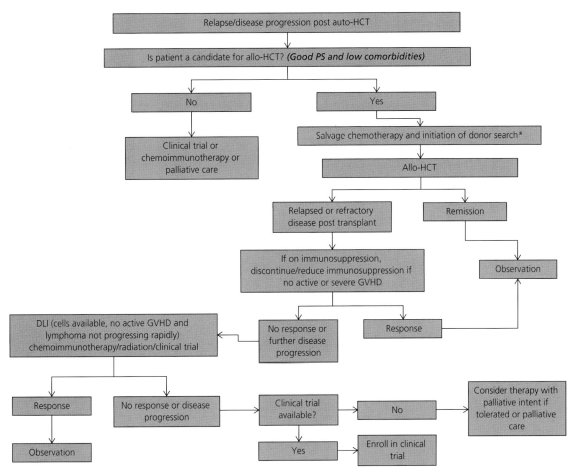

Figure 16.2 Suggested treatment algorithm for relapsed/progressive disease. DLI, donor lymphocyte infusion; GVHD, graft-versus-host disease; HCT, hematopoietic cell transplantation. Asterisk indicates that novel agents and their combinations for salvage and conditioning regimens in the context of clinical trials is recommended for allograft candidates.

importance of managing these high-risk patients on clinical trials cannot be overemphasized.

Novel therapies and their integration in transplantation for DLBCL

The development of novel "targeted therapies" that include monoclonal antibodies, cell signaling pathway inhibitors, epigenetic modulators, immunomodulators, and genetically engineered T cells has heralded a new era in cancer therapeutics. The widespread integration of rituximab into chemotherapy was indeed a turning point in the management of DLBCL. However since 2006, when the Food and Drug Administration approved

rituximab, no other novel agent has obtained approval in DLBCL. Fortunately, the field is rapidly evolving and several agents with varying mechanisms of action are being evaluated in clinical trials. Indeed, DLBCL investigators are provided the unique opportunity to integrate these agents at various stages of the disease course. The possibilities include (i) improving outcomes of initial therapy, thereby obviating the need for HCT; (ii) with salvage regimens to increase the proportion of patients eligible for HCT; (iii) optimizing conditioning regimens for auto- and allo-HCT; (iv) post-HCT consolidation and/or maintenance therapy; and (v) management of progressive disease. Another important area that requires further evaluation is the possibility of individualized therapy based on the specific histological, molecular, or genetic subtype of DLBCL. While a comprehensive review of novel agents is beyond the scope of this chapter, a few novel agents/approaches and trials are highlighted. A few excellent reviews are referenced for further reading [54,81–83].

Selected novel approaches/agents in DLBCL

Ofatumumab and obinutuzumab are next-generation high-affinity CD20 monoclonal antibodies with activity against rituximab-resistant cell lines. They have shown promising results in the relapsed/refractory setting as single-agent therapy [84–86]. Ofatumamab has shown efficacy in relapsed/refractory DLBCL as well as in combination salvage therapy [87]. Epratuzumab (anti-CD22) and MEDI-551 (anti-CD19) both have activity in DLBCL and are being evaluated in clinical trials [88,89]. The nuclear factor κ-light-chain-enhancer of activated B cells (NF-κB) signaling pathway is thought to be constitutively active in non-germinal center B-cell (non-GCB) DLBCL. A Phase II study evaluating dose-adjusted EPOCH with bortezomib showed improved response rates and median survival [90]. In combination with R-CHOP (rituximab plus cyclophosphamide, doxorubicin, vincristine, and prednisone), it was associated with 100% responses (86% CR) and 2-year PFS of 64% [91]. Randomized trials with bortezomib plus chemoimmunotherapy are underway. Carfilzomib is a next-generation proteasome inhibitor that is being evaluated as well. In Phase II studies, lenalidomide, an immunomodulator that is active in myeloma, showed response in DLBCL and interestingly seems to be more active in non-GCB subtype, with an overall response rate (ORR) of 53% in the relapsed/refractory setting [92,93]. Current trials are evaluating the role of lenalidomide in salvage and upfront settings as well. Constitutively active B-cell receptor signaling is thought to play a role in DLBCL, especially in non-GCB subtype DLBCL, and two important kinase inhibitors – Syk inhibitor (fostamatinib, 22% ORR in DLBCL) and Btk inhibitor (ibrutinib, 40% response in non-GCB DLBCL) – are currently under evaluation in clinical trials [94,95]. Attaining CR with the initial treatment for DLBCL is an important predictor of PFS and OS, even for high-risk DLBCL [96]. The standard of care for several years has remained CHOP plus rituximab. Upfront therapy with dose-adjusted EPOCH (etoposide, prednisone, vincristine, cyclophosphamide, and doxorubicin) plus rituximab has shown promise in Phase II trials in specific subsets of aggressive B-cell NHL and is currently under comparative evaluation in upfront therapy [96,97]. Although the CORAL study showed no difference between two different salvage regimens in outcomes, subgroup analyses suggested improved PFS in the R-DHAP arm in GCB DLBCL [22,98]. Maintenance therapy with rituximab after auto-HCT was evaluated in the CORAL trial, and showed no improvement in outcomes [75]. Programmed death (PD)-1 is a T-cell coreceptor that maintains an immunosuppressive tumor microenvironment and its inhibition has antitumor activity. The anti-PD-1 antibody CT-011 used as maintenance therapy after auto-HCT showed PFS of 69% and is under evaluation in clinical trials [99].

Although several new agents are under clinical evaluation, the data are not mature enough to recommend their widespread use. Moreover, the optimal timing of their integration is unknown. However, the field is rapidly expanding with the discovery of newer targets and agents and the future is exciting and promising.

Case study

A 65-year-old female with a past history of diabetes mellitus, chronic bronchitis and anxiety presents with fever, night sweats and "lumps" in the neck. Excisional biopsy of the (R) supraclavicular lymph node is consistent with diffuse large B-cell lymphoma (DLBCL), germinal center B-cell subtype. CT/PET reveals bulky lymphadenopathy above and below the diaphragm without any extranodal involvement. Bilateral bone marrow biopsies are negative for involvement with lymphoma. Lactate dehydrogenase is twice the upper limit of laboratory reference. For stage IIIB, International Prognostic Index score 3 DLBCL, six cycles of chemoimmunotherapy with R-CHOP (rituximab, cyclophosphamide, adriamycin, vincristine and prednisone) are recommended. Interim PET scan after three cycles reveals good partial remission, but end-of-therapy imaging study after completion of six cycles shows stable disease. A needle biopsy of the (L) cervical node is consistent with DLBCL. What is the most appropriate therapy for this patient?

A Administer two more cycles of R-CHOP, followed by repeat imaging in 3 months.
B Place patient on observation and repeat PET scan in 3 months.

C Administer salvage therapy with R-DHAP (rituximab, dexamethasone, cytarabine and cisplatin) followed by autologous hematopoietic cell transplantation if chemosensitivity is demonstrable.

D Administer salvage therapy with R-DHAP (rituximab, dexamethasone, cytarabine and cisplatin) followed by autologous hematopoietic cell transplantation *only* if refractory/progressive disease is noted.

E Unrelated donor allogeneic transplantation after myeloablative conditioning with cyclophosphamide and TBI.

The above vignette represents a common clinical scenario in the management of DLBCL. Since the repeat biopsy confirms the persistence of lymphoma, this represents primary refractory disease and additional cycles of R-CHOP and/or observation are both inappropriate (choices A and B). Salvage chemotherapy is recommended for disease control as well as to demonstrate chemosensitivity. If response to salvage (R-DHAP in this case) therapy were noted, high-dose therapy and autologous hematopoietic cell transplantation would be a reasonable choice for this patient and can provide durable remissions with acceptable nonrelapse mortality (choice C). Autologous transplantation is unlikely to provide any clinical benefit if progression is noted with salvage therapy (choice D) and as such a clinical trial with novel agents is recommended. Myeloablative conditioning with cyclophosphamide and TBI will be associated with prohibitive morbidity and mortality considering her age and comorbidities and is not a consideration for this patient (choice D). RIC (not an option in this question) followed by allograft may be a consideration if she were to relapse after autologous transplantation or with progressive disease; however, careful selection of the patient (comorbidities), donor and conditioning regimen is warranted.

References

1 The Non-Hodgkin's Lymphoma Classification Project. A clinical evaluation of the International Lymphoma Study Group classification of non-Hodgkin's lymphoma. *Blood* 1997;89:3909–18.

2 Fisher RI, Gaynor ER, Dahlberg S *et al.* Comparison of a standard regimen (CHOP) with three intensive chemotherapy regimens for advanced non-Hodgkin's lymphoma. *N Engl J Med* 1993;328:1002–6.

3 Coiffier B, Lepage E, Brière J *et al.* CHOP chemotherapy plus rituximab compared with CHOP alone in elderly patients with diffuse large-B-cell lymphoma. *N Engl J Med* 2002;346: 235–42.

4 Pfreundschuh M, Kuhnt E, Trümper L *et al.* CHOP-like chemotherapy with or without rituximab in young patients with good-prognosis diffuse large-B-cell lymphoma: 6-year results of an open-label randomised study of the MabThera International Trial (MInT) Group. *Lancet Oncol* 2011;12:1013–22.

5 The International Non-Hodgkin's Lymphoma Prognostic Factors Project. A predictive model for aggressive non-Hodgkin's lymphoma. *N Engl J Med* 1993;329:987–94.

6 Ziepert M, Hasenclever D, Kuhnt E *et al.* Standard International Prognostic Index remains a valid predictor of outcome for patients with aggressive CD20+ B-cell lymphoma in the rituximab era. *J Clin Oncol* 2010;28:2373–80.

7 Zhou Z, Sehn LH, Rademaker AW *et al.* An enhanced International Prognostic Index (NCCN-IPI) for patients with diffuse large B-cell lymphoma treated in the rituximab era. *Blood* 2014;123:837–42.

8 Lenz G, Wright G, Dave SS *et al.* Stromal gene signatures in large-B-cell lymphomas. *N Engl J Med* 2008;359:2313–23.

9 Savage KJ, Johnson NA, Ben-Neriah S *et al.* MYC gene rearrangements are associated with a poor prognosis in diffuse large B-cell lymphoma patients treated with R-CHOP chemotherapy. *Blood* 2009;114:3533–7.

10 Haioun C, Itti E, Rahmouni A *et al.* [18F]fluoro-2-deoxy-D-glucose positron emission tomography (FDG-PET) in aggressive lymphoma: an early prognostic tool for predicting patient outcome. *Blood* 2005;106:1376–81.

11 Coiffier B, Thieblemont C, Van Den Neste E *et al.* Long-term outcome of patients in the LNH-98.5 trial, the first randomized study comparing rituximab-CHOP to standard CHOP chemotherapy in DLBCL patients: a study by the Groupe d'Etudes des Lymphomes de l'Adulte. *Blood* 2010;116:2040–5.

12 Philip T, Guglielmi C, Hagenbeek A *et al.* Autologous bone marrow transplantation as compared with salvage chemotherapy in relapses of chemotherapy-sensitive non-Hodgkin's lymphoma. *N Engl J Med* 1995;333:1540–5.

13 Hamadani M, Craig M, Awan F, Devine S. How we approach patient evaluation for hematopoietic stem cell transplantation. *Bone Marrow Transplant* 2010;45:1259–68.

14 Jantunen E, Canals C, Rambaldi A *et al.* Autologous stem cell transplantation in elderly patients (≥60 years) with diffuse large B-cell lymphoma: an analysis based on data in the European Blood and Marrow Transplantation registry. *Haematologica* 2008;93:1837–42.

15 Wildes TM, Augustin KM, Sempek D *et al.* Comorbidities, not age, impact outcomes in autologous stem cell transplant for relapsed non-Hodgkin lymphoma. *Biol Blood Marrow Transplant* 2008;14:840–6.

16 Hamlin PA, Zelenetz AD, Kewalramani T *et al.* Age-adjusted International Prognostic Index predicts autologous stem cell transplantation outcome for patients with relapsed or primary refractory diffuse large B-cell lymphoma. *Blood* 2003;102:1989–96.

17 Derenzini E, Musuraca G, Fanti S *et al.* Pretransplantation positron emission tomography scan is the main predictor of

autologous stem cell transplantation outcome in aggressive B-cell non-Hodgkin lymphoma. *Cancer* 2008;113:2496–503.

18 Spaepen K, Stroobants S, Dupont P *et al*. Prognostic value of pretransplantation positron emission tomography using fluorine 18-fluorodeoxyglucose in patients with aggressive lymphoma treated with high-dose chemotherapy and stem cell transplantation. *Blood* 2003;102:53–9.

19 Caballero MD, Pérez-Simón JA, Iriondo A *et al*. High-dose therapy in diffuse large cell lymphoma: results and prognostic factors in 452 patients from the GEL-TAMO Spanish Cooperative Group. *Ann Oncol* 2003;14:140–51.

20 Rodriguez J, Caballero MD, Gutierrez A *et al*. Autologous stem-cell transplantation in diffuse large B-cell non-Hodgkin's lymphoma not achieving complete response after induction chemotherapy: the GEL/TAMO experience. *Ann Oncol* 2004;15:1504–9.

21 Trneny M, Bosly A, Bouabdallah K *et al*. Independent predictive value of PET-CT pre transplant in relapsed and refractory patients with CD20 diffuse large B-cell lymphoma (DLBCL) included in the CORAL study. *Blood (ASH Annual Meeting Abstracts)* 2009;114:Abstract 881.

22 Gisselbrecht C, Glass B, Mounier N *et al*. Salvage regimens with autologous transplantation for relapsed large B-cell lymphoma in the rituximab era. *J Clin Oncol* 2010;28: 4184–90.

23 Salar A, Sierra J, Gandarillas M *et al*. Autologous stem cell transplantation for clinically aggressive non-Hodgkin's lymphoma: the role of preparative regimens. *Bone Marrow Transplant* 2001;27:405–12.

24 Vose JM, Carter S, Burns LJ *et al*. Phase III randomized study of rituximab/carmustine, etoposide, cytarabine, and melphalan (BEAM) compared with iodine-131 tositumomab/BEAM with autologous hematopoietic cell transplantation for relapsed diffuse large B-cell lymphoma: results from the BMT CTN 0401 Trial. *J Clin Oncol* 2013;31:1662–8.

25 Bishop MR, Dean RM, Steinberg SM *et al*. Clinical evidence of a graft-versus-lymphoma effect against relapsed diffuse large B-cell lymphoma after allogeneic hematopoietic stem-cell transplantation. *Ann Oncol* 2008;19:1935–40.

26 Kaiser U, Uebelacker I, Abel U *et al*. Randomized study to evaluate the use of high-dose therapy as part of primary treatment for "aggressive" lymphoma. *J Clin Oncol* 2002;20: 4413–19.

27 Kluin-Nelemans HC, Zagonel V, Anastasopoulou A *et al*. Standard chemotherapy with or without high-dose chemotherapy for aggressive non-Hodgkin's lymphoma: randomized Phase III EORTC study. *J Natl Cancer Inst* 2001; 93:22–30.

28 Martelli M, Gherlinzoni F, De Renzo A *et al*. Early autologous stem-cell transplantation versus conventional chemotherapy as front-line therapy in high-risk, aggressive non-Hodgkin's lymphoma: an Italian multicenter randomized trial. *J Clin Oncol* 2003;21:1255–62.

29 Betticher D, Martinelli G, Radford J *et al*. Sequential high dose chemotherapy as initial treatment for aggressive

sub-types of non-Hodgkin lymphoma: results of the international randomized phase III trial (MISTRAL). *Ann Oncol* 2006;17:1546–52.

30 Vitolo U, Liberati A, Cabras M *et al*. High dose sequential chemotherapy with autologous transplantation versus dose-dense chemotherapy MegaCEOP as first line treatment in poor-prognosis diffuse large cell lymphoma: an "Intergruppo Italiano Linfomi" randomized trial. *Haematologica* 2005;90:793–801.

31 Milpied N, Deconinck E, Gaillard F *et al*. Initial treatment of aggressive lymphoma with high-dose chemotherapy and autologous stem-cell support. *N Engl J Med* 2004;350:1287–95.

32 Gianni AM, Bregni M, Siena S *et al*. High-dose chemotherapy and autologous bone marrow transplantation compared with MACOP-B in aggressive B-cell lymphoma. *N Engl J Med* 1997;336:1290–8.

33 Haioun C, Lepage E, Gisselbrecht C *et al*. Survival benefit of high-dose therapy in poor-risk aggressive non-Hodgkin's lymphoma: final analysis of the prospective LNH87-2 Protocol. A Groupe d'Etude des Lymphomes de l'Adulte Study. *J Clin Oncol* 2000;18:3025–30.

34 Gisselbrecht C, Lepage E, Molina T *et al*. Shortened first-line high-dose chemotherapy for patients with poor-prognosis aggressive lymphoma. *J Clin Oncol* 2002;20:2472–9.

35 Greb A, Bohlius J, Trelle S *et al*. High-dose chemotherapy with autologous stem cell support in first-line treatment of aggressive non-Hodgkin lymphoma: results of a comprehensive meta-analysis. *Cancer Treat Rev* 2007;33:338–46.

36 Le Gouill S, Milpied N, Lamy T *et al*. First-line rituximab (R) high-dose therapy (R-HDT) versus R-CHOP14 for young adults with diffuse large B-cell lymphoma: preliminary results of the GOELAMS 075 prospective multicenter randomized trial. *J Clin Oncol* 2011;29(Suppl):Abstract 8003.

37 Schmitz N, Nickelsen M, Ziepert M *et al*. Conventional chemotherapy (CHOEP-14) with rituximab or high-dose chemotherapy (MegaCHOEP) with rituximab for young, high-risk patients with aggressive B-cell lymphoma: an open-label, randomised, phase 3 trial (DSHNHL 2002-1). *Lancet Oncol* 2012;13:1250–9.

38 Tarella C, Zanni M, Di Nicola M *et al*. Prolonged survival in poor-risk diffuse large B-cell lymphoma following front-line treatment with rituximab-supplemented, early-intensified chemotherapy with multiple autologous hematopoietic stem cell support: a multicenter study by GITIL. *Leukemia* 2007;21:1802–11.

39 Stiff PJ, Unger JM, Cook JR *et al*. Autologous transplantation as consolidation for aggressive non-Hodgkin's lymphoma. *N Engl J Med* 2013;369:1681–90.

40 Philip T, Guglielmi C, Hagenbeek A *et al*. Autologous bone marrow transplantation as compared with salvage chemotherapy in relapses of chemotherapy-sensitive non-Hodgkin's lymphoma. *N Engl J Med* 1995;333:1540–5.

41 Mounier N, Canals C, Gisselbrecht C *et al*. High-dose therapy and autologous stem cell transplantation in first relapse for diffuse large B cell lymphoma in the rituximab era:

an analysis based on data from the European Blood and Marrow Transplantation Registry. *Biol Blood Marrow Transplant* 2012;18:788–93.

42 Lazarus H, Zhang M, Carreras J *et al*. A comparison of HLA-identical sibling allogeneic versus autologous transplantation for diffuse large B cell lymphoma: a report from the CIBMTR. *Biol Blood Marrow Transplant* 2010;16:35–45.

43 Fenske T, Hari P, Carreras J *et al*. Impact of pre-transplant rituximab on survival after autologous hematopoietic stem cell transplantation for diffuse large B cell lymphoma. *Biol Blood Marrow Transplant* 2009;15:1455–64.

44 Yi-Bin Chen, Hochberg EP, Feng Y *et al*. Characteristics and outcomes after autologous stem cell transplant for patients with relapsed or refractory diffuse large B-cell lymphoma who failed initial rituximab, cyclophosphamide, adriamycin, vincristine, and prednisone therapy compared to patients who failed cyclophosphamide, adriamycin, vincristine, and prednisone. *Leukemia Lymphoma* 2010;51:789–96.

45 Martín A, Conde E, Arnan M *et al*. R-ESHAP as salvage therapy for patients with relapsed or refractory diffuse large B-cell lymphoma: the influence of prior exposure to rituximab on outcome. A GEL/TAMO study. *Haematologica* 2008;93:1829–36.

46 Hamadani M, Hari PN, Zhang Y *et al*. Early failure of front-line rituximab-containing chemo-immunotherapy in diffuse large B cell lymphoma does not predict futility of autologous hematopoietic cell transplantation. *Biol Blood Marrow Transplant* 2014;20:1729–36.

47 Elstrom R, Martin P, Ostrow K *et al*. Response to second-line therapy defines the potential for cure in patients with recurrent diffuse large B-cell lymphoma: implications for the development of novel therapeutic strategies. *Clin Lymphoma Myeloma Leuk* 2010;10:192–6.

48 Mills W, Chopra R, McMillan A, Pearce R, Linch D, Goldstone A. BEAM chemotherapy and autologous bone marrow transplantation for patients with relapsed or refractory non-Hodgkin's lymphoma. *J Clin Oncol* 1995;13:588–95.

49 Stiff P, Dahlberg S, Forman S *et al*. Autologous bone marrow transplantation for patients with relapsed or refractory diffuse aggressive non-Hodgkin's lymphoma: value of augmented preparative regimens. A Southwest Oncology Group trial. *J Clin Oncol* 1998;16:48–55.

50 Philip T, Armitage JO, Spitzer G *et al*. High-dose therapy and autologous bone marrow transplantation after failure of conventional chemotherapy in adults with intermediate-grade or high-grade non-Hodgkin's lymphoma. *N Engl J Med* 1987;316:1493–8.

51 Vose JM, Zhang M, Rowlings PA *et al*. Autologous transplantation for diffuse aggressive non-Hodgkin's lymphoma in patients never achieving remission: a report from the Autologous Blood and Marrow Transplant Registry. *J Clin Oncol* 2001;19:406–13.

52 Prince HM, Crump M, Imrie K *et al*. Intensive therapy and autotransplant for patients with an incomplete response to front-line therapy for lymphoma. *Ann Oncol* 1996;7:1043–9.

53 Kewalramani T, Zelenetz AD, Hedrick EE *et al*. High-dose chemoradiotherapy and autologous stem cell transplantation for patients with primary refractory aggressive non-Hodgkin lymphoma: an intention-to-treat analysis. *Blood* 2000;96:2399–404.

54 Klyuchnikov E, Bacher U, Kroll T *et al*. Allogeneic hematopoietic cell transplantation for diffuse large B cell lymphoma: who, when and how? *Bone Marrow Transplant* 2014;49:1–7.

55 Grigg A, Ritchie D. Graft-versus-lymphoma effects: clinical review, policy proposals, and immunobiology. *Biol Blood Marrow Transplant* 2004;10:579–90.

56 Butcher B, Collins RJ. The graft-versus-lymphoma effect: clinical review and future opportunities. *Bone Marrow Transplant* 2005;36:1–17.

57 Bishop MR, Dean RM, Steinberg SM *et al*. Clinical evidence of a graft-versus-lymphoma effect against relapsed diffuse large B-cell lymphoma after allogeneic hematopoietic stem-cell transplantation. *Ann Oncol* 2008;19:1935–40.

58 Thomson KJ, Morris EC, Bloor A *et al*. Favorable long-term survival after reduced-intensity allogeneic transplantation for multiple-relapse aggressive non-Hodgkin's lymphoma. *J Clin Oncol* 2009;27:426–32.

59 Vose J, Bierman P, Anderson J *et al*. Progressive disease after high-dose therapy and autologous transplantation for lymphoid malignancy: clinical course and patient follow-up. *Blood* 1992;80:2142–8.

60 Smith SM, van Besien K, Carreras J *et al*. Second autologous stem cell transplantation for relapsed lymphoma after a prior autologous transplant. *Biol Blood Marrow Transplant* 2008;14:904–12.

61 Vandenberghe E, Pearce R, Taghipour G, Fouillard L, Goldstone AH. Role of a second transplant in the management of poor-prognosis lymphomas: a report from the European Blood and Bone Marrow Registry. *J Clin Oncol* 1997;15:1595–600.

62 Rezvani AR, Norasetthada L, Gooley T *et al*. Non-myeloablative allogeneic haematopoietic cell transplantation for relapsed diffuse large B-cell lymphoma: a multicentre experience. *Br J Haematol* 2008;143:395–403.

63 van Kampen RJW, Canals C, Schouten HC *et al*. Allogeneic stem-cell transplantation as salvage therapy for patients with diffuse large B-cell non-Hodgkin's lymphoma relapsing after an autologous stem-cell transplantation: an analysis of the European Group for Blood and Marrow Transplantation Registry. *J Clin Oncol* 2011;29:1342–8.

64 Rigacci L, Puccini B, Dodero A *et al*. Allogeneic hematopoietic stem cell transplantation in patients with diffuse large B cell lymphoma relapsed after autologous stem cell transplantation: a GITMO study. *Ann Hematol* 2012;91:931–9.

65 Dhedin N, Giraudier S, Gaulard P *et al*. Allogeneic bone marrow transplantation in aggressive non-Hodgkin's lymphoma (excluding Burkitt and lymphoblastic lymphoma): a series of 73 patients from the SFGM database. *Br J Haematol* 1999;107:154–61.

66 Hamadani M, Benson DM Jr, Hofmeister CC *et al.* Allogeneic stem cell transplantation for patients with relapsed chemorefractory aggressive non-Hodgkin lymphomas. *Biol Blood Marrow Transplant* 2009;15:547–53.

67 Peniket A, Ruiz de Elvira M, Taghipour G *et al.* An EBMT registry matched study of allogeneic stem cell transplants for lymphoma: allogeneic transplantation is associated with a lower relapse rate but a higher procedure-related mortality rate than autologous transplantation. *Bone Marrow Transplant* 2003;31:667–78.

68 Lazarus HM, Zhang M, Carreras J *et al.* A comparison of HLA-identical sibling allogeneic versus autologous transplantation for diffuse large B cell lymphoma: a report from the CIBMTR. *Biol Blood Marrow Transplant* 2010;16: 35–45.

69 Bacher U, Klyuchnikov E, Le-Rademacher J *et al.* Conditioning regimens for allotransplants for diffuse large B-cell lymphoma: myeloablative or reduced intensity? *Blood* 2012;120:4256–62.

70 El-Galaly T, Prakash V, Christiansen I *et al.* Efficacy of routine surveillance with positron emission tomography/computed tomography in aggressive non-Hodgkin lymphoma in complete remission: status in a single center. *Leukemia Lymphoma* 2011;52:597–603.

71 Ulaner GA, Lilienstein J, Gönen M, Maragulia J, Moskowitz CH, Zelenetz AD. False-positive [18F]fluorodeoxyglucose-avid lymph nodes on positron emission tomography–computed tomography after allogeneic but not autologous stem-cell transplantation in patients with lymphoma. *J Clin Oncol* 2014;32:51–6.

72 Tilly H, Dreyling M. Diffuse large B-cell non-Hodgkin's lymphoma: ESMO clinical recommendations for diagnosis, treatment and follow-up. *Ann Oncol* 2009;20(Suppl 4): 110–12.

73 Truong Q, Shah N, Knestrick M *et al.* Limited utility of surveillance imaging for detecting disease relapse in patients with non-Hodgkin lymphoma in first complete remission. *Clin Lymphoma Myeloma Leuk* 2014;14:50–5.

74 Hamadani M, Saber W, Ahn KW *et al.* Impact of pretransplantation conditioning regimens on outcomes of allogeneic transplantation for chemotherapy-unresponsive diffuse large B cell lymphoma and grade III follicular lymphoma. *Biol Blood Marrow Transplant* 2013;19:746–53.

75 Gisselbrecht C, Schmitz N, Mounier N *et al.* Rituximab maintenance therapy after autologous stem-cell transplantation in patients with relapsed CD20+ diffuse large B-cell lymphoma: final analysis of the Collaborative Trial in Relapsed Aggressive Lymphoma. *J Clin Oncol* 2012;30: 4462–9.

76 Biswas T, Dhakal S, Chen R *et al.* Involved field radiation after autologous stem cell transplant for diffuse large B-cell lymphoma in the rituximab era. *Int J Radiat Oncol Biol Phys* 2010;77:79–85.

77 Ohmachi K, Niitsu N, Uchida T *et al.* Multicenter phase II study of bendamustine plus rituximab in patients with relapsed or refractory diffuse large B-cell lymphoma. *J Clin Oncol* 2013;31:2103–9.

78 van Besien K, de Lima M, Giralt S *et al.* Management of lymphoma recurrence after allogeneic transplantation: the relevance of graft-versus-lymphoma effect. *Bone Marrow Transplant* 1997;19:977–82.

79 Morris E, Thomson K, Craddock C *et al.* Outcomes after alemtuzumab-containing reduced-intensity allogeneic transplantation regimen for relapsed and refractory non-Hodgkin lymphoma. *Blood* 2004;104:3865–71.

80 Wudhikarn K, Brunstein CG, Bachanova V, Burns LJ, Cao Q, Weisdorf DJ. Relapse of lymphoma after allogeneic hematopoietic cell transplantation: management strategies and outcome. *Biol Blood Marrow Transplant* 2011;17:1497–504.

81 Cerchietti L, Leonard J. Targeting the epigenome and other new strategies in diffuse large B-cell lymphoma: beyond R-CHOP. *Hematology Am Soc Hematol Educ Program* 2013;591–5.

82 Roschewski M, Staudt L, Wilson W. Diffuse large B-cell lymphoma: treatment approaches in the molecular era. *Nat Rev Clin Oncol* 2014;11:12–23.

83 Cai Q, Westin J, Fu K *et al.* Accelerated therapeutic progress in diffuse large B cell lymphoma. *Ann Hematol* 2014;93:541–56.

84 Coiffier B, Bosly A, Wu KL *et al.* Ofatumumab monotherapy for treatment of patients with relapsed/progressive diffuse large B-cell lymphoma: results from a multicenter Phase II study. *Blood (ASH Annual Meeting Abstracts)* 2010;116:Abstract 3955.

85 Morschhauser F, Cartron G, Thieblemont C *et al.* Obinutuzumab (GA101) monotherapy in relapsed/refractory diffuse large B-cell lymphoma or mantle-cell lymphoma: results from the phase II GAUGUIN study. *J Clin Oncol* 2013;31:2912–19.

86 Archimbaud E, Thomas X, Michallet M *et al.* Prospective genetically randomized comparison between intensive postinduction chemotherapy and bone marrow transplantation in adults with newly diagnosed acute myeloid leukemia. *J Clin Oncol* 1994;12:262–7.

87 Matasar MJ, Czuczman MS, Rodriguez MA *et al.* Ofatumumab in combination with ICE or DHAP chemotherapy in relapsed or refractory intermediate grade B-cell lymphoma. *Blood* 2013;122:499–506.

88 Micallef INM, Maurer MJ, Wiseman GA *et al.* Epratuzumab with rituximab, cyclophosphamide, doxorubicin, vincristine, and prednisone chemotherapy in patients with previously untreated diffuse large B-cell lymphoma. *Blood* 2011;118:4053–61.

89 Forero-Torres A, Hamadani M, Fanale MA *et al.* Safety profile and clinical response to MEDI-551, a humanized monoclonal anti-CD19, in a Phase 1/2 study in adults with relapsed or refractory advanced B-cell malignancies. *Blood* 2013;122:1810.

90 Dunleavy K, Pittaluga S, Czuczman MS *et al.* Differential efficacy of bortezomib plus chemotherapy within molecular subtypes of diffuse large B-cell lymphoma. *Blood* 2009;113: 6069–76.

91 Ruan J, Martin P, Furman RR *et al.* Bortezomib plus CHOP-rituximab for previously untreated diffuse large B-cell lymphoma and mantle cell lymphoma. *J Clin Oncol* 2011;29:690–7.

92 Witzig TE, Vose JM, Zinzani PL *et al.* An international phase II trial of single-agent lenalidomide for relapsed or refractory aggressive B-cell non-Hodgkin's lymphoma. *Ann Oncol* 2011;22:1622–7.

93 Hernandez-Ilizaliturri FJ, Deeb G, Zinzani PL *et al.* Higher response to lenalidomide in relapsed/refractory diffuse large B-cell lymphoma in nongerminal center B-cell-like than in germinal center B-cell-like phenotype. *Cancer* 2011;117: 5058–66.

94 Friedberg JW, Sharman J, Sweetenham J *et al.* Inhibition of Syk with fostamatinib disodium has significant clinical activity in non-Hodgkin lymphoma and chronic lymphocytic leukemia. *Blood* 2010;115:2578–85.

95 Brown JR, Sharman JP, Harb WA *et al.* Phase Ib trial of AVL-292, a covalent inhibitor of Bruton's tyrosine kinase (Btk), in chronic lymphocytic leukemia (CLL) and B-non-Hodgkin lymphoma (B-NHL). *J Clin Oncol* 2012;30(Suppl): Abstract 8032.

96 Dunleavy K, Pittaluga S, Maeda LS *et al.* Dose-adjusted EPOCH-rituximab therapy in primary mediastinal B-cell lymphoma. *N Engl J Med* 2013;368:1408–16.

97 Dunleavy K, Pittaluga S, Shovlin M *et al.* Low-intensity therapy in adults with Burkitt's lymphoma. *N Engl J Med* 2013;369:1915–25.

98 Thieblemont C, Briere J, Mounier N *et al.* The germinal center/activated B-cell subclassification has a prognostic impact for response to salvage therapy in relapsed/refractory diffuse large B-cell lymphoma: a Bio-CORAL study. *J Clin Oncol* 2011;29:4079–87.

99 Gordon L, Weller E, Armand P *et al.* A Phase II study of CT-011, an anti-PD-1 antibody, after auSCT in recurrent/refractory DLBCL: first analysis of progression-free-survival (PFS), overall survival (OS) and toxicity (TOX). *Ann Oncol* 2011;22(Suppl 4):iv102–iv103.

100 Rodriguez R, Nademanee A, Ruel N *et al.* Comparison of reduced-intensity and conventional myeloablative regimens for allogeneic transplantation in non-Hodgkin's lymphoma. *Biol Blood Marrow Transplant* 2006;12: 1326–34.

101 Sirvent A, Dhedin N, Michallet M *et al.* Low nonrelapse mortality and prolonged long-term survival after reduced-intensity allogeneic stem cell transplantation for relapsed or refractory diffuse large B cell lymphoma: report of the Société Française de Greffe de Moelle et de Thérapie Cellulaire. *Biol Blood Marrow Transplant* 2010;16: 78–85.

102 Kim J, Kim S, Tada K *et al.* Allogeneic stem cell transplantation in patients with de novo diffuse large B-cell lymphoma who experienced relapse or progression after autologous stem cell transplantation: a Korea-Japan collaborative study. *Ann Hematol* 2014;93:1345–51.

CHAPTER 17

Mantle cell lymphoma

Sascha Dietrich and Peter Dreger

Indications for transplantation in mantle cell lymphoma

With an incidence of less than 0.5 per 100,000 inhabitants per year in Europe, mantle cell lymphoma (MCL) is a rare subtype, comprising less than 5% of all newly diagnosed lymphomas [1]. However, because of its poor prognosis under conventional chemoimmunotherapy, hematopoietic stem cell transplantation (HSCT) plays a predominant role in MCL treatment algorithms, and with more than 1000 transplants per year MCL is among the most frequent lymphoma transplant indication in the European Society for Blood and Marrow Transplantation (EBMT) registry (EBMT, data on file).

Autologous HSCT
Autologous HSCT consolidation is considered a standard part of first-line treatment of younger (less than 60–65 years) patients with MCL [2,3] (Table 17.1). This is based on several uncontrolled studies and one prospective randomized trial comparing autologous (auto)-HSCT consolidation with interferon maintenance in patients with MCL in first remission [4]. This trial demonstrated that auto-HSCT provides a significant progression-free survival (PFS) benefit and, after longer follow-up, also an overall survival (OS) benefit over interferon [5]. Recent epidemiologic data from Scandinavia considering primary treatment strategies confirmed that auto-HSCT is an independent predictor of improved survival [6]. The results of upfront auto-HSCT in MCL can be further improved by

incorporation of rituximab and high-dose ara-C into the induction regimen as observed in prospective randomized trials and cohort studies [7,8]. A registry analysis suggested that the benefit of auto-HSCT may also be relevant in fit elderly patients (65–70 years) [9]. Current prognostic criteria do not permit risk-adapted therapy (i.e., omission of auto-HSCT in "low-risk" patients as defined by clinical and/or genetic criteria) [3,10,11].

The prognosis of patients with relapsed or refractory MCL is generally poor. Although the results of salvage auto-HSCT are inferior to first-line transplants, auto-HSCT remains a salvage option for transplant-naive patients [3,12,13].

Allogeneic HSCT
Albeit merely supported by retrospective studies, in the absence of reasonable alternative treatment options, allogeneic (allo)-HSCT seems to be the only modality capable of providing long-term disease control in patients with relapsed and even refractory MCL [12,14–16]. Therefore the consensus is to recommend allo-HSCT to patients with MCL who relapse or become refractory after auto-HSCT or an appropriately intensive pretreatment [2,3] (Table 17.1). In contrast, there is no evidence to support upfront allo-HSCT in MCL outside of clinical trials. It remains to be shown if novel molecular drugs, such as B-cell receptor kinase inhibitors, will affect HSCT indications in MCL or other B-cell malignancies in the future [17,18].

Clinical Guide to Transplantation in Lymphoma, First Edition. Edited by Bipin N. Savani and Mohamad Mohty.
© 2015 John Wiley & Sons, Ltd. Published 2015 by John Wiley & Sons, Ltd.

Table 17.1 HSCT indications in mantle cell lymphoma.

Disease risk	Donor			
	HLA-identical sibling	WMUD	MMUD <10/10	Auto-HSCT
First remission	D	D	NR	S
CR >1, previous auto no	CO	CO	D	S
CR >1, previous auto yes	S	S	CO	NR
Refractory	CO	CO	D	NR

Auto, auto-HSCT; CO, clinical option (can be carried out after careful assessment of risks and benefits in experienced centers); CR, complete remission; D, developmental (only in studies); MMUD <10/10, mismatched unrelated donor (1 or more allele difference); NR, not recommended; S, standard of care (generally indicated in suitable patients); WMUD, well-matched unrelated donor.
Source: Sureda *et al.* [56].

Timing and preparation of patients for transplantation in mantle cell lymphoma

Autologous HSCT

In keeping with the indications described above, the optimum timing of auto-HSCT is first-line consolidation after an adequate induction therapy. Although not significant in all studies [12,14], it seems that the depth of remission achieved at the time of auto-HSCT is correlated with transplant outcome [7,19,20]. This effect was even more pronounced if sensitive disease detection techniques such as positron emission tomography (PET) and molecular minimal residual disease (MRD) assessment were employed [20,21]. Thus, based on the evidence available, induction therapy should contain high-dose ara-C and rituximab as mandatory treatment elements in order to achieve maximum response [3,7,8]. However, there is no consensus that, prior to auto-HSCT, induction treatment should be continued until PET/MRD negativity is reached [3,22].

The same principles apply for patients who are considered for second-line auto-HSCT even if evidence-based data supporting this recommendation are sparse.

Allogeneic HSCT

Because of the excellent results of first-line sequential intensification strategies comprising high-dose ara-C, rituximab, and auto-HSCT as key treatment elements

on the one hand and the unavoidable toxicity of allo-HSCT on the other hand, it appears that allografting for consolidating MCL in first remission is at least not superior to auto-HSCT [13]. Thus, first-line allo-HSCT is not supported by current guidelines [2,3]. In contrast, allo-HSCT has a role in salvage treatment of MCL as the prognosis of MCL relapse on auto-HSCT or nontransplant first-line therapies is poor [14,15,23]. Again, sustained disease control at allo-HSCT seems to be a prerequisite for successful outcome [24]. Therefore according to disease history and the individual situation, appropriate salvage regimens should be considered for achieving stable remission prior to transplant. These comprise high-dose ara-C or other intensive salvage regimens in use for treating aggressive lymphoma, bortezomib-based schedules [25], temsirolimus [26], bendamustine [23], immuno-modulatory drugs [27] or, most promising, molecular pathway inhibitors such as ibrutinib [28]. However, allo-HSCT can provide long-term remissions even in a fraction of patients who undergo transplantation in a refractory disease status [16], implying that failure to achieve response should not preclude allo-HSCT in refractory patients who otherwise fulfil the eligibility criteria for transplant.

Autologous hematopoietic stem cell transplantation for mantle cell lymphoma

Results of first-line auto-HSCT

As documented by large prospective trials, modern first-line sequential intensification strategies comprising auto-HSCT are associated with excellent disease control as reflected by 5-year PFS of 65% or higher if induction contains high-dose ara-C and rituximab (Table 17.2). Despite this, relapses continuously occur, discouraging hopes that high-dose therapy could be curative in a significant fraction of patients with MCL. A PFS plateau was initially seen in the Nordic MCL2 trial but disappeared after more advanced follow-up, suggesting that high-dose chemotherapy alone is not likely to cure the vast majority of patients with MCL [8,29]. Factors adversely affecting outcome of auto-HSCT include a high MCL International Prognostic Index (MIPI); poor disease control at transplant by clinical criteria, PET, or MRD;

Table 17.2 Selected prospective clinical trials of auto-HSCT as part of first-line treatment of mantle cell lymphoma.

	Dreyling et al. [4]	Dreger et al. [32]	Tam et al. [12]	Geisler et al. [8,29,54]	Kolstad et al. [20]	Hermine et al. [7]	Hoster et al. [10]
N	62	34	50	160	160	235	234
MIPI (low/intermediate/high)	NA	NA	40%/33%/28%	51%/26%/23%	48%/31%/21%	60%/25%/15%	64%/23%/13%
Proportion of patients in CR at auto-HSCT	35%	24%	46%*	54%	51%	25%	36%
Proportion of patients having received ara-C + rituximab-based induction	29%	17%	26%	100%	100%	0	100%
High-dose regimen	TBI/CY	R-TBI/CY	TBI/CY/R-TBI/CY	BEAM	BEAM/Z-BEAM	TBI/CY	TBI/ara-C/melphalan
High-dose regimen TBI-based	100%	100%	74%	0	0	100%	100%
Progression-free survival	54% (3 years)	83% (4 years)	39% (6 years)	66% (6 years) 43% (10 years)	71% (4 years)	65% (5 years)[†]	40% (5 years)[†]
Overall survival	83% (3 years)	87% (4 years)	61% (6 years)	70% (6 years) 58% (10 years)	78% (4 years)	75% (5 years)[†]	68% (5 years)[†]
Factors significantly affecting progression-free survival	—	R-TBI/CY[‡]	Marrow graft, B symptoms	MIPI, Ki-67, R + ara-C induction[§]	MIPI, pre-HSCT PET, post-HSCT MRD	R + ara-C induction, MIPI	
Follow-up (years)	? 1	? 7 (0.5–6.8)	6.0	6.5	4.4	4.3	

*Including CRu.
[†]Measured from start of induction therapy.
[‡]In comparison to 34 historical patients who had received TBI/CY without peritransplant rituximab.
[§]In comparison to 41 historical patients who had received induction without ara-C + rituximab.
BEAM, BCNU, etoposide, ara-C, melphalan; CR, complete remission; CY, cyclophosphamide; HSCT, hematopoietic stem cell transplantation; MIPI, Mantle Cell Lymphoma International Prognostic Index; MRD, minimal residual disease; NA, not available; PET, positron emission tomography; R, rituximab; TBI, total body irradiation.

a high proliferation rate; and using an induction treatment devoid of rituximab and high-dose ara-C (Table 17.2). The latter factor may explain why the outcome results reported in registry analyses seem to be less good (Table 17.3). Several studies have addressed the effect of type of high-dose regimen but have failed to resolve general significant benefits of total body irradiation (TBI)-based myeloablation over high-dose chemotherapy, although TBI tended to provide superior disease control in subset analyses [30,31]. Similarly, in the Nordic MCL3 trial the incorporation of radioimmunotherapy into the high-dose regimen did not improve outcome of patients who proceeded to auto-HSCT with less than partial remission compared to historical controls from the MCL2 trial [20]. In a small study on largely rituximab-naive patients receiving TBI-based high-dose therapy, *in*

vivo purging with peritransplant rituximab was associated with a significant PFS benefit compared to historical controls without peritransplant rituximab [32]. In contrast, evidence that *ex vivo* purging of the autograft can improve the outcome of auto-HSCT in MCL is lacking [33].

In contrast to follicular lymphoma [34], in MCL rituximab maintenance after auto-HSCT is not an established treatment strategy, although it proved to be of significant benefit in elderly patients responding to standard chemoimmunotherapy [35]. Preliminary data suggest that rituximab maintenance could be an effective tool for preventing relapse after autografting for MCL as well [36]. Preliminary results of a prospective LYMA trial have confirmed these findings [37]. Similarly, sound evidence that preemptive rituximab treatment on MRD persistence or recurrence after

Table 17.3 Selected registry studies on auto-HSCT as part of first-line treatment of mantle cell lymphoma.

	Rubio *et al.* [30]	Budde *et al.* [55]	Fenske *et al.* [13]	Touzeau *et al.* [31]
N	488	85	249	396
MIPI (low/intermediate/high)	NA	55%/31%/14%	NA	NA
Proportion of patients in CR at auto-HSCT	68%	66%	71%	53%*
Proportion of patients having received ara-C + rituximab-based induction	35%	48%	NA	NA
High-dose regimen	Various	NA	Various	Various
High-dose regimen TBI-based	33%	NA	22%	48%
Progression-free survival	47% (5 year)	NA	52% (5 year)	66% (3 year)
Overall survival	73% (5 year)	NA	61% (5 year)	83% (3 year)
Factors significantly affecting progression-free survival	No CR at HSCT	MIPI	No CR at HSCT	No CR at HSCT, age, rituximab exposure
Follow-up (years)	2.5	2.4 (0.1–12.6)	3.5 (0.3–13.2)	3.0 (0.1–16.3)

*Including CRu.
BEAM, BCNU, etoposide, ara-C, melphalan; CR, complete remission; CY, cyclophosphamide; HSCT, hematopoietic stem cell transplantation; MIPI, Mantle Cell Lymphoma International Prognostic Index; NA, not available; R, rituximab; TBI, total body irradiation.

auto-HSCT for MCL may prolong remission and survival is lacking [38], implying that MRD monitoring after autologous transplantation is not mandatory [3].

Results of salvage auto-HSCT

In contrast to the first-line setting, structured analyses of auto-HSCT as part of salvage therapy for MCL are sparse. The largest prospective study has been published by investigators from the M.D. Anderson Cancer Center, showing on 36 patients that rescue auto-HSCT is feasible but results in PFS and OS rates (10% and 35% at 6 years) which are significantly inferior to those achieved after first-line auto-HSCT [12]. Similarly, 5-year PFS and OS after rescue autotransplant were significantly worse compared to first-line auto-HSCT (29% and 44% vs. 52% and 61%, respectively) in 132 patients autografted after first-line treatment failure in a comprehensive registry study by the Center for International Blood and Marrow Transplant Research (CIBMTR) [13]. Nevertheless, in this study the results of auto-HSCT were at least similar to those of allo-HSCT in transplant-naive patients in the salvage setting. In contrast, a second auto-HSCT after a previous autografting failure seems to be of limited value in MCL, while a large proportion of patients who undergo allo-HSCT as second transplant can become long-term survivors in this setting [15].

In conclusion, whereas it is unclear if autologous or allogeneic transplantation should be preferred in transplant-naive patients with MCL needing salvage treatment, of patients who have relapsed after a previous auto-HSCT only those who manage to undergo allo-HSCT may enjoy long-term survival. Accordingly, allo-HSCT should be offered to eligble patients who have MCL recurrence after previous autologous transplantation [2,3].

Allogeneic hematopoietic stem cell transplantation for mantle cell lymphoma

Despite continuous improvement of therapeutic strategies, allo-HSCT remains the only curative treatment option for patients with MCL. In contrast to auto-HSCT, where autologous stem cells are infused to compensate for hematologic toxicity of high-dose chemotherapy, the rationale for allo-HSCT encompasses a completely different biological mode of action. An allogeneic stem cell transplant has the capability to mediate a durable immune-therapeutic process that targets the lymphoma cells (graft-versus-lymphoma activity, GVL). The downside of this powerful donor T-cell-mediated effect is graft-versus-host disease (GVHD), which accounts for the substantially increased mortality and morbidity of allo-HSCT in comparison with auto-HSCT. To define indications for allo-HSCT in a disease like MCL, its beneficial effects and curative potential have to be weighed against the risk of transplant-related morbidity and mortality. For this purpose the following key questions need to be addressed.

1 Is GVL effective in MCL?
2 Does the beneficial effect of allo-HSCT justify the toxicity of the procedure?
3 What is the best timing for allo-HSCT in MCL?

Evidence for GVL efficacy in mantle cell lymphoma

Despite very long remissions of up to 16 years [14], convincing plateaus of PFS curves are generally not present in long-term follow-up studies of patients who have undergone auto-HSCT for MCL. In contrast, long-term lymphoma-free survival after allo-HSCT for MCL could be demonstrated by a number of reports, including chemotherapy-refractory patients who experienced prolonged remissions after allo-HSCT [12,15,39,40]. However, it might be argued that stem cells infused for allo-HSCT do not contain contaminating tumor cells and it thus remains debatable whether the GVL effect or the absence of contaminating tumor cells is responsible for these sustained remissions. Khouri *et al.* [41] reported results on 16 heavily pretreated patients who had undergone myeloablative allo-HSCT with a PFS of 55% at 3 years. Three patients in this study continued to have MRD as determined by lymphoma-specific polymerase chain reaction (PCR) shortly after transplant but converted to negative status several months after allo-HSCT [41]. This observation suggests that a low tumor burden can be effectively eradicated by the donor immune system, thereby providing evidence for a GVL effect. Moreover, the fact that allo-HSCT based on reduced-intensity conditioning (RIC) can result in durable disease control even in patients who have failed a myeloablative auto-HSCT is in keeping with effective GVL activity in MCL [12,14,15].

Further evidence for the existence of a GVL effect in MCL comes from findings that the occurrence of chronic GVHD is associated with reduced relapse risk and the efficacy of donor lymphocyte infusions (DLI) [24], and that the use of antithymocyte globulin (ATG) may be complicated by an increased risk of relapse [42].

Taken together, there is some indirect evidence that GVL activity targeting MCL cells exists and has clinical relevance, but further characterization of this effect is needed. Nevertheless, in the EBMT European Mantle Cell Lymphoma Network Consensus Project, MRD

relapse post allo-HSCT was considered an indication for rapid withdrawal of immunosuppression and DLI if GVHD is absent [3].

Outcome of allo-HSCT in mantle cell lymphoma

Patients with MCL who have relapsed after intensive front-line therapies have only limited options for long-term disease control. In this setting, allo-HSCT has proven to provide long-term disease control even for refractory patients [43–45]. The traditional myeloablative conditioning regimens evaluated in these initial studies in heavily pretreated patients were associated with a very high treatment-related mortality of up to 40%. Subsequently, RIC procedures (Table 17.4) were used in patients with MCL to lower initially observed high nonrelapse mortality (NRM) rates but at the same time maintaining the beneficial GVL effect. Maris *et al.* [46] updated results of 33 heavily pretreated MCL patients who received conditioning with fludarabine and low-dose TBI. Compared to myeloablative

Table 17.4 Outcome of selected RIC studies in mantle cell lymphoma.

Center and RIC regimen	N	Results
M.D. Anderson Cancer Center [12] FCR (85%), PFA (14%)	35	6-year OS, 53% 6-year PFS, 46% 1-year NRM, 9%
EBMT (on file 2011) Various regimens	279	3-year OS, 45% 3-year PFS, 34% 3-year NRM, 38%
British Society of Blood and Marrow Transplantion [24] Various fludarabine–alkylator combinations, mostly alemtuzumab-based (82%)	70	5-year OS, 14% 5-year PFS, 37% 5-year NRM, 23%
Fred Hutchison Cancer Center [46] Fludarabine and 2-Gy TBI	53	5-year OS, 58% 5-year PFS, 52% 5-year NRM, 27%
CIBMTR (allo-HSCT in first remission) [13] Various	50	5-year OS, 62% 5-year PFS, 55% 1-year NRM, 25%
CIBMTR (allo-HSCT beyond first remission) [13] Various	88	5-year OS, 31% 5-year PFS, 24% 1-year NRM, 17%

FCR, fludarabine, cyclophosphamide, rituximab; NRM, nonrelapse mortality; OS, overall survival; PFA, cisplatin, fludarabine, cytarabine; PFS, progression-free survival; TBI, total body irradiation.

regimens, 5-year NRM could be slightly reduced but was still as high as 27%. An impressively low NRM of only 9% after 1 year was reported in a study by the M.D. Anderson Cancer Center, suggesting a benefit in favor of RIC. Accordingly, because of its better tolerability, which allows its use also in elderly and frail patients, RIC conditioning is now the preferred choice for allografting patients with MCL [3].

The overall survival of patients with MCL after allo-HSCT varies slightly among reports, most likely depending on patients included in the different studies. Single-center experiences with advanced-disease patients reported a 2-year OS of 59% in Heidelberg [14] and 65% in Seattle [46], and a 6-year OS of 53% at the M.D. Anderson Cancer Center [40]. In contrast, multicenter studies report worse OS rates of 20–30% after 5 years [13,42]. Taken together, these studies suggest that allo-HSCT in MCL is capable of providing long-term disease control, but no comparative studies have been performed to answer the question if the risk of the disease-related mortality justifies the risk of NRM associated with allo-HSCT.

Post-transplantation disease monitoring for mantle cell lymphoma

As pointed out earlier, sound evidence that preemptive treatment with rituximab or any other agent on MRD persistence or recurrence after auto-HSCT for MCL may prolong remission and survival is lacking [38]. Therefore MRD monitoring after autologous transplantation is not accepted as a standard strategy [3].

There is some consensus that MRD persistence or recurrence after allo-HSCT for MCL should trigger preemptive immune-modulating interventions, such as immunosuppression tapering or DLI [3]. However, unlike in chronic lymphocytic leukemia (CLL) where this practice can help to navigate GVL toward effective disease eradication [47], the real-life situation in MCL is more complicated. This is due to the fact that molecular MRD assessment needed for MCL is much more time-consuming than MRD-flow as used in CLL, and because disease kinetics can be very dynamic in MCL, thereby outpacing MRD-based preemptive therapy. Therefore MRD monitoring after allo-HSCT for MCL is not a generally accepted policy [3].

Management of mantle cell lymphoma relapse after transplantation

Relapse after autologous HSCT

The prognosis of MCL patients has improved considerably during recent years. However, despite the merits of modern aggressive first-line therapy including auto-HSCT, a continuous pattern of relapse can be observed in MCL (Figure 17.1).

A large retrospective study of the EBMT analyzed salvage therapies and outcome of 360 patients with MCL who had relapsed after auto-HSCT. Median OS after disease recurrence was considerably poor, only 19 months in this study [15]. In a small retrospective study of three referral centers in Germany the median OS after auto-HSCT failure was comparably dismal with 23 months [14]. However, the EBMT study also demonstrated that outcome of MCL relapse after auto-HSCT has improved significantly over the last decade, suggesting that salvage strategies for this condition have significantly improved. Beside chemotherapy refractoriness, the most important prognostic factor determining prognosis after relapse is a short PFS interval of less than 12 months after auto-HSCT. This observation corroborates findings of the retrospective study of three German referral centers [14] and parallels results in patients with follicular lymphoma [48] or aggressive B-cell lymphoma relapsing after auto-HSCT [49]. An important feature of MCL that contributes substantially to its poor prognosis is the development of chemorefractory disease in many patients after relapse. As many as 40% of patients in the EBMT study were refractory to their first salvage treatment after auto-HSCT failure, which is significantly inferior to only 8% of chemotherapy-refractory patients prior to auto-HSCT within the same patient cohort. Alternative and chemotherapy-free approaches – such as lenalidomide [27] and, most promising, ibrutinib [28] – are therefore highly warranted to improve the unfavorable outcome of patients with chemorefractory disease.

No general consensus exists on how to treat patients with MCL relapse after auto-HSCT. The choice of the most suitable therapeutic regimen for patients with relapsed disease intuitively depends on multiple parameters, such as performance status and/or biological age, remission duration after auto-HSCT, chemotherapy sensitivity, and biological features of the disease. However, to

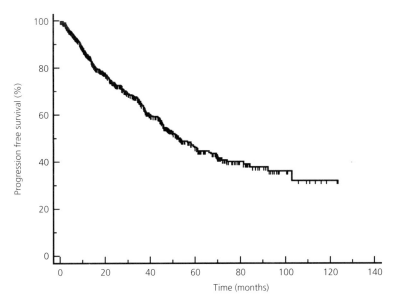

Figure 17.1 Progression-free survival of patients with mantle cell lymphoma who received an autologous stem cell transplantation between 2000 and 2008 and were registered with the EBMT database (*N* = 786).

date a risk-stratified rescue approach is lacking. Because of its registry design, the previously mentioned EBMT study represents current practice in many centers and showed that first salvage regimens after relapse were predominantly chemotherapy-based in more than 80% of patients. As for most other lymphomas, noncross-resistant salvage regimens should generally be used in MCL. If for instance R-CHOP (rituximab plus cyclophosphamide, doxorubicin, vincristine, and prednisone), in combination with high-dose ara-C, was used to induce first remission prior to auto-HSCT, a reasonable choice for treatment of relapse could be bendamustine plus rituximab, which showed an impressive 84% overall response rate (ORR) with 53% complete remissions in a recent Spanish retrospective study [23]. Other options include bortezomib-based or lenalidomide-based regimens [25,27] and ibrutinib [28]. The only compound which has been positively evaluated in a Phase III study in the MCL relapse setting is temsirolimus, but its ORR in this approval trial was only 22% [50].

Second transplantation after auto-HSCT failure

Despite success with new drugs in highly refractory cases of MCL, relapses will occur inevitably after all currently available treatment approaches. The

question of whether a second stem cell transplant might be used to consolidate response after salvage treatment seems reasonable. In the previously mentioned EBMT study, approximately one-quarter of patients received a second stem cell transplantation. Only 4% of patients received a second auto-HSCT and although conclusions on only seven patients are difficult to draw, only one long-term survivor was observed in the auto-HSCT2 group. A second auto-HSCT can therefore not be recommended based on the available data. The majority of patients (20%) evaluated in the EBMT study who received a second transplant underwent allo-HSCT, showing a significant number of long-term remissions with a 2-year OS of 48%. The most important prognostic factor for outcome after allo-HSCT was the duration of remission after the first auto-HSCT. Almost all patients who relapsed within the first year after auto-HSCT and subsequently received an allo-HSCT died quickly thereafter. In contrast, patients with longer remission duration achieved a plateau after second allo-HSCT at approximately 50%. It is important to mention that patients evaluated in this study were mostly chemotherapy sensitive [15]. These results suggest that allo-HSCT might be a valuable option for young and eligible patients who have a chemotherapy-sensitive relapse after auto-HSCT. For details of the allo-HSCT procedure, see Chapter 4.

Relapse after allo-HSCT

Data on how to treat MCL relapse after allo-HSCT is sparse. Generally, the same concepts as for relapse after auto-HSCT could be applied. However, a prior allo-HSCT provides a unique opportunity to take advantage of the GVL effect. To stimulate GVL, withdrawal of immunosuppression or the administration of DLI could be used. In a report by Wudhikarn *et al.* [51] on 72 patients with lymphoma relapse after allo-HSCT, such immunomodulating interventions were successful in individual patients, resulting in 43% OS after 2 years of the seven patients with MCL included in this analysis. In selected patients a second allo-HSCT might be an option. In a recent EBMT registry analysis on 140 allografted patients with lymphoma (including 22 patients with MCL) who underwent a second allo-transplant because of lymphoma relapse, 3-year PFS and OS were around 20% and 30%, respectively, with no significant differences between individual lymphoma subsets [52]. Thus, a second allo-HSCT might be an option for eligble patients, in particular if the interval between first allotransplant and relapse has not been too short.

Novel therapies and their integration in transplantation for mantle cell lymphoma

Novel agents are currently changing the landscape of MCL treatment. First examples of successful targeted therapeutics in the treatment of MCL comprise temsirolimus (mTOR inhibitor) and bortezomib (proteasome inhibitor). Temsirolimus was approved in Europe for the treatment of relapsed MCL based on a prospective trial that evaluated two dose regimens of temsirolimus in comparison with investigator-choice single-agent therapy in relapsed or refractory disease. Patients treated with temsirolimus 175/75 mg had significantly longer PFS than those treated with investigator-choice therapy [50]. Objective response rates were significantly higher in the 175/75-mg group (22%) compared with the investigator-choice group (2%). However, despite the superiority of temsirolimus over alternative therapies the median PFS

was still poor, only 4.8 months in the temsirolimus arm with the highest dose.

In the United States, the proteasome inhibitor bortezomib was approved for treatment of MCL in the salvage setting based on results that demonstrated responses in approximately 30% of relapsed or refractory patients [25]. However, median time to progression was also quite poor, only 6.2 months. Both agents have also been evaluated within combination regimens with improved response rates up to 50% for both drugs. In 2013 the Food and Drug Administration (FDA) approved two new promising drugs (lenalidomide and ibrutinib) for the treatment of relapsed MCL. The Phase II EMERGE trial, which included 134 patients, showed that single-agent lenalidomide has substantial activity against relapsed and refractory MCL. The ORR was 28% and median response duration was approximately 17 months [53]. Another drug with breakthrough status which was recently approved by the FDA based on the results of a Phase II trial in relapsed or refractory MCL is the Bruton's tyrosine kinase inhibitor ibrutinib. Even as single agent this drug has proven to have a much higher efficacy than the drugs described previously. An ORR of 68% and complete remission (CR) in 21% of patients were observed after the first reported follow-up, but on longer follow-up the CR rate improved even further to 40%, although the ORR did not change. Estimated response duration in this initial trial was 17.5 months and thus clearly better than that observed with any other new drug.

However, curing patients with any of these single-agent approaches seems unlikely so far. Future studies exploring these agents in combination treatments will show if these exciting results can be improved further. The European MCL Network is currently planning to conduct a study where ibrutinib is incorporated before and after auto-HSCT and will finally be compared to a nontransplant arm which also involves ibrutinib. This study aims to answer the question of whether auto-HSCT is still beneficial in the area of targeted therapies. Patients with refractory MCL prior to allo-HSCT have a rather poor prognosis and lymphomas are often growing before the immune effect can contribute to disease control. Novel agents such as ibrutinib could help to induce better remissions prior to allo-HSCT and might thereby improve outcome, but this has to be tested in future trials.

References

1 Sant M, Allemani C, Tereanu C *et al*. Incidence of hematologic malignancies in Europe by morphologic subtype: results of the HAEMACARE project. *Blood* 2010;**116**:3724–34.

2 Dreyling M, Thieblemont C, Gallamini A *et al*. ESMO Consensus conferences: guidelines on malignant lymphoma. Part 2: marginal zone lymphoma, mantle cell lymphoma, peripheral T-cell lymphoma. *Ann Oncol* 2013;**24**:857–77.

3 Robinson S, Dreger P, Caballero D *et al*. The EBMT/EMCL consensus project on the role of autologous and allogeneic stem cell transplantation in mantle cell lymphoma. *Leukemia* 2015;**29**:464–73.

4 Dreyling M, Lenz G, Hoster E *et al*. Early consolidation by myeloablative radiochemotherapy followed by autologous stem cell transplantation in first remission significantly prolongs progression-free survival in mantle-cell lymphoma: results of a prospective randomized trial of the European MCL Network. *Blood* 2005;**105**:2677–84.

5 Hoster E, Metzner B, Forstpointner R *et al*. Autologous stem cell transplantation and addition of rituximab independently prolong response duration in advanced stage mantle cell lymphoma. *Blood (ASH Annual Meeting Abstracts)* 2009;**114**:Abstract 880.

6 Abrahamsson A, Albertsson-Lindblad A, Brown PN *et al*. Real world data on primary treatment for mantle cell lymphoma: a Nordic Lymphoma Group observational study. *Blood* 2014;**124**:1288–95.

7 Hermine O, Hoster E, Walewski J *et al*. Alternating courses of 3× CHOP and 3× DHAP plus rituximab followed by a high dose ara-c containing myeloablative regimen and autologous stem cell transplantation (ASCT) increases overall survival when compared to 6 courses of CHOP plus rituximab followed by myeloablative radiochemotherapy and ASCT in mantle cell lymphoma: final analysis of the MCL Younger Trial of the European Mantle Cell Lymphoma Network (MCL net). *Blood (ASH Annual Meeting Abstracts)* 2012;**120**:Abstract 151.

8 Geisler CH, Kolstad A, Laurell A *et al*. Long-term progression-free survival of mantle cell lymphoma following intensive front-line immunochemotherapy with in vivo-purged stem cell rescue: a non-randomized phase-II multicenter study by the Nordic Lymphoma Group. *Blood* 2008;**112**:2687–93.

9 Jantunen E, Canals C, Attal M *et al*. Autologous stem-cell transplantation in patients with mantle cell lymphoma beyond 65 years of age: a study from the European Group for Blood and Marrow Transplantation (EBMT). *Ann Oncol* 2012;**23**:166–71.

10 Hoster E, Klapper W, Hermine O *et al*. Confirmation of the mantle-cell lymphoma International Prognostic Index in randomized trials of the European Mantle-Cell Lymphoma Network. *J Clin Oncol* 2014;**32**:1338–46.

11 Fernandez V, Salamero O, Espinet B *et al*. Genomic and gene expression profiling defines indolent forms of mantle cell lymphoma. *Cancer Res* 2010;**70**:1408–18.

12 Tam CS, Bassett R, Ledesma C *et al*. Mature results of the M.D. Anderson Cancer Center risk-adapted transplantation strategy in mantle cell lymphoma. *Blood* 2009;**113**:4144–52.

13 Fenske TS, Zhang MJ, Carreras J *et al*. Autologous or reduced-intensity conditioning allogeneic hematopoietic cell transplantation for chemotherapy-sensitive mantle-cell lymphoma: analysis of transplantation timing and modality. *J Clin Oncol* 2013;**32**:273–81.

14 Dietrich S, Tielesch B, Rieger M *et al*. Patterns and outcome of relapse after autologous stem cell transplantation for mantle cell lymphoma. *Cancer* 2011;**117**:1901–10.

15 Dietrich S, Boumendil A, Finel H *et al*. Outcome and prognostic factors in patients with mantle-cell lymphoma relapsing after autologous stem cell transplantation: a retrospective study of the European Group for Blood and Marrow Transplantation (EBMT). *Ann Oncol* 2014;**25**:1053–8.

16 Hamadani M, Saber W, Ahn KW *et al*. Allogeneic hematopoietic cell transplantation for chemotherapy-unresponsive mantle cell lymphoma: a cohort analysis from the Center for International Blood and Marrow Transplant Research. *Biol Blood Marrow Transplant* 2013;**19**:625–31.

17 Wang ML, Rule S, Martin P *et al*. Targeting BTK with ibrutinib in relapsed or refractory mantle-cell lymphoma. *N Engl J Med* 2013;**369**:507–16.

18 Kahl BS, Spurgeon SE, Furman RR *et al*. Results of a phase I study of idelalisib, a PI3Kdelta inhibitor, in patients with relapsed or refractory mantle cell lymphoma (MCL). *Blood* 2014;**123**:3398–405.

19 Vandenberghe E, Ruiz dE, Loberiza FR *et al*. Outcome of autologous transplantation for mantle cell lymphoma: a study by the European Blood and Bone Marrow Transplant and Autologous Blood and Marrow Transplant Registries. *Br J Haematol* 2003;**120**:793–800.

20 Kolstad A, Laurell A, Jerkeman M *et al*. Nordic MCL-3 study: BEAM/C conditioning intensified with 90Y-ibritumomab-tiuxetan in responding non-CR patients followed by autologous transplant in mantle cell lymphoma. *Blood* 2014;**123**:2953–9.

21 Pott C, Hoster E, Delfau-Larue M-H *et al*. Molecular remission is an independent predictor of clinical outcome in patients with mantle cell lymphoma after combined immunochemotherapy: a European MCL intergroup study. *Blood* 2010;**115**:3215–23.

22 Metzeler KH, Heilmeier B, Edmaier KE *et al*. High expression of lymphoid enhancer-binding factor-1 (LEF1) is a novel favorable prognostic factor in cytogenetically normal acute myeloid leukemia. *Blood* 2012;**120**:2118–26.

23 Garcia-Noblejas A, Martinez CC, Navarro MB *et al*. Bendamustine as salvage treatment for patients with relapsed or refractory mantle cell lymphoma patients: a retrospective study of the Spanish experience. *Ann Hematol* 2014;**93**:1551–8.

24 Cook G, Smith GM, Kirkland K *et al*. Outcome following reduced intensity allogeneic stem cell transplantation (RIC AlloSCT) for relapsed and refractory mantle-cell lymphoma

(MCL): a study of the British Society for Blood and Marrow Transplantation. *Biol Blood Marrow Transplant* 2010;**16**:1419–27.

25 Fisher RI, Bernstein SH, Kahl BS *et al.* Multicenter phase II study of bortezomib in patients with relapsed or refractory mantle cell lymphoma. *J Clin Oncol* 2006;**24**:4867–74.

26 Witzig TE, Geyer SM, Ghobrial I *et al.* Phase II trial of single-agent temsirolimus (CCI-779) for relapsed mantle cell lymphoma. *J Clin Oncol* 2005;**23**:5347–56.

27 Zaja F, De Luca S, Vitolo U *et al.* Salvage treatment with lenalidomide and dexamethasone in relapsed/refractory mantle cell lymphoma: clinical results and effects on microenvironment and neo-angiogenic biomarkers. *Haematologica* 2012;**97**:416–22.

28 Wang ML, Rule S, Martin P *et al.* Targeting BTK with ibrutinib in relapsed or refractory mantle-cell lymphoma. *N Engl J Med* 2013;**369**:507–16.

29 Geisler CH, Kolstad A, Laurell A *et al.* Nordic MCL2 trial update: six-year follow-up after intensive immunochemotherapy for untreated mantle cell lymphoma followed by BEAM or BEAC + autologous stem-cell support: still very long survival but late relapses do occur. *Br J Haematol* 2012;**158**:355–62.

30 Rubio MT, Boumendil A, Luan JJ *et al.* Is there still a place for total body irradiation (TBI) in the conditioning regimen of autologous stem cell transplantation in mantle cell lymphoma? A retrospective study from the Lymphoma Working Party of the EBMT. *Blood (ASH Annual Meeting Abstracts)* 2010;**116**:Abstract 688.

31 Touzeau C, Leux C, Bouabdallah R *et al.* Autologous stem cell transplantation in mantle cell lymphoma: a report from the SFGM-TC. *Ann Hematol* 2014;**93**:233–42.

32 Dreger P, Rieger M, Seyfarth B *et al.* Incorporation of rituximab into the ablative regimen improves the outcome of first-line autologous stem cell transplantation for mantle cell lymphoma: a controlled phase-II study. *Haematologica* 2007;**92**:42–9.

33 Andersen NS, Donovan JW, Borus JS *et al.* Failure of immunologic purging in mantle cell lymphoma assessed by polymerase chain reaction detection of minimal residual disease. *Blood* 1997;**90**:4212–21.

34 Pettengell R, Schmitz N, Gisselbrecht C *et al.* Rituximab purging and/or maintenance in patients undergoing autologous transplantation for relapsed follicular lymphoma: a prospective randomized trial from the Lymphoma Working Party of the European Group for Blood and Marrow Transplantation. *J Clin Oncol* 2013;**31**:1624–30.

35 Chien JW, Zhang XC, Fan W *et al.* Evaluation of published single nucleotide polymorphisms associated with acute GVHD. *Blood* 2012;**119**:5311–19.

36 Dietrich S, Weidle J, Rieger M *et al.* Rituximab maintenance therapy after autologous stem cell transplantation prolongs progression free survival in patients with mantle cell lymphoma. *Leukemia* 2014;**28**:708–9.

37 Le Gouill S, Thieblemont C, Oberic L *et al.* Rituximab maintenance versus wait and watch after four courses of R-DHAP followed by autologous stem cell transplantation in previously untreated young patients with mantle cell lymphoma: first interim analysis of the Phase III Prospective Lyma Trial, a Lysa Study. *Blood (ASH Annual Meeting Abstracts)* 2014;**124**:Abstract 3070.

38 Andersen NS, Pedersen LB, Laurell A *et al.* Pre-emptive treatment with rituximab of molecular relapse after autologous stem cell transplantation in mantle cell lymphoma. *J Clin Oncol* 2009;**27**:4365–70.

39 Adkins D, Brown R, Goodnough LT *et al.* Treatment of resistant mantle cell lymphoma with allogeneic bone marrow transplantation. *Bone Marrow Transplant* 1998;**21**:97–9.

40 Khouri IF, Lee MS, Saliba RM *et al.* Nonablative allogeneic stem-cell transplantation for advanced/recurrent mantle-cell lymphoma. *J Clin Oncol* 2003;**21**:4407–12.

41 Khouri IF, Lee MS, Romaguera J *et al.* Allogeneic hematopoietic transplantation for mantle-cell lymphoma: molecular remissions and evidence of graft-versus-malignancy. *Ann Oncol* 1999;**10**:1293–9.

42 Le Gouill S, Kroger N, Dhedin N *et al.* Reduced-intensity conditioning allogeneic stem cell transplantation for relapsed/refractory mantle cell lymphoma: a multicenter experience. *Ann Oncol* 2012;**23**:2695–703.

43 Ganti AK, Bierman PJ, Lynch JC *et al.* Hematopoietic stem cell transplantation in mantle cell lymphoma. *Ann Oncol* 2005;**16**:618–24.

44 Milpied N, Gaillard F, Moreau P *et al.* High-dose therapy with stem cell transplantation for mantle cell lymphoma: results and prognostic factors, a single center experience. *Bone Marrow Transplant* 1998;**22**:645–50.

45 Peniket AJ, Ruiz de Elvira MC, Taghipour G *et al.* An EBMT registry matched study of allogeneic stem cell transplants for lymphoma: allogeneic transplantation is associated with a lower relapse rate but a higher procedure-related mortality rate than autologous transplantation. *Bone Marrow Transplant* 2003;**31**:667–78.

46 Maris MB, Sandmaier BM, Storer BE *et al.* Allogeneic hematopoietic cell transplantation after fludarabine and 2 Gy total body irradiation for relapsed and refractory mantle cell lymphoma. *Blood* 2004;**104**:3535–42.

47 Dreger P, Döhner H, Ritgen M *et al.* Allogeneic stem cell transplantation provides durable disease control in poor-risk chronic lymphocytic leukemia: long-term clinical and MRD results of the GCLLSG CLL3X trial. *Blood* 2010;**116**:2438–47.

48 Kornacker M, Stumm J, Pott C *et al.* Characteristics of relapse after autologous stem cell transplantation for follicular lymphoma: a long-term follow-up. *Ann Oncol* 2009;**20**:722–8.

49 Gisselbrecht C, Schmitz N, Mounier N *et al.* Rituximab maintenance therapy after autologous stem-cell transplantation in patients with relapsed CD20(+) diffuse large B-cell lymphoma: final analysis of the collaborative trial in relapsed aggressive lymphoma. *J Clin Oncol* 2012;**30**:4462–9.

50 Hess G, Herbrecht R, Romaguera J *et al.* Phase III study to evaluate temsirolimus compared with investigator's choice

therapy for the treatment of relapsed or refractory mantle cell lymphoma. *J Clin Oncol* 2009;**27**:3822–9.

51 Wudhikarn K, Brunstein CG, Bachanova V *et al.* Relapse of lymphoma after allogeneic hematopoietic cell transplantation: management strategies and outcome. *Biol Blood Marrow Transplant* 2011;**17**:1497–504.

52 Horstmann K, Boumendil A, Finel H *et al.* Second allogeneic stem cell transplantation in patients with lymphoma relapse after a first allogeneic transplantation. A retrospective study of the EBMT Lymphoma Working Party. *Bone Marrow Transplant* 2015.

53 Goy A, Sinha R, Williams ME *et al.* Single-agent lenalidomide in patients with mantle-cell lymphoma who relapsed or progressed after or were refractory to bortezomib: phase II MCL-001 (EMERGE) study. *J Clin Oncol* 2013;**31**:3688–95.

54 Geisler CH, Kolstad A, Laurell A *et al.* The Mantle Cell Lymphoma International Prognostic Index (MIPI) is superior to the International Prognostic Index (IPI) in predicting survival following intensive first-line immunochemotherapy and autologous stem cell transplantation (ASCT). *Blood* 2010;**115**:1530–3.

55 Budde LE, Guthrie KA, Till BG *et al.* Mantle cell lymphoma international prognostic index but not pretransplantation induction regimen predicts survival for patients with mantle-cell lymphoma receiving high-dose therapy and autologous stem-cell transplantation. *J Clin Oncol* 2011;**29**:3023–9.

56 Sureda A, Bader P, Cesaro S *et al.* Indications for allogeneic and autologous stem cell transplantation for haematological diseases, solid tumours and immune disorders: current practice in Europe 2015. *Bone Marrow Transplant* 2015.

CHAPTER 18

Hodgkin lymphoma

Eva Domingo-Domenech and Anna Sureda

Indications for transplantation in Hodgkin lymphoma

Hodgkin lymphoma (HL) is one of the most curable hematologic malignancies, with 7000–7500 new cases diagnosed annually in the United States. HL displays a bimodal curve in incidence and most of the patients present with early-stage disease. The dual-peak incidence supports the hypothesis that HL may be a common result of two distinct pathogenic processes: an infectious agent, such as Epstein–Barr virus (EBV), may have an impact in development of the disease in young adults, while a mechanism shared with other lymphomas may account for the pathogenesis of HL in the older age group [1].

Mortality of HL has significantly decreased over the last 30 years. Patients with early-stage HL have an overall survival (OS) of over 90% with modern first-line therapies [2]; however, in patients being diagnosed in advanced stages, 10-year OS is only above 50% [3]. Consolidation with high-dose chemotherapy/autologous stem cell transplantation (HDC/ASCT) is not a recommended procedure in patients with HL in first complete remission (CR) after conventional first-line chemoradiotherapy [4].

The number of patients with primary resistant or relapsed HL is low, although they represent a clinical challenge. The use of ASCT is now considered the standard of care for relapsed HL patients. Two randomized trials showed significant benefit in terms of freedom from treatment failure (FFTF) for ASCT over conventional chemotherapy for relapsed disease [5,6]. These trials have resulted in the recommendation of ASCT at time of first relapse for even the most favorable patients, although salvage radiotherapy can offer an effective treatment for selected subsets of patients with relapsed or refractory HL.

Patients with HL who relapse after ASCT have a very poor long-term outcome; there is little information about prognostic factors in this setting. A retrospective analysis of the Lymphoma Working Party (LWP) of the European Society for Blood and Marrow Transplantation (EBMT) and Gruppo Italiano Trapianto di Midollo Osseo (GITMO) [7] including 511 adult patients with relapsed HL after ASCT indicates that after a median follow-up of 49 months, OS of these patients was 32% at 5 years. Independent risk factors for OS were early relapse after ASCT, stage IV disease and bulky disease at the time of relapse, poor performance status, and age 50 years and over. For patients with no risk factors, OS at 5 years was 62% compared with 37% and 12% for those having one and two or more factors, respectively. Relapsed disease after ASCT represents a clear unmet need. Therapeutic options in this subgroup of patients are very heterogeneous and include salvage chemotherapy and/or radiotherapy followed or not by a second stem cell transplantation, palliative care, new drugs, or biological agents. HDC supported by allogeneic stem cell transplantation (allo-SCT) is a suitable approach for patients relapsing after ASCT and with early relapsed or refractory HL. A broad spectrum of evidence supports the existence of a graft-versus-Hodgkin lymphoma (GVHL) effect [8] and some studies show a lower rate of relapse after allo-SCT compared with ASCT.

Clinical Guide to Transplantation in Lymphoma, First Edition. Edited by Bipin N. Savani and Mohamad Mohty.
© 2015 John Wiley & Sons, Ltd. Published 2015 by John Wiley & Sons, Ltd.

Autologous hematopoietic stem cell transplantation for Hodgkin lymphoma

The first randomized trial compared ASCT with BEAM (BCNU, etoposide, ara-C, melphalan) to mini-BEAM without any stem cell support in patients with active HL, in whom conventional therapy had failed [5]. Twenty patients were assigned treatment with BEAM plus ASCT and 20 with mini-BEAM. Five BEAM recipients died compared with nine mini-BEAM recipients. Both 3-year event-free survival (EFS) and progression-free survival (PFS) showed significant differences in favor of BEAM plus ASCT (P = 0.025 and P = 0.005, respectively). No differences in terms of OS were seen.

The second randomized trial (HD01 Trial) was published 10 years later [6]. A total of 161 patients were assigned two cycles of Dexa-BEAM and either two further courses of Dexa-BEAM or BEAM. There was a significant improvement in 3-year FFTF for patients undergoing ASCT compared to four cycles of Dexa-BEAM (55% vs. 34%, P = 0.019). The 3-year FFTF was significantly better for patients treated with BEAM, regardless of whether the first relapse had occurred early (<12 months) (41% vs. 12%, P = 0.007) or late (>12 months) (75% vs. 44%, P = 0.02). Of note, there was no statistically significant difference in OS for any subgroup of patients.

Prognostic factors for long-term outcome after ASCT

The impact of ASCT in the long-term outcome of patients with relapsed/refractory HL is not the same in all subgroups of patients. Time to relapse (<12 months vs. ≥12 months) [9–11], extranodal disease at relapse [9,11], advanced stage and anemia at relapse [10], B symptoms [11,12], and refractory disease [12] were found to be important adverse prognostic factors. The German Hodgkin Lymphoma Study Group (GHSG) was able to construct a retrospective risk factor score from patients that were included in a Phase III prospective clinical trial [13]. The presence of significant anemia at relapse, early or multiple relapses, and stage IV translated into a dismal overall outcome and a 3-years PFS less than 20%. More recently, a positive fluorodeoxyglucose positron emission tomography (FDG-PET) scan at the end of salvage chemotherapy and before ASCT has also been considered an adverse prognostic factor;

in a group of 101 patients with both non-Hodgkin lymphoma and HL, both FDG-PET after two cycles of chemotherapy and clinical risk score were independent prognostic factors for failure-free survival after ASCT [14]. Two other studies have added additional information to the prognostic value of FDG-PET; a pretransplant positive PET/gallium scan was able to predict poor outcome after ASCT [15]. Finally, in a group of 189 HL patients prospectively included in transplantation protocols, functional imaging status before ASCT was the only factor significant for EFS and OS by multivariate analysis and clearly identified poor-risk patients (5-year EFS 31% and 75% for functional imaging-positive and -negative patients, respectively) [16].

Debulking therapy before ASCT and preparative regimen before ASCT

The best debulking regimen before HDC/ASCT remains to be defined; there are no published prospective randomized clinical trials comparing efficacy and toxicity of the different strategies used. The most commonly used regimens, such as DHAP (dexamethasone, cytarabine, cisplatin) [17], ICE (ifosfamide, carboplatin, etoposide) [18], ESHAP (etoposide, methylprednisolone, high-dose cytarabine, and cisplatin) [19], and IGEV (ifosfamide, gemcitabine, vinorelbine) [20], have been shown to be effective in reducing bulky disease, mobilizing stem cells into the peripheral blood, and testing chemosensitivity before the high-dose procedure.

A wide variety of HDC regimens has been used with ASCT for HL. No prospective clinical trials have been performed, although regimens have been compared retrospectively. HDC regimens are frequently divided into those that use total body irradiation (TBI) and those that contain only drugs. The use of TBI may be associated with increased pulmonary toxicity, particularly in patients who have received prior mediastinal irradiation. Spanish registry results showed that the use of TBI-containing regimens prior to ASCT was associated with a significantly higher risk of transplant-related mortality [21], basically related to a higher incidence of secondary malignancies after the autologous procedure.

One of the most common HDC regimens used prior to ASCT is the CBV (cyclophosphamide, carmustine, etoposide) regimen developed at the M.D. Anderson Cancer Center. The original CBV regimen has been modified and individual institutions have used widely differing schedules. No prospective trials have examined whether variations in the CBV regimen lead to different outcomes, although higher doses of carmustine have been associated with an increased risk of pulmonary toxicity, particularly in patients who have received prior chest irradiation. Another HDC regimen is the BEAM protocol, which was developed by investigators from London and has also been widely modified. Retrospective analyses have failed to show significant differences in survival when CBV-type and BEAM-type were compared [22,23].

Can we improve the results of an autologous transplantation procedure?

The GHSG developed a sequential HDC protocol that was used before the transplant conditioning itself [24]. Treatment consisted of two cycles of DHAP to reduce tumor burden. Patients achieving a complete or partial remission went on to receive an HDC program including high-dose cyclophosphamide (4 g/m^2 i.v.), methotrexate (8 g/m^2 i.v.), vincristine (1.4 mg/m^2 i.v.), and etoposide (2 g/m^2 i.v.). Patients were then autografted using BEAM. Response rate after the final evaluation was 80%. FFTF and OS for patients with early relapse were 62% and 78%, respectively, and for patients with late relapse 63% and 79%, respectively. These promising results prompted the GHSG to develop a prospective Phase III clinical trial that randomized the conventional salvage approach (DHAP ×2 cycles plus ASCT) compared to DHAP plus high-dose sequential protocol plus ASCT. Interestingly, there were no significant differences in terms of PFS, FFTF, or OS between the study arms [13]. Potential reasons to explain the lack of effectiveness of this more intensive procedure were the higher toxicity of the intensive arm, the increased length to reach the transplantation procedure, as well as the significantly higher percentage of patients in the intensive arm who were not able to receive 100% of the expected chemotherapy dose.

Tandem ASCT has also been explored in a limited number of nonrandomized studies in order to improve results in those patients with adverse prognostic factors at the time of relapse. In the H96 trial [25], with 245 HL patients included, tandem ASCT was used in patients with two or more adverse factors (time to relapse <12 months, stage III or IV at relapse, and relapse within previously irradiated sites) and single BEAM-conditioned ASCT in the intermediate-risk group (up to one adverse prognostic factor). The 5-year freedom

from second failure and OS estimates were 73% and 85%, respectively, for the intermediate-risk group and 46% and 57%, respectively, for the poor-risk group. With this data, tandem ASCT cannot currently be recommended outside of clinical trials, although long-term outcome of patients with adverse prognosis disease seems better when treatment includes two cycles of HDT and ASCT.

Allogeneic hematopoietic stem cell transplantation for Hodgkin lymphoma

Compared to the number of autologous transplants, few patients with HL have undergone an allo-SCT (Figure 18.1). One of the major obstacles was the unfavorable outcome of allo-SCT in patients with HL reported in all early series. Two large registry-based studies gave disappointing results regarding the role of myeloablative allo-SCT in the high nonrelapse mortality (NRM) of the procedure. A total of 100 HL patients allografted from HLA-identical siblings were reported by the International Bone Marrow Transplant Registry (IBMTR) [26]. The 3-year-rates for OS, DFS, and probability of relapse were only 21%, 15%, and 65%, respectively. Major problems were persistent or recurrent disease or respiratory complications, which accounted for 35–51% of deaths. A case-matched analysis including 45 allografts and 45 autografts reported to the EBMT [27] did not find significant differences in actuarial probabilities of OS, PFS, and relapse rate (RR) between allo-SCT and ASCT (25%, 15%, and 61% vs. 37%, 24%, and 61%, respectively). NRM at 4 years was significantly higher for allografts than for autografts (48% vs. 27%). A potential beneficial effect of allo-SCT was not discernible at this point as results of both studies were hampered by an exceedingly high NRM.

Nonetheless, RR after allo-SCT compared favorably with that after ASCT in most instances and gave rise to speculations that there may be a GVHL effect similar to what had been described as the graft-versus-leukemia effect in the early 1980s. Reduced-intensity conditioning (RIC) became clinical practice in the mid 1990s. It has certainly been a major factor in the constant rise in the number of patients undergoing allo-SCT for HL in recent years.

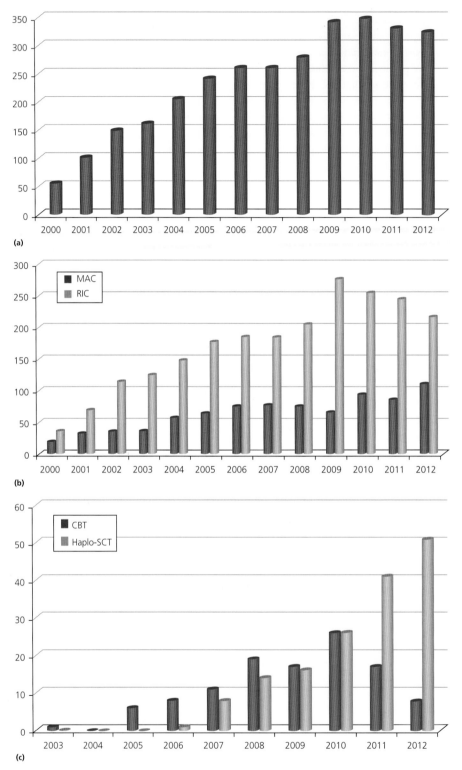

Figure 18.1 Allogeneic stem cell transplants for relapsed/refractory Hodgkin lymphoma: **a)** evolution of allogeneic stem cell transplantation over time; **b)** myeloablative conditioning (MAC) vs. reduced-intensity conditioning (RIC) regimens in allogeneic stem cell transplantation recipients; **c)** evolution of cord blood transplants (CBT) and haploidentical transplants (haplo-SCT) over time. The experience of the Lymphoma Working Party (LWP) of the European Society for Blood and Marrow Transplantation (EBMT) (personal communication).

The EBMT was the first group to retrospectively compare the outcomes after reduced-intensity or myeloablative conditioning in patients with relapsed/refractory HL [28] (Figure 18.2). NRM was significantly decreased in the RIC/allo-SCT group (23% vs. 46% at 1 year). The development of chronic graft-versus-host disease (GVHD) decreased the incidence of relapse after transplantation, which translated into a better PFS and OS. This analysis indicated that RIC/allo-SCT was able to reduce NRM and improve the long-term outcome of these patients.

Allogeneic transplantation in patients failing after an ASCT

Allo-SCT has basically been used in ASCT failures. Unfortunately, the information we have in this setting is based on Phase II prospective clinical trials that include reduced numbers of patients with short follow-up. In addition, the transplantation procedure is heterogeneous among different studies and comparisons are impossible to perform (Table 18.1). There are no Phase III randomized prospective clinical trials comparing the role of allo-SCT ahead of other therapeutic strategies in this setting.

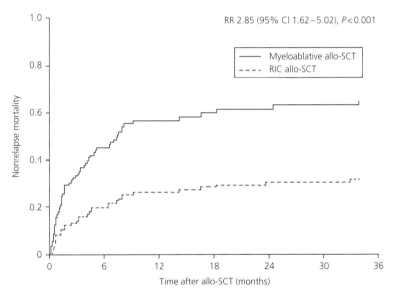

Figure 18.2 Nonrelapse mortality after allogeneic stem-cell transplantation (allo-SCT) for Hodgkin lymphoma according to the type of conditioning regimen, based on a Cox model. From Sureda *et al.* [28]. Reproduced with permission of American Society of Clinical Oncology.

Table 18.1 Review of outcomes of reduced-intensity allogeneic stem cell transplantation for relapsed/refractory Hodgkin lymphoma.

	No. of patients	Chemosensitivity (%)	PFS (%)	OS (%)	NRM (%)	RR (%)
Robinson *et al.* (2002) [62]	52	67	42 (2 years)	56 (2 years)	17 (2 years)	45 (2 years)
Peggs *et al.* (2005) [8]	49	67	39 (4 years)	55 (4 years)	15 (2 years)	33 (4 years)
Alvarez *et al.* (2006) [31]	40	50	32 (2 years)	48 (2 years)	25 (1 year)	NA
Todisco *et al.* (2007) [63]	14	57	25 (2 years)	57 (2 years)	0	NA
Corradini *et al.* (2007) [64]	32	62	NA	32 (3 years)	3 (3 years)	81 (3 years)
Anderlini *et al.* (2008) [41]	58	52	20 (2 years)	48 (2 years)	15 (2 years)	61 (2 years)
Devetten *et al.* (2009) [42]	143	44	20 (2 years)	37 (2 years)	33 (2 years)	47 (2 years)
Robinson *et al.* (2009) [29]	285	59	29 (4 years)	25 (4 years)	19 (1 year)	53 (3 years)
Sureda *et al.* (2012) [32]	92	67	24 (4 years)	43 (4 years)	15 (1 year)	59 (4 years)

PFS, progression-free survival; OS, overall survival; NRM, nonrelapse mortality; RR, relapse rate; NA, not available.

The LWP of the EBMT has also reported the largest retrospective analysis looking at 285 multiply relapsed HL patients [29]; 47 patients (17%) were in CR, 123 patients (43%) had chemosensitive disease, and 115 patients (40%) had chemoresistant disease. The NRM was 12% at 100 days, 20% at 12 months, and to 22% at 3 years; refractory disease was significantly associated with a higher NRM. The 2-year PFS was 29% and it was also significantly worse for patients with chemoresistant disease (P < 0.001). Development of either acute or chronic GVHD was associated with a lower RR. A total of 40 patients with relapsed/refractory HL undergoing RIC/allo-SCT from an HLA-identical sibling (N = 20) or a matched unrelated donor (N = 20) were reported by Anderlini et al. [30]. The 2-year OS and PFS were 64% and 32%, respectively; the 2-year projected risk of disease progression was 55%. There was a trend for the response status prior to allo-SCT to favorably impact PFS (P = 0.07) and disease progression (P = 0.049), but not OS. Partial responders and patients with stable refractory disease did similarly with regard to OS and PFS. Response rate 3 months after the allo-SCT was 67% in the Spanish experience [31]; 40 HL patients with multiply relapsed disease and adverse prognostic factors were treated with intravenous fludarabine (150 mg/m²) and melphalan (140 mg/m²) with cyclosporine A and methotrexate as GVHD prophylaxis. The 2-year OS and PFS were 48% and 32%, respectively. Refractoriness to chemotherapy was the only adverse prognostic factor for both OS and PFS. The *in vivo* T-cell depletion with alemtuzumab was the basis of the RIC protocol used by the UK Cooperative Group [8]. NRM was 16% at 2 years and projected 4-year OS and PFS were 56% and 39%, respectively. Finally, the largest Phase II trial including 78 patients with multiply relapsed HL and with adverse prognostic factors has been a joint effort of the Spanish Group for Lymphomas and Stem Cell Transplantation (GELTAMO) and the LWP of the EBMT [32]. Median follow-up of the whole series was 4 years. NRM was 8% at 100 days and 15% at 1 year. Relapse was the major cause of failure. Patients that were allografted in CR had a significantly better outcome. PFS was 48% at 1 year and 24% at 4 years and OS 71% at 1 year and 43% at 4 years (Figure 18.3). Chronic GVHD was associated with a lower relapse incidence and a better PFS.

Allo-SCT has been retrospectively compared with other treatment strategies; the UK group identified a group of patients who had relapsed following a BEAM autograft who were chemosensitive at relapse and had survived at least 12 months from relapse and who would therefore have been eligible for a reduced-intensity transplant [33]. This was a highly selected group, representing 44% of all relapses who were predicted to have the best survival. These conventionally treated patients were compared to more recently treated ones who received a reduced-intensity allograft. OS from time of diagnosis and time of autograft were significantly improved following allo-SCT, when compared to the historical control group. The estimated current PFS for the allografted patients was 34% at 5 years and 42% if in chemosensitive relapse at the time of transplant, suggesting the early promising results might translate into a favorable long-term outcome. A recently published study had similar outcomes and showed an advantage for allogeneic transplant over chemotherapy alone in patients with poor-risk HL who had relapsed following ASCT [34].

The role of dose intensity in the conditioning regimen of an allogeneic transplant

RIC regimens have allowed allo-SCT to be performed more safely; relapse is now the commonest cause of treatment failure. Conditioning intensity/anti-lymphoma activity may be an important factor in determining RR. Some of the truly nonmyeloablative regimens have been associated with particularly high RR values [35,36]. This concept of regimen intensity being important is also supported by the EBMT analysis, which showed an RR of 32% following myeloablative conditioning compared to 58% with RIC regimens [28]. Furthermore, within the RIC group, there was a higher RR and lower OS in patients who were conditioned with low-dose TBI, which is one of the regimens with the least toxicity (P < 0.04). Other studies have also shown a better outcome using more intensive regimens like the combination of fludarabine and melphalan when compared to less intensive regimens [30] and the BEAM–alemtuzumab regimen has also been demonstrated to give good disease control in the medium term [37]. An EBMT retrospective analysis performed in children and adolescents [38] indicated that RIC protocols give at the end a poorer outcome because the decreased NRM seen in this setting is not able to

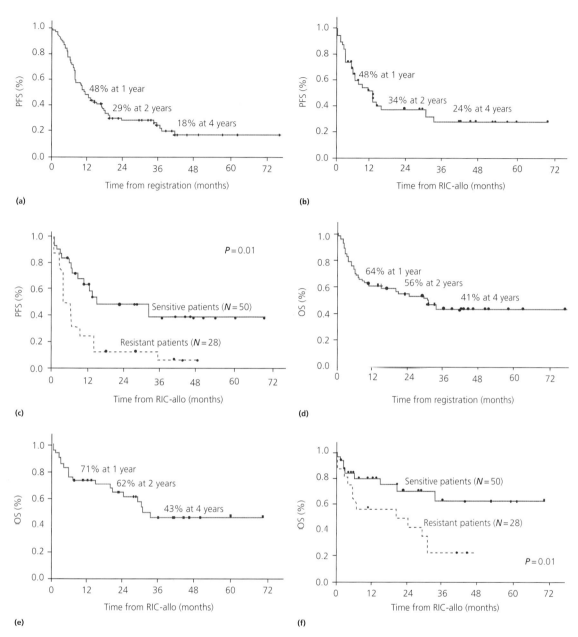

Figure 18.3 Progression-free survival (PFS) from entry into the trial. OS, overall survival. From Sureda *et al.* [32]. Reproduced with permission of Ferrata Storti Foundation.

counterbalance the higher RR after the transplant. In this sense, efforts should be made to try to personalize the conditioning regimen, taking into consideration the clinical characteristics of the patients. Recently, the LWP of the EBMT has undertaken a second retrospective analysis comparing long-term outcome of patients with

HL undergoing a myeloablative allo-SCT (*N* = 99) and those receiving RIC/allo-SCT (*N* = 215) in recent years, from January 2006 to December 2010 (S. Stavrik, personal communication). With a median follow-up of 34 months, NRM did not show significant differences between both groups of patients (11% at 36 months), RR was significantly higher in the RIC group (55% vs. 40% at 36 months, $P = 0.05$) giving a significant advantage in terms of PFS for the myeloablative group (50% vs. 33% at 36 months, $P = 0.02$) with no differences in OS (53% vs. 50% at 36 months).

Moving allogeneic transplantation to earlier phases of the disease

The more recent investigation of a response-adjusted transplantation algorithm identifies a further potential strategy for evaluation of allo-SCT in those deemed to be at high risk of failure of ASCT, targeting the intensification to those who have residual FDG-avid disease following salvage therapy [39]. The 3-year PFS of 68% in this high-risk group was encouraging, with 80% current PFS following donor lymphocyte infusion (DLI). Such approaches may require refinement according to delineation of number of lines of salvage, and according to the outcome of prospective studies evaluating maintenance strategies following ASCT and it is recommended that they be evaluated within the context of prospective national studies. These results have constituted the basis for a Phase II prospective clinical trial (CRUK-PAIReD, EUDRACT-2008-004956-60) already closed for recruitment that is analyzing long term outcome of relapsed/refractory HL patients who do not achieve a metabolic CR with first-line salvage chemotherapy and undergo an allo-SCT with BEAM protocol as conditioning regimen and the use of Campath 1H as GVHD prophylaxis. Final results of this trial are eagerly awaited by the transplant community.

Do we have any evidence of a GVHL effect?

Despite the theoretical reliance of reduced-intensity transplantation on a GVHL effect, there are relatively few studies which convincingly demonstrate this activity in HL. In the context of RIC transplantation, there is some evidence of a reduction in relapse in association with GVHD.

The most convincing evidence of GVHL activity in HL comes from the use of DLI to treat patients who relapse following allo-SCT (Table 18.2). Response rates to DLI have been reported to be between 15 and 60%, with complete responses seen in around 30% of patients. Many of these patients had received concurrent chemotherapy or radiotherapy but responses have been seen to DLI alone and some of these have been durable. There appears to be a higher

Table 18.2 Review of response rates after donor lymphocyte infusions.

	No. of patients	RR (%)	No. of patients receiving DLI	ORR (%)
Alvarez et al. (2006) [31]	40	NA	11	54
Anderlini et al. (2008) [41]	58	61 (2 years)	14	43
Peggs et al. (2011) [40]	76	33 (4 years)	24/31	79
Sureda et al. (2012) [32]	92	59 (4 years)	20/40	50

RR, relapse rate; DLI, donor lymphocyte infusion; ORR, overall response rate; NA, not available.

response rate in the UK series and it is not known whether the high incidence of mixed chimerism seen in patients who received Campath 1H promotes GVHL responses as it does in some animal models. The optimal T-cell dose for GVHL remains unclear, although many groups use an escalating dose schedule to try to reduce the risk of severe GVHD. Unlike follicular lymphoma, there is preliminary evidence that in relapsed HL, GVHL responses are unlikely in the absence of GVHD. However, when DLI is given for mixed chimerism, there appears to be a GVHL effect that is independent of GVHD [40]. Although the DLI responses are impressive in some patients, the majority of patients will not achieve long-term benefit from DLI and further study is needed to optimize this potential effect.

Increasing the pool of donors for HL patients having an allo-SCT

In Europe and North America, only around one-third of patients will have an HLA-matched sibling donor, so the use of alternative donors is essential to expand the number of patients eligible for the procedure. The advent of molecular techniques has improved the accuracy of tissue typing reports but the associated increase in HLA polymorphism has made finding an exact molecularly matched donor more difficult. However, the continual increase in unrelated donor numbers, the availability of cord blood, and the use of T-cell depletion has allowed a rise in the number of alternative donor transplants performed.

Although the number of published studies using unrelated donors remains limited at present, the transplant outcomes appear similar to those using sibling donors [8,28,41,42]. Not surprisingly, rates of GVHD may be higher and many groups have used T-cell depletion strategies with either alemtuzumab or anti-thymocyte globulin to reduce the incidence of this complication. Interestingly, unrelated donor transplants in patients with HL appear to have a similar OS and PFS to sibling donor transplants [8,28]. Therefore, given the lack of effective therapeutic options for patients who relapse post autologous transplantation, consideration of an unrelated allogeneic transplant is mandatory.

The published experience with cord blood donors in HL is much more limited but may be feasible [43,44]. A Eurocord–Netcord study showed a 30% PFS at 1 year in patients with relapsed HL [45]. A recently published French study showed that use of a cord blood donor was associated with inferior survival [46]. Longer-term follow-up of these patients will obviously be necessary to determine whether the GVHL activity of the cord blood obviates the need for post-transplant DLI. Finally, haploidentical donors have been used in small series indicating that this may also be a useful donor source, although follow-up is too short to determine the long-term impact of this approach [36,47]. Raiola *et al.* [47] recently published the results of a group of 26 multiply relapsed HL patients treated with a related HLA haploidentical allo-SCT, following RIC conditioning with low-dose TBI, as proposed by the Baltimore group. GVHD prophylaxis consisted of high-dose post-transplantation cyclophosphamide, mycophenolate, and a calcineurin inhibitor. The incidence of grade II–IV acute GVHD and of chronic GVHD was 24% and 8%, respectively. With a median follow-up of 24 months, 21 patients were alive and 20 disease-free. Cumulative incidences of NRM and relapse were 4% and 31%, respectively, and actuarial 3-year OS and PFS 77% and 63%, respectively. These preliminary results have significantly increased the interest in performing haploidentical allo-SCT in this setting.

Post-transplantation disease monitoring for Hodgkin lymphoma

Follow-up of patients with HL after an ASCT is based on medical visits, physical examinations, and basic analysis. Many centers also include computed tomography (CT)

scan every 6 months or every year up to 5 years after the ASCT. Nevertheless, there is no universal consensus regarding this latter point. PET/CT is not routinely recommended after an ASCT. The role of PET/CT in patients with HL is clearly established at diagnosis and at the end of treatment but not after an intensive procedure. As already discussed, PET positivity before an ASCT is an adverse prognostic factor for the long-term outcome of the procedure [14–16].

Disease monitoring after an allo-SCT should follow the same guidelines already described for the autologous setting. In a prospective study of 80 patients undergoing RIC/allo-SCT, pretransplantation PET status had no significant impact on either RR or OS; 34 relapses were observed, of which 17 were PET-positive with a normal CT scan at relapse. DLIs were administered in 26 episodes of relapse and were guided by PET alone in 14 patients. Post-transplant surveillance PET allowed early treatment of patients otherwise CT negative [48].

Management of relapses after transplantation for Hodgkin lymphoma

Relapses after ASCT

Despite the use of ASCT in patients with primary refractory or relapsed disease, up to 50% of patients will ultimately relapse after ASCT. These patients are likely incurable with standard therapies. Some of these patients can be considered candidates for an allo-SCT (young patients with a HLA compatible donor and with chemosensitive disease). The possibility of using "new" drugs such as brentuximab vedotin as salvage therapy for patients relapsing after an ASCT will potentially increase the candidates for an allogeneic procedure due to the high percentage of objective responses and the low toxicity profile of the drug. On the contrary, some patients might not consider allo-SCT as a treatment option due to transplantation side effects and the possibility of attaining a durable CR with brentuximab vedotin and will eventually be retreated with the drug if they suffer relapse or disease progression. Some patients achieve good outcomes following a second autologous transplant; these patients represent a highly selected group who relapsed more than 3 years post first autologous transplant [49].

However, in a considerable number of cases, the treatment plan will not be curative. In the noncurative setting, there are many conventional agents that may be used in sequence or combination to provide disease control; gemcitabine and vinblastine are frequently used [50,51]. It would be more appealing to use novel agents that exploit alternative mechanisms of action because patients have already been exposed to multiple standard agents. Brentuximab vedotin has shown excellent results administered as a single drug at a dose of 1.8 mg/kg i.v. every 3 weeks in this setting [52]. A pilot study of the monoclonal anti-CD20 antibody rituximab has shown a response rate of 22% in classic HL and was associated with resolution of B symptoms [53]. Additional data suggest several classes of agents –histone deacetylase inhibitors, mammalian target of rapamycin inhibitors, and immunomodulatory agents – are potentially worthy of further study in relapsed/refractory HL [54–56]. Other principles to follow for patients relapsing after an ASCT in the palliative setting are involved or extended field radiation if the disease is localized, other investigational agents or inclusion in prospective clinical trials if possible, and sequential single-agent chemotherapy for patients with advanced stage and/or significant comorbidities. In any case, patient preference should also be an important factor in clinical decision-making.

Relapses after an allo-SCT

Disease relapse is the leading cause of treatment failure in patients with HL treated with an allo-SCT, with relapse rate increasing from 45 to 55%. There are no standard treatment options for patients failing an allo-SCT. If the patient does not have active GVHD and has already stopped immunosuppressive therapy, DLI has been extensively used. Although a significant proportion of patients achieve a complete or partial remission with DLI, only a small proportion of them are long-term responders. An exception to the rule is those patients receiving alemtuzumab as part of the GVHD prophylaxis.

Brentuximab vedotin has also been used in the post-allo-SCT setting as a single drug [57] or in combination with DLI. This latter approach has been reported by Theurich *et al.* [58] in four HL patients with disease relapse after an allo-SCT who showed marked clinical and metabolic responses with a median duration of disease control of at least 349 days after treatment initiation, still ongoing in three of them.

The bifunctional alkylator bendamustine hydrochloride may be considered an attractive agent for use in this clinical setting because of a variety of mechanistic differences compared to other alkylating agents employed in HL. Anastasia *et al.* [59] have reported on the use of bendamustine as single agent in 67 HL patients with a median age of 34 years who had failed either an ASCT ($N = 45$, 67%) or an autologous/allogeneic SCT ($N = 22$, 33%). Bendamustine was administered at 90 or 120 mg/m^2 on days 1 and 2 of each 28-day cycle for a median of three cycles. The overall response rate (ORR) for the 67 patients was 57%. After a median follow-up of 13 months, PFS was 49% and OS was 70% at 1 year; 49 (73%) patients survived and 18 (27%) patients died. Bendamustine has also been combined with DLI in a small group of patients.

Patients relapsing after an allo-SCT represent a clear unmet need. Patient performance status and comorbidities as well as patient preference should also be considered important factors in clinical decision-making.

Novel therapies and their integration in transplantation for Hodgkin lymphoma

CD30 is a member of the tumor necrosis factor cell receptor superfamily that is highly expressed in Reed–Sternberg cells, but with highly restricted expression in normal cells. After several failed attempts to develop naked anti-CD30 antibody therapy, remarkable progress was achieved by conjugating the naked antibody SGN30 to antitubulin monomethyl auristatin E to generate the antibody–drug conjugate brentuximab vedotin (BV). BV represents the only so-called "new" drug that has entered the market in the HL arena. It has been granted approval by both the Food and Drug Administration (FDA) and the European Medicines Agency (EMA) for those patients with HL who relapse after an ASCT and for those patients failing at least two lines of chemotherapy and who are not being considered candidates for an intensive procedure. The interesting results seen in the Phase I trial with BV as a single drug in CD30-positive hematologic malignancies led to a Phase II trial that evaluated the efficacy and safety of BV (1.8 mg/kg by intravenous infusion every 3 weeks up to a maximum of 16 cycles) in 102 patients with relapsed or refractory

HL after ASCT [60]. ORR was 75%, with a 34% CR. The median PFS for all patients was 5.6 months, and the median duration of response for those in CR was 20.5 months. After a median observation time of more than 1.5 years, 31 patients were alive and free of documented progressive disease. The drug was quite well tolerated, the most common treatment-related adverse events being peripheral sensory neuropathy, nausea, fatigue, neutropenia, and diarrhea. Similarly, BV resulted in an ORR of 71% and a CR of 34% in 14 transplantation-naive patients, resulting in a 56% conversion rate to transplantation eligibility after therapy.

BV is being used in the pre-allo-SCT setting, as a "bridge to allo," and in the post-allogeneic setting to treat patients with relapsed/progressive disease after the allogeneic procedure. Chen *et al.* [61] have recently published their experience with 18 patients with multiply relapsed HL undergoing RIC/allo-SCT after being treated with BV as salvage therapy. NRM and acute and chronic GVHD incidence after the allogeneic procedure were not significantly different from that previously described. Although median follow-up was only 12 months, PFS was 100%. A retrospective analysis comparing outcomes after allo-SCT in relapsed/refractory HL patients who received BV and underwent RIC allo-SCT versus those who did not receive BV and still underwent RIC allo-SCT also found that the administration of BV as a bridge to transplant significantly increased the percentage of patients achieving a CR before the procedure, thus improving the comorbidity index of the patients before the procedure, decreasing NRM, RR after the procedure, and improving the overall outcome of the patients. The widespread use of BV in patients with HL relapsing after an ASCT will most certainly change the treatment paradigm of this subgroup of patients, either by allowing some patients to avoid the allogeneic procedure or by increasing the pool of potential candidates for allogeneic transplant and thus acting as a "bridge to allo." Additional information on long-term outcome of patients being treated with this drug or the development of prospective clinical trials in this setting will most probably shed some light on this question.

HL relapsing after an allo-SCT represents a major clinical challenge. Gopal *et al.* [57] have used BV in 25 HL patients with recurrent disease after allo-SCT. Patients were over 100 days after allo-SCT, had no active GVHD, and received a median of nine prior regimens. Patients received BV 1.2 or 1.8 mg/kg i.v. every 3 weeks (median, eight cycles; range, 1–16). Overall and complete response rates were 50% and 38%, respectively, among 24 evaluable patients. Median time to response was 8.1 weeks, median PFS was 7.8 months, and median OS was not reached.

Finally, BV is also being integrated in the ASCT setting with the objective to improve PET-negative CR rates before the procedure or to decrease the relapse rate after ASCT. Patients with relapsed/refractory HL who had failed one prior regimen were enrolled in a Phase II clinical trial, receiving weekly BV followed by PET. Patients who achieved normalization of PET proceeded to ASCT while patients with PET scores of Deauville 3 or higher received two cycles of augmented ICE prior to consideration for ASCT. In a preliminary analysis recently presented that included 28 evaluable patients, this therapeutic approach was able to produce high CR rates, adequate stem cell collection, and facilitated referral to ASCT for virtually all patients. The AETHERA Trial (NCT01100502) is a randomized, double-blind, placebo-controlled Phase III study of SGN-35 and best supportive care versus placebo and best supportive care in the treatment of patients at high risk of residual HL following ASCT. This trial is closed for recruitment. Positive results for the experimental arm will indicate the potential for using maintenance therapy in this subset of high-risk HL patients.

References

1 Hjalgrim H, Engels EA. Infectious aetiology of Hodgkin and non-Hodgkin lymphomas: a review of the epidemiological evidence. *J Intern Med* 2008;**264**:537–48.

2 Armitage JO. Early stage Hodgkin's lymphoma. *N Engl J Med* 2010;**363**:653–62.

3 Canellos GP, Anderson JR, Propert KJ. Chemotherapy of advanced Hodgkin's disease with MOPP, ABVD, or MOPP alternating with ABVD. *N Engl J Med* 1992;**327**:1478–84.

4 Ljungman P, Bregni M, Brune M *et al.* Allogeneic and autologous transplantation for haematological diseases, solid tumours and immune disorders: current practice in Europe 2009. *Bone Marrow Transplant* 2010;**45**:219–34.

5 Linch DC, Winfield D, Goldstone AH *et al.* Dose intensification with autologous bone-marrow transplantation in relapsed and resistant Hodgkin's disease: results of a BNLI randomised trial. *Lancet* 1993;**341**:1051–4.

6 Schmitz N, Pfistner B, Sextro M *et al.* Aggressive conventional chemotherapy compared with high-dose chemotherapy with autologous haemopoietic stem-cell transplantation for relapsed chemosensitive Hodgkin's disease: a randomised trial. *Lancet* 2002;**359**:2065–71.

7 Martínez C, Canals C, Sarina B *et al.* Identification of prognostic factors predicting outcome in Hodgkin's lymphoma patients relapsing after autologous stem cell transplantation. *Ann Oncol* 2013;**24**:2430–4.

8 Peggs KS, Hunter A, Chopra R. Clinical evidence of a graft-versus-Hodgkin's-lymphoma effect after reduced-intensity allogeneic transplantation. *Lancet* 2005;**365**:1934–41.

9 Brice P, Bouabdallah R, Moreau P *et al.* Prognostic factors for survival after high-dose therapy and autologous stem cell transplantation for patients with relapsing Hodgkin's disease: analysis of 280 patients from the French registry. *Bone Marrow Transplant* 1997;**20**:21–6.

10 Josting A, Engert A, Diehl V, Canellos GP. Prognostic factors and treatment outcome in patients with primary progressive and relapsed Hodgkin's disease. *Ann Oncol* 2002;**13**(Suppl 1):112–16.

11 Moskowitz CH, Nimer SD, Zelenetz AD *et al.* A 2-step comprehensive high-dose chemoradiotherapy second-line program for relapsed and refractory Hodgkin disease: analysis by intent to treat and development of a prognostic model. *Blood* 2001;**97**:616–23.

12 Tarella C, Cuttica A, Vitolo U *et al.* High-dose sequential chemotherapy and peripheral blood progenitor cell autografting in patients with refractory and/or recurrent Hodgkin lymphoma: a multicenter study of the Intergruppo Italiano Linfomi showing prolonged disease free survival in patients treated at first recurrence. *Cancer* 2003;**97**:2748–59.

13 Josting A, Mueller H, Borchmann P *et al.* Dose intensity of chemotherapy in patients with relapsed Hodgkin's lymphoma. *J Clin Oncol* 2010;**28**:5074–80.

14 Schot BW, Zijlstra JM, Sluiter WJ *et al.* Early FDG-PET assessment in combination with clinical risk scores determines prognosis in recurrent lymphoma. *Blood* 2007;**109**:486–91.

15 Jabbour E, Hosing C, Ayers G *et al.* Pretransplant positive positron emission tomography/gallium scans predict poor outcome in patients with recurrent/refractory Hodgkin lymphoma. *Cancer* 2007;**109**:2481–9.

16 Moskowitz AJ, Yahalom J, Kewalramani T *et al.* Pretransplantation functional imaging predicts outcome following autologous stem cell transplantation for relapsed and refractory Hodgkin lymphoma. *Blood* 2010;**116**:4934–7.

17 Josting A, Rudolph C, Reiser M. Time-intensified dexamethasone/cisplatin/cytarabine: an effective salvage therapy with low toxicity in patients with relapsed and refractory Hodgkin's disease. *Ann Oncol* 2002;**13**:1628–35.

18 Moskowitz CH, Nimer SD, Zelenetz AD. A 2-step comprehensive high-dose chemoradiotherapy second-line program for relapsed and refractory Hodgkin disease: analysis by intent to treat and development of a prognostic model. *Blood* 2001;**97**:616–23.

19 Aparicio J, Segura A, Garcerá S. ESHAP is an active regimen for relapsing Hodgkin's disease. *Ann Oncol* 1999;**10**:593–5.

20 Santoro A, Magagnoli M, Spina M. Ifosfamide, gemcitabine, and vinorelbine: a new induction regimen for refractory and relapsed Hodgkin's lymphoma. *Haematologica* 2007;**92**:35–41.

21 Sureda A, Arranz R, Iriondo A *et al.* Autologous stem-cell transplantation for Hodgkin's disease: results and prognostic factors in 494 patients from the Grupo Español de Linfomas/Transplante Autólogo de Médula Osea Spanish Cooperative Group. *J Clin Oncol* 2001;**19**:1395–404.

22 Brice P, Bouabdallah R, Moreau P *et al.* Prognostic factors for survival after high-dose therapy and autologous stem cell transplantation for patients with relapsing Hodgkin's disease: analysis of 280 patients from the French Registry. *Bone Marrow Transplant* 1997;**20**:21–6.

23 Czyz J, Dziadziusko R, Knopiska-Postuszuy W *et al.* Outcome and prognostic factors in advanced Hodgkin's disease treated with high-dose chemotherapy and autologous stem cell transplantation: a study of 341 patients. *Ann Oncol* 2004;**15**:1222–30.

24 Josting A, Rudolph C, Mapara M *et al.* Cologne high-dose sequential chemotherapy in relapsed and refractory Hodgkin lymphoma: results of a large multicenter study of the German Hodgkin Lymphoma Study Group (GHSG). *Ann Oncol* 2005;**16**:116–23.

25 Morschhauser F, Brice P, Fermé C *et al.* Risk-adapted salvage treatment with single or tandem autologous stem-cell transplantation for first relapse/refractory Hodgkin's lymphoma: results of the prospective multicenter H96 trial by the GELA/SFGM study group. *J Clin Oncol* 2008;**26**:5980–7.

26 Gajewski JL, Phillips GL, Sobocinski KA *et al.* Bone marrow transplants from HLA-identical siblings in advanced Hodgkin's disease. *J Clin Oncol* 1996;**14**:572–8.

27 Milpied N, Fielding AK, Pearce RM *et al.* Allogeneic bone marrow transplant is not better than autologous transplant for patients with relapsed Hodgkin's disease. European Group for Blood and Bone Marrow Transplantation. *J Clin Oncol* 1996;**14**:1291–6.

28 Sureda A, Robinson S, Canals C *et al.* Reduced-intensity conditioning compared with conventional allogeneic stem-cell transplantation in relapsed or refractory Hodgkin's lymphoma: an analysis from the Lymphoma Working Party of the European Group for Blood and Marrow Transplantation. *J Clin Oncol* 2008;**26**:455–62.

29 Robinson SP, Sureda A, Canals C *et al.* Reduced intensity conditioning allogeneic stem cell transplantation for Hodgkin's lymphoma: identification of prognostic factors predicting outcome. *Haematologica* 2009;**94**:230–8.

30 Anderlini P, Saliba R, Acholonu S *et al* Reduced-intensity allogeneic stem cell transplantation in relapsed and refractory Hodgkin's disease: low transplant-related mortality and impact of intensity of conditioning regimen. *Bone Marrow Transplant* 2005;**35**:943–51.

31 Alvarez I, Sureda A, Caballero MD *et al.* Nonmyeloablative stem cell transplantation is an effective therapy for refractory or relapsed Hodgkin lymphoma: results of a Spanish prospective cooperative protocol. *Biol Blood Marrow Transplant* 2006;**12**:172–83.

32 Sureda A, Canals C, Arranz R *et al.* Allogeneic stem cell transplantation after reduced intensity conditioning in patients with relapsed or refractory Hodgkin's lymphoma. Results of the HDR-ALLO study: a prospective clinical trial by the Grupo Español de Linfomas/Trasplante de Médula Osea (GEL/TAMO) and the Lymphoma Working Party of the European Group for Blood and Marrow Transplantation. *Haematologica* 2012;**97**:310–17.

33 Thomson KJ, Peggs KS, Smith P *et al.* Superiority of reduced-intensity allogeneic transplantation over conventional treatment for relapse of Hodgkin's lymphoma following autologous stem cell transplantation. *Bone Marrow Transplant* 2008;**41**:765–70.

34 Sarina B, Castagna L, Farina L *et al.* Allogeneic transplantation improves the overall and progression-free survival of Hodgkin lymphoma patients relapsing after autologous transplantation: a retrospective study based on the time of HLA typing and donor availability. *Blood* 2010;**115**:3671–7.

35 Corradini P, Zallio F, Mariotti J *et al.* Effect of age and previous autologous transplantation on nonrelapse mortality and survival in patients treated with reduced-intensity conditioning and allografting for advanced hematologic malignancies. *J Clin Oncol* 2005;**23**:6690–8.

36 Burroughs LM, O'Donnell PV, Sandmaier BM *et al.* Comparison of outcomes of HLA-matched related, unrelated, or HLA-haploidentical related hematopoietic cell transplantation following nonmyeloablative conditioning for relapsed or refractory Hodgkin lymphoma. *Biol Blood Marrow Transplant* 2008;**14**:1279–87.

37 Faulkner RD, Craddock C, Byrne JL *et al.* BEAM–alemtuzumab reduced-intensity allogeneic stem cell transplantation for lymphoproliferative diseases: GVHD, toxicity, and survival in 65 patients. *Blood* 2004;**103**:428–34.

38 Claviez A, Canals C, Dierickx D *et al.* Allogeneic hematopoietic stem cell transplantation in children and adolescents with recurrent and refractory Hodgkin lymphoma: an analysis of the European Group for Blood and Marrow Transplantation. *Blood* 2009;**114**:2060–7.

39 Thomson KJ, Kayani I, Ardeshna K *et al.* A response-adjusted PET-based transplantation strategy in primary resistant and relapsed Hodgkin lymphoma. *Leukemia* 2013;**27**:1419–22.

40 Peggs KS, Kayani I, Edwards N *et al.* Donor lymphocyte infusions modulate relapse risk in mixed chimeras and induce durable salvage in relapsed patients after T-cell-depleted allogeneic transplantation for Hodgkin's lymphoma. *J Clin Oncol* 2011;**29**:971–8.

41 Anderlini P, Saliba R, Acholonu S *et al.* Fludarabine–melphalan as a preparative regimen for reduced-intensity conditioning allogeneic stem cell transplantation in relapsed and refractory Hodgkin's lymphoma: the updated M.D. Anderson Cancer Center experience. *Haematologica* 2008;**93**:257–64.

42 Devetten MP, Hari PN, Carreras J *et al.* Unrelated donor reduced-intensity allogeneic hematopoietic stem cell transplantation for relapsed and refractory Hodgkin lymphoma. *Biol Blood Marrow Transplant* 2009;**15**:109–17.

43 Majhail NS, Weisdorf DJ, Wagner JE *et al.* Comparable results of umbilical cord blood and HLA-matched sibling donor hematopoietic stem cell transplantation after reduced-intensity preparative regimen for advanced Hodgkin lymphoma. *Blood* 2006;**107**:3804–7.

44 Rodrigues CA, Sanz G, Brunstein CG *et al.* Analysis of risk factors for outcomes after unrelated cord blood transplantation in adults with lymphoid malignancies: a study by the Eurocord–Netcord and Lymphoma Working Party of the European Group for Blood and Marrow Transplantation. *J Clin Oncol* 2009;**27**:256–63.

45 Rodrigues CA, Rocha V, Dreger P *et al.* Alternative donor hematopoietic stem cell transplantation for mature lymphoid malignancies after reduced-intensity conditioning regimen: similar outcomes with umbilical cord blood and unrelated donor peripheral blood. *Haematologica* 2014;**99**:370–7.

46 Marcais A, Porcher R, Robin M *et al.* Impact of disease status and stem cell source on the results of reduced intensity conditioning transplant for Hodgkin's lymphoma: a retrospective study from the French Society of Bone Marrow Transplantation and Cellular Therapy (SFGM-TC). *Haematologica* 2013;**98**:1467–75.

47 Raiola A, Dominietto A, Varaldo R *et al.* Unmanipulated haploidentical BMT following non-myeloablative conditioning and post-transplantation CY for advanced Hodgkin's lymphoma. *Bone Marrow Transplant* 2014;**49**:190–4.

48 Lambert JR, Bomanji JB, Peggs KS *et al.* Prognostic role of PET scanning before and after reduced-intensity allogeneic stem cell transplantation for lymphoma. *Blood* 2010;**115**:2763–8.

49 Thomson KJ, Peggs KS, Blundell E, Goldstone AH, Linch DC. A second autologous transplant may be efficacious in selected patients with Hodgkin's lymphoma relapsing after a previous autograft. *Leukemia Lymphoma* 2007;**48**:881–4.

50 Little R, Wittes RE, Longo DL, Wilson WH Vinblastine for recurrent Hodgkin's disease following autologous bone marrow transplant. *J Clin Oncol* 1998;**16**:584–8.

51 Zinzani PL, Bendandi M, Stefoni V *et al.* Value of gemcitabine treatment in heavily pretreated Hodgkin's disease patients. *Haematologica* 2000;**85**:926–9.

52 Younes A. Novel treatment strategies for patients with relapsed classical Hodgkin lymphoma. *Hematology Am Soc Hematol Educ Program* 2009;**507–19**.

53 Younes A, Romaguera J, Hagemeister F *et al.* A pilot study of rituximab in patients with recurrent, classic Hodgkin disease. *Cancer* 2003;**98**:310–14.

54 Johnston PB, Inwards DJ, Colgan JP *et al* A Phase II trial of the oral mTOR inhibitor everolimus in relapsed Hodgkin lymphoma. *Am J Hematol* 2010;**85**:320–4.

55 Younes A, Sureda A, Ben-Yehuda D *et al.* Panobinostat in patients with relapsed/refractory Hodgkin's lymphoma after autologous stem-cell transplantation: results of a phase II study. *J Clin Oncol* 2012;**30**:2197–203.

56 Fehniger TA, Larson S, Trinkaus K *et al.* A phase II multi-center study of lenalidomide in relapsed or refractory classical Hodgkin lymphoma. *Blood (ASH Annual Meeting Abstracts)* 2009;**114**:Abstract 3693.

57 Gopal AK, Ramchandren R, O'Connor OA *et al.* Safety and efficacy of brentuximab vedotin for Hodgkin lymphoma recurring after allogeneic stem cell transplantation. *Blood* 2012;**120**:560–8.

58 Theurich S, Malcher J, Wennhold K *et al.* Brentuximab vedotin combined with donor lymphocyte infusions for early relapse of Hodgkin lymphoma after allogeneic stem-cell transplantation induces tumor-specific immunity and sustained clinical remission. *J Clin Oncol* 2013;**31**:e59–63.

59 Anastasia A, Carlo-Stella C, Corradini P *et al.* Bendamustine for Hodgkin lymphoma patients failing autologous or autologous and allogeneic stem cell transplantation: a retrospective study of the Fondazione Italiana Linfomi. *Br J Haematol* 2014;**166**:140–2.

60 Younes A, Gopal AK, Smith SE *et al.* Results of a pivotal phase II study of brentuximab vedotin for patients with relapsed or refractory Hodgkin's lymphoma. *J Clin Oncol* 2012;**30**:2183–9.

61 Chen R, Palmer JM, Thomas SH *et al.* Brentuximab vedotin enables successful reduced-intensity allogeneic hematopoietic cell transplantation in patients with relapsed or refractory Hodgkin lymphoma. *Blood* 2012;**119**:6379–81.

62 Robinson SP, Goldstone AH, Mackinnon S *et al.* Chemoresistant or aggressive lymphoma predicts for a poor outcome following reduced-intensity allogeneic progenitor cell transplantation: an analysis from the Lymphoma Working Party of the European Group for Blood and Bone Marrow Transplantation. *Blood* 2002;**100**:4310–16.

63 Todisco E, Castagna L, Sarina B *et al.* Reduced-intensity allogeneic transplantation in patients with refractory or progressive Hodgkin's disease after high-dose chemotherapy and autologous stem cell infusion. *Eur J Haematol* 2007;**78**:322–9.

64 Corradini P, Dodero A, Farina L *et al.* Allogeneic stem cell transplantation following reduced-intensity conditioning can induce durable clinical and molecular remissions in relapsed lymphomas: pre-transplant disease status and histotype heavily influence outcome. *Leukemia* 2007;**21**:2316–23.

CHAPTER 19

Peripheral T-cell lymphomas

Giulia Perrone, Chiara De Philippis, Lucia Farina and Paolo Corradini

Indication for transplantation in T-cell lymphoma

Peripheral T-cell lymphomas (PTCLs) represent a rare subtype of non-Hodgkin lymphoma (NHL) that includes several diseases derived from mature T lymphocytes and natural killer (NK) cells. Consequently, patients affected by PTCL have been historically treated as those affected by B-cell NHL [1]. Unfortunately, with the exception of anaplastic lymphoma kinase (ALK)-positive large cell lymphoma (ALCL), PTCL response to CHOP (cyclophosphamide, doxorubicin, vincristine, prednisone) is much less satisfactory than that of B-cell NHL, with high relapse rate and a 5-year overall survival (OS) of about 30% [2]. To improve the outcomes, hematopoietic stem cell transplantation (SCT) has been included in the therapeutic strategy of PTCL.

Prospective Phase II studies and retrospective analyses have investigated the role of SCT in PTCL, but randomized trials are lacking. The interpretation of the results of these studies is challenging for the following reasons:

1 Multiple histologies were often analyzed together due to the rarity of this lymphoma subtype; in particular, most of the studies that we discuss enrolled nodal and extranodal PTCLs, but in some cases also adult T-cell leukemia/lymphoma (ATLL) and cutaneous T-cell lymphoma (CTCL) were included.

2 Some analyses included both patients receiving transplant in first or subsequent remission.

3 Different pretransplant treatments and conditioning regimens were applied.

Taking into account these limitations, some indications can be driven by the available data.

Autologous stem cell transplantation (ASCT) has been studied at relapse or as consolidation of the first remission. Although consolidation in first remission remains an area of controversy, several institutional and national guidelines (European Society for Medical Oncology [3], British Committee for Standards in Haematology [4], SIE-SIES-GITMO [5]) recommend ASCT after induction chemotherapy in PTCL patients, excluding ALK-positive ALCL and low-risk disease (Table 19.1). In fact, ALK-positive ALCL is a unique subtype of PTCL that carries a more favorable prognosis and response rates similar to those of diffuse large B-cell lymphoma (DLBCL) after conventional chemotherapy. Patients with ALK-positive status have already shown a significant superior outcome with ASCT, either as frontline or salvage therapy, compared to other PTCL subtypes [6–8]. It is questionable, particularly in low-risk ALK-positive ALCL, whether ASCT upfront can further improve the outcome compared to standard chemotherapy alone, but prospective studies addressing this point are lacking. With regard to patients with ALK-negative ALCL treated with ASCT, as consolidation, they seem to have a better outcome compared to other histologic subtypes [9–12].

In order to identify high-risk patients the International Prognostic Index (IPI) was applied and shown to be predictive also for patients affected by T-cell NHL [13]. Other prognostic score systems were designed and validated in retrospective studies such as the Prognostic Index for PTCL (PIT score) and, more recently, a

Clinical Guide to Transplantation in Lymphoma, First Edition. Edited by Bipin N. Savani and Mohamad Mohty.
© 2015 John Wiley & Sons, Ltd. Published 2015 by John Wiley & Sons, Ltd.

Table 19.1 Guideline recommendations.

British Committee for Standards in Haematology [4]	European Society for Medical Oncology [3]	SIE-SIES-GITMO [5]
First-line therapy *PTCL-NOS* CHOP remains the standard therapy. Consolidation with ASCT should be considered *AITL* Outside a clinical trial, CHOP or FC would be considered standard therapy. Consolidation with ASCT should be considered *ALCL* Patients with limited stage ALCL and no adverse prognostic features by IPI should be treated with three to four cycles of CHOP chemotherapy and involved-field radiotherapy. All other patients should receive six to eight cycles of CHOP chemotherapy. ALK-negative patients should be treated as for PTCL-NOS *EATL* CHOP-like therapy, with or without upfront autograft is the standard approach outside trial, but evidence of efficacy is lacking and adoption of a more intensive approach, such as NCRI/SNLG protocol, is a reasonable option in fitter patients	First-line treatment of all T-cell NHL subtypes should be based on anthracycline-containing regimens such as CHOP/CHOEP and CHOP-like regimens. An exception to this assumption could probably be made for EATL that has been treated with a specific regimen according to the Scottish Lymphoma Group. For patients with poor-risk T-cell NHL (IPI or PIT ≥2) with chemosensitive disease (in CR or PR), after induction chemotherapy ASCT should be delivered	In patients aged 65 years or younger, with nodal, intestinal, or hepatosplenic T-cell lymphomas, except for ALK-positive ALCL, six courses of CHOP or CHOEP (induction phase) followed by ASCT (consolidation phase) is the recommended therapy. For ALK-positive ALCL patients with an IPI score <3, the induction phase with CHOP or CHOEP for six courses without the consolidation phase is recommended. For patients older than 65 years, CHOP or CHOP-like regimens are the first therapeutic options. In patients fit for intensive chemotherapy, the approach used in the younger patient can be considered
Relapsed or refractory disease *PTCL* Relapsed or refractory disease should be treated with relapse-schedule chemotherapy and considered for allo-SCT *AITL* Consolidation with ASCT should be considered for chemosensitive diseases after relapse if not already used in first remission	Second-line treatment of refractory/relapsed T-cell NHL should contain one or more among the following drugs: platinum, gemcitabine. ASCT should be considered for relapsed/refractory PTCL-NOS, ALK-negative ALCL and AITL. Allo-SCT in relapsed/refractory T-cell NHL (PTCL-NOS, ALK-negative ALCL, and AITL) proved to be the only curative treatment of this patient subset (by retrospective studies). Refractory or relapsed T-cell NHL should be enrolled, whenever possible, in Phase I or II prospective clinical trials aimed at exploring the efficacy of new drugs that have shown activity in preclinical studies	In patients with refractory or relapsed PTCL (excluding ALCL), platinum-based, ifosfamide-based, gemcitabine-containing chemotherapy, pralatrexate, romidepsin, or bendamustine are the recommended therapies. The current evidence does not allow a choice among these agents. In refractory or relapsed ALCL, brentuximab should be preferred. Patients with chemosensitive disease should receive consolidation with allo-SCT. In the absence of a donor, ASCT can be used. In nontransplant eligible patients, novel agents should be recommended, but these therapies should be considered as experimental and should be done within clinical trials

prognostic index that takes into account the expression of Ki-67 protein [14,15]. In general, a high-risk score (PIT score or IPI ≥2) can identify those patients who may benefit from a consolidation strategy with ASCT.

There are limited data on the use of allogeneic (allo)-SCT in patients with PTCL, as upfront therapy. Because of the poor prognosis of the disease, it might have a role in particular settings, but allo-SCT upfront has to be evaluated only in the context of clinical trials.

Regarding treatment of relapsed or refractory disease, patients responding to further therapy are usually considered for SCT. Whether ASCT or allo-SCT should be preferred remains a critical issue, at least in those patients who have received only conventional chemotherapy during the first line. Comparative studies of ASCT versus myeloablative allo-SCT failed to demonstrate a survival benefit of allo-SCT due to the higher nonrelapse mortality (NRM), but they showed a lower relapse rate suggesting the existence of the so-called graft-versus-lymphoma (GVL) effect in PTCL [6,16]. Reduced-intensity conditioning (RIC) regimens could be offered as an alternative to conventional high-dose chemoradiotherapy in order to reduce organ toxicity and NRM [17,18]. The benefit of allo-SCT has been demonstrated by the survival curves, which usually reach a plateau after 24–36 months, suggesting the potential curability of about 40–50% of relapsed and refractory T-cell NHL patients [6,19–22]. Therefore, RIC allo-SCT can be considered a therapeutic option in the setting of relapsed PTCL.

Timing and preparation of patients for transplantation in T-cell lymphoma

ASCT should be offered to eligible patients achieving at least a partial response (PR) after induction treatment and it could be considered in those patients with a chemosensitive relapse who did not receive ASCT upfront. In the majority of prospective and retrospective studies, after four to six cycles of chemotherapy, responding patients received a mobilizing treatment in preparation for the subsequent ASCT. Interestingly, while bone marrow involvement at diagnosis recurs as an independent predictor of negative outcome in at least two prospective studies, no study has confirmed its negative impact on outcome at the time of ASCT harvest [7,23]. We currently do not know if achieving complete remission (CR) versus PR, or normalized functional imaging (^{18}F-fluorodeoxyglucose positron emission tomography, FDG-PET), before ASCT significantly improves long-term outcome. Nevertheless, several studies have already shown that patients in CR at transplantation have a better long-term outcome

compared to patients achieving less than CR or less than PR [10,24–28].

In relapsed patients, an allo-SCT should be considered as consolidation after salvage therapy, so the donor search should be started as soon as the relapse has been demonstrated in patients aged 65 years or younger. In the practical clinical setting, there are two main points to consider:

1 The interval from diagnosis to the allogeneic procedure may significantly impair the results, suggesting that allo-SCT should be planned during the chemosensitive phase, as soon as the patient achieves CR or at least PR status.

2 Since most of the patients eligible for an allo-SCT have already failed ASCT, RIC regimens should be preferred; myeloablative regimens could probably be chosen in selected cases, such as in young fit patients with a low comorbidity score (HCT-CI) not in CR at transplant or who do not receive high-dose chemotherapy. In addition, the absence of effective alternative treatment suggests initiation of donor search for all young and fit patients achieving less than PR during first-line treatment.

Autologous hematopoietic stem cell transplantation for T-cell lymphoma

Front-line autologous stem cell transplantation

Several Phase II prospective trials have suggested the benefit of upfront ASCT (Table 19.2). The Spanish Lymphoma/Autologous Bone Marrow Transplant Study Group (GELTAMO) initially published a retrospective analysis of 74 patients undergoing ASCT after achievement of CR with first-line anthracycline-based induction chemotherapy [11]. After a median follow-up of 67 months, 5-year OS and progression-free survival (PFS) were 68% and 63%, respectively, and the main cause of death was disease progression. In multivariate analysis only the PIT score was significantly associated with OS and PFS. Although data about ALK expression were lacking, patients affected by ALCL had a significantly better outcome than the others. The same authors published the results of a prospective study in 26 high-risk nodal PTCL patients excluding those with ALK-positive ALCL [29]. The treatment plan included ASCT after four cycles of Mega-CHOP in patients who were

Table 19.2 Prospective studies of front-line autologous stem cell transplant in PTCL patients.

Study	PTCL	ALK positive	Induction therapy	Status at transplant	Transplant rate	Conditioning regimens	TRM	Response rate	PFS	OS
Corradini et al. (2006) [10]	62	19 (31%)	HDS	CR1 56% PR1 16% PD 24%	74%	Mitox/mel or BEAM	5%	CR 89% PR 11%	30% (12 years) 60% if in CR before ASCT	34% (12 years)
Rodriguez et al. (2007) [29]	26	No	Mega-CHOP	CR 46% PR 27%	73%	BEAM	0%	CR 89% PR 5%	53% (3 years)	73% (3 years)
Mercadal et al. (2008) [24]	41	No	HD-CHOP/ESHAP	CR1 49% PR1 10%	41%	BEAM/BEAC	ND	CR 51% PR 7%	30% (4 years)	39% (4 years) 58% for ASCT (5 years)
Reimer et al. (2009) [30]	83	No	CHOP	CR1 39% PR1 40%	66%	TBI/CY	4%	CR 58% PR 8%	36% (3 years)	48% (3 years) 71% for ASCT 11% not ASCT
D'Amore et al. (2012) [12]	166	No	CHOEP-14 CHOP-14 (>60 years)	ORR 82% PD 16%	72%	BEAM/BEAC	4%	At 3 months CR/uCR 54% PR 8%	44% (5 years)	51% (5 years) 61% for ASCT 28% not ASCT

BEAC, carmustine, etoposide, cytarabine, cyclophosphamide; BEAM, carmustine, etoposide, cytarabine, melphalan; CHOEP, cyclophosphamide, doxorubicin, vincristine, etoposide, and prednisone; CHOP, cyclophosphamide, doxorubicin, vincristine, prednisone; CR1, first complete remission; ESHAP, etoposide, cytarabine, cisplatin, methylprednisolone; HDS, high-dose sequential chemotherapy; Mitox/mel, mitoxantrone, melphalan; ORR, overall response rate; OS, overall survival; PD, progressive disease; PFS, progression-free survival; PR1, first partial remission; PTCL, peripheral T-cell lymphoma; TBI/CY, total body irradiation, cyclophosphamide; TRM, transplant-related mortality.

gallium-scan negative after three courses and in those who were gallium-scan positive but achieved a response after salvage therapy. After a median follow-up of 3 years, OS and PFS of the entire cohort were 73% and 53%, respectively; 73% of the patients were autografted and they achieved 2-year OS and PFS of 84% and 56%, respectively. The authors suggested that salvage treatment before ASCT could rescue part of the primary resistant or early progressive patients.

An Italian multicenter Phase II prospective study employed high-dose sequential chemotherapy followed by ASCT as first-line treatment in 62 patients affected by high-risk PTCL (stage III–IV and/or age-adjusted IPI >1), including 19 ALK-positive ALCL [10]. Similar to the GELTAMO results, on an-intent-to-treat analysis only 46 of 62 patients (74%) completed the whole program. Progressive disease during the induction phase was the main obstacle for proceeding to the autografting phase and the main reason for treatment failure. The high progression rate led to disappointing 12-year OS and event-free survival (EFS) curves (34% and 30%, respectively). However, in the cohort of patients who underwent ASCT, the response rate was high; 89% of them reached CR, with a 12-year disease-free survival (DFS) curve projected at 55%. When patients with PTCL-NOS (not otherwise specified) were in CR at transplant, EFS achieved 62% compared with 10% of those not in CR. In fact, the CR status remained a significant predictor of long-term outcome in multivariate analysis, suggesting that consolidation of CR with ASCT offers a greater chance of long-term survival. As with the Spanish data, patients with ALCL had the most favorable OS and EFS (62% and 54%, respectively, compared to 21% and 18% in non-ALCL).

More recently, the German group published the results of a prospective multicenter study employing myeloablative cyclophosphamide and total body irradiation as the conditioning regimen for 83 ALK-negative PTCL patients who were at least in PR after six CHOP cycles [30]. Similarly to the Italian and Spanish studies, 34% of the patients did not complete the study protocol due to progressive disease. The estimated 3-year OS was 71% for patients who underwent ASCT compared to 11% for those who did not. The PIT score was the only parameter correlated with survival.

To increase the number of patients undergoing transplant in CR or at least PR, some trials have been designed with an intensive pretransplant phase [12,24]. In 2008,

Mercadal *et al.* [24] reported a Phase II study on 41 ALK-negative PTCL patients who were treated with three CHOP cycles alternating with three ESHAP (etoposide, cytarabine, cisplatin, methylprednisolone) cycles and followed by ASCT. Only 59% of patients had chemosensitive disease and because of the high rate of severe hematologic toxicity and mobilization failure, only 41% eventually received ASCT. After a median follow-up of 3.2 years, 4-year OS and PFS were 39% and 30%, respectively, for the entire cohort. No difference in terms of OS was observed in patients in CR who were candidates for ASCT, whether ASCT was carried out or not, suggesting that achieving CR after induction significantly impacts OS. The Nordic Lymphoma Group designed a dose-dense induction phase for 160 ALK-negative PTCL patients; after 6 courses of 2-weekly CHOEP (cyclophosphamide, doxorubicin, vincristine, etoposide, and prednisone) cycles, 53% of the patients achieved CR and 72% could undergo ASCT at the last follow-up [12]. The 5-year OS and PFS were 51% and 44%, respectively. Anaplastic histology and IPI score had the major impact on outcome.

From the studies reported here several important messages emerge clearly: (i) approximately one-third of patients display primary resistant or early progressive disease, consequently becoming ineligible for transplant; (ii) treatment strategy including ASCT upfront can result in long-term duration of response in chemosensitive patients; (iii) to validate the results in larger cohorts of patients and with longer follow-up, all ALK-negative PTCL patients should be enrolled in prospective trials including ASCT as first-line treatment; and (iv) clinical protocols should be designed with an innovative pretransplant phase in order to achieve the best disease response before transplant and increase the number of patients able to be autografted.

Autologous stem cell transplantation in relapsed/refractory PTCL

A number of retrospective studies have been published on the use of ASCT as salvage treatment. GELTAMO reported the results of 123 patients who received an ASCT in the salvage setting; 5-year OS and PFS were 45% and 34%, respectively. In this analysis, having more than one factor of the adjusted IPI or a high β_2-microglobulin at transplant were identified as adverse prognostic factors [25]. Moreover, PFS and OS of patients in second or subsequent CR at transplant (35% and 57%, respectively) were superior to PFS and OS in those in more than second PR (23% and 33%) or with refractory disease (10% and 9%). In other retrospective studies [26,27], the importance of being in CR at the time of transplant, in order to achieve long-term survival, was emphasized.

Some studies have focused on the different results between PTCL-NOS and ALCL after ASCT for relapsed disease. The Toronto group compared relapsed and refractory PTCL patients with those affected by DLBCL, who were transplanted for the same indications over the same period; 3-year OS and EFS were 48% and 37%, respectively, for PTCL compared to 53% and 42%, respectively, for DLBCL [31]. A significantly different outcome has been demonstrated in patients with PTCL-NOS (3-year EFS 23%) as compared to patients with ALCL who had a similar outcome to DLBCL. These results were in line with the data from a retrospective study from the Memorial Sloan-Kettering Cancer Center of New York that reported a 5-year PFS of 24% for relapsed or refractory ALK-negative PTCL [32], whereas the better prognosis of ALCL after ASCT has been confirmed by studies from northern Europe investigators [7,8].

In recent years, efforts have been made to define the role of ASCT in specific subtypes. Angioimmunoblastic T-cell lymphoma (AITL) patients have a median survival of 18 months after conventional chemotherapy, with less than 50% of patients achieving CR. Federico *et al.* [33] retrospectively analysed 243 patients with AITL on behalf of the International Peripheral T-cell Lymphoma Project. Only 17% of patients were treated with ASCT. The 5-year OS of the whole population was 32%, confirming the poor outcome of AITL. A retrospective analysis by the European Society for Blood and Marrow Transplantation (EBMT) of 146 AITL patients demonstrated an OS and PFS of 59% and 42% at 4 years after ASCT [28]. The PFS was higher in patients who received ASCT in CR, achieving 56% at 4 years, as compared to 23% in cases of chemorefractory disease. Enteropathy-associated T-cell lymphoma (EATL) is another very poor prognosis PTCL subtype, commonly correlated with celiac disease. Because of its rarity, very few data are available, mainly from surgery and anthracycline-based chemotherapy. In a prospective observational study, EATL patients were treated upfront with alternating courses of IVE (ifosfamide, vincristine, etoposide) and

methotrexate followed by ASCT [34]. The survival curves showed a 5-year OS of 60% compared to a historical control of 22% with conventional chemotherapy, supporting the role of intense upfront regimens as a bridge to transplant. The retrospective study from the EBMT on 44 EATL patients treated with ASCT demonstrated 4-year PFS and OS of 54% and 59%, respectively, confirming the possibility of long-term disease control [35].

In conclusion, the prognosis of ALK-negative PTCL seems poor when ASCT is used for relapsed disease and long-term remissions have been observed in less than one-third of patients. Those who benefit the most are the patients with ALK-positive ALCL, in CR at the time of transplant, and/or with a low IPI score.

Allogeneic hematopoietic stem cell transplantation for T-cell lymphoma

Allo-SCT provides several advantages over ASCT, including a lymphoma-free graft and the potentially active GVL effect; yet, few studies have specifically addressed the role of allo-SCT in the setting of PTCL.

Survival after myeloablative allo-SCT has been influenced by the high NRM, mainly related to graft-versus-host disease (GVHD), infections, and organ toxicities. Retrospective comparative analyses of ASCT versus allo-SCT in aggressive lymphomas presented some selection bias because usually patients in the allograft cohort had more advanced disease, more prior therapies, and/or bone marrow involvement [36]. However, these studies demonstrated that allografting induced a lower relapse risk as compared to ASCT, but the high NRM offset any survival benefit. A first small retrospective comparative study by the GELTAMO group evaluated the outcome of patients receiving ASCT ($N = 29$) or allo-SCT ($N = 7$) for PTCL; the 3-year OS was 39% and 29%, respectively. However, the majority of patients in the allograft group died in CR because of transplant-related complications [16]. In 2006, a Japanese group published the first large analysis on the outcome of T-cell NHL after myeloablative allo-SCT from matched related and unrelated donors [37]; 51 patients were retrospectively described and, in univariate analysis, OS was better for PTCL as compared to B-cell NHL or other T-cell NHLs.

During the last 15 years, RIC regimens have been increasingly used in relapsed NHL in order to reduce

NRM, thus making this strategy feasible in elderly or heavily pretreated patients (Table 19.3) [17]. In 2004, one of the first papers on RIC allo-SCT reported six patients affected by PTCL who had a favorable survival after transplant [38]. The first prospective study evaluated the outcome of 17 relapsed PTCL patients after a fludarabine-based RIC regimen; 14 of 17 enrolled patients were alive (12 in CR) after a median follow-up of 28 months with an estimated 3-year NRM, OS, and PFS of 6%, 81%, and 64%, respectively [39]. In this study there were some data suggesting the existence of the GVL effect in PTCL: (i) the achievement of durable responses with allografting in patients who had already failed a previous ASCT; (ii) the demonstration of clinical responses to donor lymphocyte infusion (DLI). These preliminary results were then supported by a larger Italian multicenter retrospective study with a longer follow-up [19]. In this study, the 5-year outcome showed NRM, OS, and PFS of 12%, 50%, and 40%, respectively, and a plateau in the survival curves after 36 months, suggesting that these patients have been cured by allo-SCT. In multivariate analysis, age over 45 years and refractory disease were independent prognostic factors, underlying that the timing of allo-SCT can significantly influence the final results. Similarly, in a French retrospective study of 77 T-cell NHL patients allografted with RIC or myeloblative regimens, those patients with chemorefractory disease or who were heavily pretreated experienced a worse outcome [20]. Registry data from the Center for International Blood and Marrow Transplant Research (CIBMTR) confirmed the importance of having chemosensitive disease and having received less than two lines of chemotherapy in improving survival after allo-SCT [6]. In both the Italian and French studies, the survival was not significantly different among the histologic subtypes of T-cell NHL (note that the majority of ALCL had an unknown ALK mutational status), although AITL did slightly better. In support of this finding, an EBMT retrospective analysis of 45 AITL patients undergoing allo-SCT between 1998 and 2005 showed a relapse risk of 20% at 3 years, with a PFS of 53% and an OS of 64% [40].

In the last few years a growing number of studies have demonstrated the feasibility and efficacy of allo-SCT in relapsed and refractory T-cell NHL, including the extranodal subtypes [41–48]. A retrospective study on 52 patients treated with allo-SCT from 1997 to 2009 at the Dana Farber Cancer Institute showed that nodal PTCL had a better prognosis (OS and PFS) compared to extranodal T-cell NHL in multivariate analysis [42]. In another retrospective analysis on 37 patients, including 13 CTCL, Zain *et al.* [43] did not show a different outcome when comparing CTCL with PTCL treated with either RIC or myeloablative allo-SCT. In fact, in larger studies allo-SCT in CTCL offered an estimated OS of about 50% at 3 years, primarily driven by donor type, disease phase, and type of conditioning [44,45]. The prognosis of 12 patients with advanced and refractory extranodal NK/T-cell lymphoma treated with allo-SCT as salvage treatment was specifically addressed by Ennishi *et al.* [46], with 3-year OS and EFS of 53% and 55%, respectively.

Based on the encouraging results shown by allo-SCT in the salvage setting, a Phase II trial by Corradini *et al.* [49] was designed to evaluate the role of upfront treatment intensification in PTCL, including allo-SCT. Induction chemotherapy employing CHOP–alemtuzumab, high-dose methotrexate, cytarabine, and cyclophosphamide was followed by consolidation with either allo-SCT or ASCT, based on the availability of an HLA-identical sibling or matched unrelated donor. Despite the intensive chemotherapy program, 30% of the patients did not undergo transplantation because of progressive disease. With a median follow-up of 40 months, the estimated 4-year OS and PFS were 49% and 44%, respectively. On multivariate analysis the achievement of CR maintained for at least 6 months had a dominant effect on PFS and OS, regardless of patient age, IPI, or extranodal involvement. Patients who received a transplant had an advantage in OS. The sample size did not allow assessment of the superiority of allo-SCT versus ASCT, but the results showed 4-year OS and PFS to both be 69% in allografted patients.

In conclusion, allo-SCT can be offered in relapsed and refractory T-cell NHL based on the following observations:

1 In all studies the survival curves seem to reach a plateau after 24–36 months, suggesting the potential curability of the disease.

2 Delaying the allogeneic procedure too long from diagnosis may significantly impair the results, and thus allo-SCT should be performed at an early stage and during the chemosensitive disease course.

3 RIC regimens have increased the feasibility of allo-SCT by reducing the NRM, and may be the best choice, at least in old and heavily pretreated patients.

Table 19.3 Retrospective and prospective studies on reduced-intensity conditioning allo-SCT in PTCL.

Study	PTCL	Disease status	Previous ASCT	Chemosensitive at transplant	Conditioning regimen	NRM	Relapse rate	PFS	OS
Corradini et al. (2004) [39] Phase II	17	Relapsed/refractory	47%	82%	RIC Thiotepa-based	6% (2 years)	12%	64% (3 years)	81% (3 years)
Faulkner et al. (2004) [38]	65 NHL patients 6 PTCL	Relapsed/refractory	11%	67%	RIC BEAM–alemtuzumab	13% (2 years)	20% (2 years)	54% (3 years)	63% (3 years)
Wulf et al. (2005) [41]	10	Relapsed/refractory	2/10	6/10	RIC FluBuCy	1/10 at 100 days	2/10	—	—
Shustov et al. (2010) [47]	17 including CTCL,NKL,ATLL	Relapsed/refractory	35%	76%	RIC TBI-based	19% (3 years)	26% (3 years)	53% (3 years)	59% (3 years)
Zain et al. (2011) [43]	37, including 13 CTCL	Relapsed/refractory	1 patient	32%	65% RIC 35% Myeloablative	28% (5 years)	24% (5 years)	46.5 (5 years)	52% (5 years)
Delioukina et al. (2012) [22]	27 including 11 CTCL	Relapsed/refractory	0%	59%	RIC FluMel	22% (2 years)	30% (2 years)	47% (2 years)	55% (2 years)
Dodero et al. (2012) [19]	52	Relapsed/refractory	52%	75%	RIC Thiotepa-based	12% (5 years)	49% (5 years)	40% (5 years)	50% (5 years)
Corradini et al. (2014) [49] Phase II	61	Upfront	0%	65%	RIC	13% (3 years)	42% (3 years)	44% (4 years)	49% (4 years)
Le Gouill et al. (2008) [20]	77	Relapsed/refractory	25%	74%	Myeloablative (57 patients) Nonmyeloablative (20 patients)	33% (5 years)	NA	53% (5 years) (EFS)	57% (5 years)

ATLL, acute T-cell leukemia/lymphoma; BEAM, carmustine, etoposide, cytarabine, melphalan; CTCL, cutaneous T-cell lymphoma; FluBuCy, fludarabine, busulfan, cyclophosphamide; FluMel, fludarabine, melphalan; NHL, non-Hodgkin lymphoma; NKL, NK lymphoma; NRM, nonrelapse mortality; OS, overall survival; PFS, progression-free survival; PTCL, peripheral T-cell lymphoma; RIC, reduced-intensity conditioning; TBI, total body irradiation.

The future will hopefully see the combination of new agents and allo-SCT improve results in the significant proportion of refractory T-cell NHL patients who, at the moment, are not considered eligible for SCT.

Post-transplant disease monitoring in T-cell lymphoma

T-cell NHL patients are at high risk of relapse and development of refractory disease. Relapse risk mainly depends on histologic subtypes, risk scores at diagnosis, and response to first-line chemotherapy. Monitoring disease status after transplantation is critical for prompt discovery of early relapses and for driving post-transplantation therapies. Disease assessment should be done according to the revised response criteria for malignant lymphoma [50] and remembering that the relapse risk is higher during the first 2 years after transplant.

According to clinical practice, post-transplantation computed tomography (CT) of neck, chest, and abdomen, as well as bone marrow evaluation if positive before transplantation, should be performed after transplant. Thereafter, routine follow-up by imaging studies should be done every 3 months for the first 2 years, every 6 months for the following 3 years, and then yearly or whenever clinically appropriate.

FDG-PET is highly sensitive and specific in the imaging of B-cell lymphomas. However, its role in the diagnostic evaluation of PTCL is less defined, but potentially useful due to the high incidence of extranodal disease. In a recent study the impact of PET on response assessment and survival prediction after ASCT was retrospectively evaluated [51]; 41 patients with T-cell NHL underwent both contrast-enhanced CT and PET for response assessment. Of 41 patients, 11 showed a discordant response between the two image modalities and in six of these eleven patients the additional PET study changed the post-ASCT response. Moreover, a positive PET scan after transplant was associated with lower EFS and OS rates.

The identification of a molecular marker based on a lymphoma-specific translocation, for example t(2;5) in ALK-positive ALCL, or gene rearrangement of the tumor T-cell receptor may be useful in monitoring minimal residual disease (MRD) in patients with bone marrow involvement at diagnosis. In the post-allo-SCT setting, MRD techniques would allow early intervention when tumor burden is low and immunotherapy can be potentially more effective. At the moment, no relevant data have been published on this topic except for patients affected by ALK-positive ALCL [52].

Management of relapse after transplantation for T-cell lymphoma

Relapse after autologous transplantation

As already mentioned, patients relapsed after ASCT, who are less than 65–70 years old, should initiate search for a donor. Eligibility for allo-SCT should be based not only on age but also on comorbidities and performance status. Eligible patients should proceed to allo-SCT as soon as CR, or at least PR, is achieved after salvage treatment. The role of a second ASCT is unknown and not recommended outside clinical trials.

Salvage treatment is usually based on a combination of chemotherapy drugs, including platinum, gemcitabine and, more recently, bendamustine [53–57]. In a retrospective study including 40 patients with relapsed/refractory PTCL, those treated with DHAP (cisplatin, cytarabine, desamethasone) or ESHAP displayed an overall response rate (ORR) of 62% [53]. Dexa-BEAM (dexamethasone, carmustine, etoposide, cytarabine, melphalan) was retrospectively compared with ICE (ifosfamide, carboplatin, etoposide) in relapsed/refractory PTCL [54]. The results showed a higher ORR (69% vs. 20%), CR (38% vs. 7%), and PFS (6.4 vs. 2 months) with dexa-BEAM, although treatment toxicities were more frequent with this schedule. Gemcitabine has also been shown to be active in relapsed PTCL [55,56]. In a single institution Phase II study, 39 patients with relapsed/refractory PTCL ($N = 20$) or CTCL ($N = 19$) received gemcitabine 1200 mg/m² on days 1, 8, and 15 every 28 days. ORR in PTCL was 55%, with 30% CR [55]. Gemcitabine was also used in combination with other antineoplastic agents. The combination of gemcitabine (1000 mg/m² on days 1, 8, and 15), cisplatin (100 mg/m² on day 15), and methylprednisolone (1000 mg daily for 5 days) delivered to 16 previously treated patients showed an ORR of 69% and a CR of 19% [56]. Unfortunately, these studies included only patients relapsed before ASCT, and the specific efficacy of these chemotherapy combinations in the setting of post-ASCT relapse remains uncertain. Recently, a Phase II trial, including 60 patients, evaluated the use of bendamustine in relapsed or refractory T-cell NHL. Bendamustine was given at 120 mg/m^2 on days 1 and 2 every 3 weeks for six cycles. The ORR of 50%, with 28% CR, highlighted that this drug can be effective in PTCL [57]. Notably, in this study 12% of the patients were relapsed after an ASCT, but there was no difference in the ORR based on previous treatment. In addition, two of the responding patients were able to proceed to allo-SCT.

The CD30-directed antibody–drug conjugate brentuximab represents a valid treatment option in ALCL patients. In a recent Phase II study, 58 patients with relapsed/refractory ALCL achieved an ORR of 86% (57% CR) after brentuximab [58]. This study included 15 patients who received a prior ASCT (26%), but specific outcomes for this subgroup have not been published. The median duration of response was 13.2 months for the six subjects who received a subsequent allo-SCT. More recently, brentuximab has shown to produce CRs and PRs also in PTCL-NOS and AITL (ORR 33% and 54%, respectively). Interestingly, responses were not correlated with CD30 expression, suggesting potential efficacy of this drug in non-ALCL patients [59]. These data suggest that both bendamustine and brentuximab can be considered as a bridge to allografting.

When patients fail to achieve a response to salvage chemotherapy or are chemorefractory, experimental agents should be used and, whenever possible, patients should be considered for inclusion in clinical trials based on such agents.

Relapse after allogeneic transplantation

About 50–60% of patients usually relapse within 2–3 years after allo-SCT [19–22,41,49]. Therapy in this population of patients is challenging, and patients should be considered for inclusion in clinical trials with new drugs.

Based on the supposed GVL effect, immune manipulation after allo-SCT may be pursued at least in those patients who show limited and/or slowly progressive disease. In the absence of active and severe GVHD, the first step is the reduction or withdrawal of immunosuppressive therapy. In a retrospective study including 14 patients, Hamadani *et al.* [60] showed a prolonged response with tapering of immunosuppressive medications. The second step is the use of escalating DLI in patients who are not on immunosuppressive therapy and in those without GVHD. Dodero *et al.* [19]

administered DLIs to 12 PTCL patients relapsing after allo-SCT; eight patients responded, including five CRs. Median survival of patients achieving CR after DLI was 5 years, and no subsequent relapses were reported. In a retrospective study including 35 patients who experienced progression of ATLL after a first allo-SCT, nine were treated with DLI and four of these achieved CR [61]. DLI-induced remissions were durable, with three cases of remission lasting more than 3 years.

While DLI appears to be a good choice in relapsed T-cell NHL, no data are available to support whether it is best administered alone or following cytoreductive therapies. In general, in patients with widespread, organ-threatening or bulky relapse, DLI should be administered after cytoreductive systemic therapy or involved-field radiation.

Novel therapies and their integration in transplantation for T-cell lymphoma

In the past few years, the identification of cell surface molecular markers and the better understanding of the mechanisms of PTCL pathogenesis have led to the development of novel therapies that may potentially be integrated in transplant programs. We have already mentioned the anti-CD30 monoclonal antibody brentuximab that is commercially available for relapsed ALK-positive ALCL, but it also displayed significant clinical responses in other PTCLs [58,59]. Similarly, the anti-CD52 monoclonal antibody alemtuzumab has been approved for the treatment of relapsed PTCL irrespective of CD52 expression level [62]. Nevertheless, after preliminary encouraging results, this antibody has been progressively less used due to the high incidence of viral and opportunistic infections.

Another drug that is already available is pralatrexate. Pralatrexate is a folate analog metabolic inhibitor, designed to have a higher affinity for reduced folate carrier type 1 (RFC-1), leading to enhanced intracellular uptake compared with methotrexate. The multicenter Phase II PROPEL study evaluated the efficacy of pralatrexate (30 mg/m^2 per week for 6 weeks followed by 1 week of rest) in 115 patients with relapsed or refractory T-cell NHL, including 16% relapsed after ASCT [63]. Treatment was continued until evidence of disease progression, development of unacceptable toxicity, or physician discretion. ORR was 29%, comprising 11% CR. Interestingly, 19% of primary refractory patients had evidence of response. The most common grade 3/4 adverse events were thrombocytopenia (32%), mucositis (22%), neutropenia (22%), and anemia (18%).

Other drugs are under investigation in T-cell NHL and for some of them interesting results are already published and summarized in the following sections.

Histone deacetylase inhibitors

Histone deacetylase (HDAC) inhibitors are epigenetic therapies that induce acetylation of histones and other proteins, resulting in antitumor-suppressor gene transcription, growth inhibition, and apoptosis. Among this new class of agents, romidepsin has been the most studied in T-cell NHL. Two published Phase II trials studied romidepsin in refractory/relapsed CTCL and PTCL, including patients relapsed after ASCT [64,65]. Romidepsin was administered at a dose of 14 mg/m^2 i.v. on days 1, 8 and 15 every 28 days. ORR was 25–38%, with a median duration of response of 9–17 months. The most common nonhematologic adverse events were nausea, infections, and fatigue (most being grade 1–2). The major hematologic adverse event was essentially thrombocytopenia. In addition to their activity in T-cell NHL, HDAC inhibitors have already been shown to prevent acute GVHD and this suggests the feasibility of administering these drugs in the context of relapse after allo-SCT [66].

Lenalidomide

Lenalidomide is an immunomodulatory agent with several potential mechanisms of action (direct cytotoxicity, enhanced NK/T-cell function, alteration of microenvironment). Limited data suggest antitumor activity in T-cell NHL. The ORR was about 30% in two published studies [67,68]. Since lenalidomide seems to increase the risk of GVHD, its use should be carefully evaluated in relapsed T-cell NHL after allo-SCT.

Mogamulizumab

Mogamulizumab is a humanized anti-CCR4 (CC chemokine receptor 4) IgG1 monoclonal antibody with a defucosylated Fc region, thereby enhancing antibody-dependent cellular toxicity. Since CCR4 is expressed in most patients with ATLL and based on encouraging preclinical results, early-phase trials were conducted on patients with this subgroup of T-cell NHL. In a Phase II study, 28 patients were enrolled with relapsed/refractory

CCR4-positive ATLL [69]. Mogamulizumab was administered at a dose of 1.0 mg/kg as weekly infusion. ORR was 50%, including eight CRs.

Crizotinib

Crizotinib is a small molecule competitive inhibitor of ALK and MET kinase activity. Recent data showed that 10 of 11 patients affected by relapsed and refractory ALK-positive NHL showed a response after crizotinib, with four of them achieving a durable CR [70].

References

1 Vose J, Armitage J, Weisenburger D. International peripheral T-cell and natural killer/T-cell lymphoma study: pathology findings and clinical outcomes. *J Clin Oncol* 2008;**26**:4124–30.

2 Coiffier B, Brousse N, Peuchmaur M *et al.* Peripheral T-cell lymphomas have a worse prognosis than B-cell lymphomas: a prospective study of 361 immunophenotyped patients treated with the LNH-84 regimen. *Ann Oncol* 1990;**1**:45–50.

3 Dreyling M, Thieblemont C, Gallamini A *et al.* ESMO Consensus conferences: guidelines on malignant lymphoma. Part 2: marginal zone lymphoma, mantle cell lymphoma, peripheral T-cell lymphoma. *Ann Oncol* 2013;**24**:857–77.

4 Dearden CE, Johnson R, Pettengell R *et al.* Guidelines for the management of mature T-cell and NK-cell neoplasms (excluding cutaneous T-cell lymphoma). *Br J Haematol* 2011;**153**:451–85.

5 Corradini P, Marchetti M, Barosi G *et al.* SIE-SIES-GITMO guidelines for the management of adult peripheral T- and NK-cell lymphomas, excluding mature T-cell leukemias. *Ann Oncol* 2014;**25**:2339–50.

6 Smith SM, Burns LJ, van Besien K *et al.* Hematopoietic cell transplantation for systemic mature T-cell non-Hodgkin lymphoma. *J Clin Oncol* 2013;**31**:3100–9.

7 Blystad AK, Enblad G, Kvaloy S *et al.* High-dose therapy with autologous stem cell transplantation in patients with peripheral T cell lymphomas. *Bone Marrow Transplant* 2001;**27**:711–16.

8 Jantunen E, Wiklund T, Juvonen E *et al.* Autologous stem cell transplantation in adult patients with peripheral T-cell lymphoma: a nation-wide survey. *Bone Marrow Transplant* 2004;**33**:405–10.

9 Savage KJ, Harris NL, Vose JM *et al.* ALK-anaplastic large-cell lymphoma is clinically and immunophenotypically different from both ALK+ ALCL and peripheral T-cell lymphoma, not otherwise specified: report from the International Peripheral T-Cell Lymphoma Project. *Blood* 2008;**111**:5496–504.

10 Corradini P, Tarella C, Zallio F *et al.* Long-term follow-up of patients with peripheral T-cell lymphomas treated up-front with high-dose chemotherapy followed by autologous stem cell transplantation. *Leukemia* 2006;**20**:1533–8.

11 Rodríguez J, Conde E, Gutiérrez A *et al*. The results of consolidation with autologous stem-cell transplantation in patients with peripheral T-cell lymphoma (PTCL) in first complete remission: the Spanish Lymphoma and Autologous Transplantation Group experience. *Ann Oncol* 2007;**18**:652–7.

12 D'Amore F, Relander T, Lauritzsen G *et al*. Up-front autologous stem-cell transplantation in peripheral T-cell lymphoma: NLG-T-01. *J Clin Oncol* 2012;**30**:3093–9.

13 Ansell SM, Habermann TM, Kurtin PJ *et al*. Predictive capacity of the International Prognostic Factor Index in patients with peripheral T-cell lymphoma. *J Clin Oncol* 1997;**15**:2296–301.

14 Gallamini A, Stelitano C, Calvi R *et al*. Peripheral T-cell lymphoma unspecified (PTCL-U): a new prognostic model from a retrospective multicentric clinical study. *Blood* 2004; **103**:2474–9.

15 Went P, Agostinelli C, Gallamini A *et al*. Marker expression in peripheral T-cell lymphoma: a proposed clinical-pathologic prognostic score. *J Clin Oncol* 2006;**24**:2472–9.

16 Rodriguez J, Munsell M, Yazji S *et al*. Impact of high-dose chemotherapy on peripheral T-cell lymphomas. *J Clin Oncol* 2001;**19**:3766–70.

17 Barrett AJ, Savani BN. Stem cell transplantation with reduced-intensity conditioning regimens: a review of ten years experience with new transplant concepts and new therapeutic agents. *Leukemia* 2006;**20**:1661–72.

18 Rodriguez R, Nademanee A, Ruel N *et al*. Comparison of reduced-intensity and conventional myeloablative regimens for allogeneic transplantation in non-Hodgkin's lymphoma. *Biol Blood Marrow Transplant* 2006;**12**:1326–34.

19 Dodero A, Spina F, Narni F *et al*. Allogeneic transplantation following a reduced-intensity conditioning regimen in relapsed/refractory peripheral T-cell lymphomas: long-term remissions and response to donor lymphocyte infusions support the role of a graft-versus-lymphoma effect. *Leukemia* 2012;**26**:520–6.

20 Le Gouill S, Milpied N, Buzyn A *et al*. Graft-versus-lymphoma effect for aggressive T-cell lymphomas in adults: a study by the Societe Francaise de Greffe de Moelle et de Therapie Cellulaire. *J Clin Oncol* 2008;**26**:2264–71.

21 Goldberg JD, Chou JF, Horwitz S *et al*. Long-term survival in patients with peripheral T-cell non-Hodgkin lymphomas after allogeneic hematopoietic stem cell transplant. *Leukemia Lymphoma* 2012;**53**:1124–9.

22 Delioukina M, Zain J, Palmer JM, Tsai N, Thomas S, Forman S. Reduced-intensity allogeneic hematopoietic cell transplantation using fludarabine-melphalan conditioning for treatment of mature T-cell lymphomas. *Bone Marrow Transplant* 2012;**47**:65–72.

23 Chen AI, Mcmillan A, Negrin RS, Horning SJ, Laport GG. Long-term results of autologous hematopoietic cell transplantation for peripheral T cell lymphoma: the Stanford experience. *Biol Blood Marrow Transplant* 2008;**14**:741–7.

24 Mercadal S, Briones J, Xicoy B *et al*. Intensive chemotherapy (high-dose CHOP/ESHAP regimen) followed by autologous stem-cell transplantation in previously untreated patients with peripheral T-cell lymphoma. *Ann Oncol* 2008;**19**:958–63.

25 Rodriguez J, Conde E, Gutierrez A *et al*. The adjusted International Prognostic Index and beta-2-microglobulin predict the outcome after autologous stem cell transplantation in relapsing/refractory peripheral T-cell lymphoma. *Haematologica* 2007;**92**:1067–74.

26 Yang DH, Kim WS, Kim SJ *et al*. Prognostic factors and clinical outcomes of high-dose chemotherapy followed by autologous stem cell transplantation in patients with peripheral T cell lymphoma, unspecified: complete remission at transplantation and the prognostic index of peripheral T cell lymphoma are the major factors predictive of outcome. *Biol Blood Marrow Transplant* 2009;**15**:118–25.

27 Numata A, Miyamoto T, Ohno Y *et al*. Long-term outcomes of autologous PBSCT for peripheral T-cell lymphoma: retrospective analysis of the experience of the Fukuoka BMT group. *Bone Marrow Transplant* 2010;**45**:311–16.

28 Kyriakou C, Canals C, Goldstone A *et al*. High-dose therapy and autologous stem-cell transplantation in angioimmunoblastic lymphoma: complete remission at transplantation is the major determinant of outcome. Lymphoma Working Party of the European Group for Blood and Marrow Transplantation. *J Clin Oncol* 2008;**26**:218–24.

29 Rodriguez J, Conde E, Gutierrez A *et al*. Frontline autologous stem cell transplantation in high-risk peripheral T-cell lymphoma: a prospective study from the Gel-Tamo Study Group. *Eur J Haematol* 2007;**79**:32–8.

30 Reimer P, Rudiger T, Geissinger E *et al*. Autologous stem-cell transplantation as first-line therapy in peripheral T-cell lymphomas: results of a prospective multicenter study. *J Clin Oncol* 2009;**27**:106–13.

31 Song KW, Mollee P, Keating A, Crump M. Autologous stem cell transplant for relapsed and refractory peripheral T-cell lymphoma: variable outcome according to pathological subtype. *Br J Haematol* 2003;**120**:978–85.

32 Kewalramani T, Zelenetz AD, Teruya-Feldstein J *et al*. Autologous transplantation for relapsed or primary refractory peripheral T-cell lymphoma. *Br J Haematol* 2006;**134**:202–7.

33 Federico M, Rudiger T, Bellei M *et al*. Clinicopathologic characteristics of angioimmunoblastic T-cell lymphoma: analysis of the International Peripheral T-cell Lymphoma Project. *J Clin Oncol* 2013;**31**:240–6.

34 Sieniawski M, Angamuthu N, Boyd K *et al*. Evaluation of enteropathy-associated T-cell lymphoma comparing standard therapies with a novel regimen including autologous stem cell transplantation. *Blood* 2010;**115**:3664–70.

35 Jantunen E, Boumendil A, Finel H *et al*. Autologous stem cell transplantation for enteropathy-associated T-cell lymphoma: a retrospective study by the EBMT. *Blood* 2013;**121**:2529–32.

36 Mollee P, Lazarus HM, Lipton J. Why aren't we performing more allografts for aggressive non-Hodgkin's lymphoma? *Bone Marrow Transplant* 2003;**31**:953–60.

37 Kim SW, Tanimoto TE, Hirabayashi N *et al*. Myeloablative allogeneic hematopoietic stem cell transplantation for non Hodgkin lymphoma: a nationwide survey in Japan. *Blood* 2006;**108**:382–9.

38 Faulkner RD, Craddock C, Byrne JL *et al*. BEAM–alemtuzumab reduced-intensity allogeneic stem cell transplantation for lymphoproliferative diseases: GVHD, toxicity, and survival in 65 patients. *Blood* 2004;**103**:428–34.

39 Corradini P, Dodero A, Zallio F *et al*. Graft-versus-lymphoma effect in relapsed peripheral T-cell non-Hodgkin's lymphomas after reduced-intensity conditioning followed by allogeneic transplantation of hematopoietic cells. *J Clin Oncol* 2004;**22**:2172–6.

40 Kyriakou C, Canals C, Finke J *et al*. Allogeneic stem cell transplantation is able to induce long-term remissions in angioimmunoblastic T-cell lymphoma: a retrospective study from the Lymphoma Working Party of the European Group for Blood and Marrow Transplantation. *J Clin Oncol* 2009;**27**:3951–8.

41 Wulf GG, Hasenkamp J, Jung W, Chapuy B, Truemper L, Glass B. Reduced intensity conditioning and allogeneic stem cell transplantation after salvage therapy integrating alemtuzumab for patients with relapsed peripheral T-cell non-Hodgkin's lymphoma. *Bone Marrow Transplant* 2005;**36**:271–3.

42 Jacobsen ED, Kim HT, Ho VT *et al*. A large single-center experience with allogeneic stem-cell transplantation for peripheral T-cell non-Hodgkin lymphoma and advanced mycosis fungoides/Sezary syndrome. *Ann Oncol* 2011;**22**:1608–13.

43 Zain J, Palmer JM, Delioukina M *et al*. Allogeneic hematopoietic cell transplant for peripheral T-cell non-Hodgkin lymphoma results in long-term disease control. *Leukemia Lymphoma* 2011;**52**:1463–73.

44 Duarte RF, Canals C, Onida F *et al*. Allogeneic hematopoietic cell transplantation for patients with mycosis fungoides and Sézary syndrome: a retrospective analysis of the Lymphoma Working Party of the European Group for Blood and Marrow Transplantation. *J Clin Oncol* 2010;**28**:4492–9.

45 Duvic M, Donato M, Dabaja B *et al*. Total skin electron beam and non-myeloablative allogeneic hematopoietic stem-cell transplantation in advanced mycosis fungoides and Sezary syndrome. *J Clin Oncol* 2010;**28**:2365–72.

46 Ennishi D, Maeda Y, Fujii N *et al*. Allogeneic hematopoietic stem cell transplantation for advanced extranodal natural killer/T-cell lymphoma, nasal type. *Leukemia Lymphoma* 2011;**52**:1255–61.

47 Shustov AR, Gooley TA, Sandmaier BM *et al*. Allogeneic haematopoietic cell transplantation after nonmyeloablative conditioning in patients with T-cell and natural killer-cell lymphomas. *Br J Haematol* 2010;**150**:170–8.

48 Suzuki R, Suzumiya J, Nakamura S *et al*. Hematopoietic stem cell transplantation for natural killer-cell lineage neoplasms. *Bone Marrow Transplant* 2006;**37**:425–31.

49 Corradini P, Vitolo U, Rambaldi A *et al*. Intensified chemoimmunotherapy with or without stem cell transplantation in newly diagnosed patients with peripheral T-cell lymphoma. *Leukemia* 2014;**28**:1885–91.

50 Cheson BD, Pfistner B, Juweid ME *et al*. Revised response criteria for malignant lymphoma. *J Clin Oncol* 2007;**25**:579–86.

51 Sohn BS, Yoon DH, Kim KP *et al*. The role of 18F-fluorodeoxyglucose positron emission tomography at response assessment after autologous stem cell transplantation in T-cell non-Hodgkin's lymphoma patients. *Ann Hematol* 2013;**92**:1369–77.

52 Damm-Welk C, Mussolin L, Zimmermann M *et al*. Early assessment of minimal residual disease identifies patients at very high relapse risk in NPM-ALK-positive anaplastic large-cell lymphoma. *Blood* 2014;**123**:334–7.

53 Puig N, Wang L, Seshadri T *et al*. Treatment response and overall outcome of patients with relapsed and refractory peripheral T-cell lymphoma compared to diffuse large B-cell lymphoma. *Leukemia Lymphoma* 2013;**54**:507–13.

54 Mikesch JH, Kuhlmann M, Demant A *et al*. DexaBEAM versus ICE salvage regimen prior to autologous transplantation for relapsed or refractory aggressive peripheral T cell lymphoma: a retrospective evaluation of parallel patient cohorts of one center. *Ann Hematol* 2013;**92**:1041–8.

55 Zinzani Pl, Venturini F, Stefoni V *et al*. Gemcitabine as single agent in pretreated T-cell lymphoma patients: evaluation of the long-term outcome. *Ann Oncol* 2010;**21**:860–3.

56 Arkenau HT, Chong G, Cunningham D *et al*. Gemcitabine, cisplatin and methylprednisolone for the treatment of patients with peripheral T-cell lymphoma: the Royal Marsden Hospital experience. *Haematologica* 2007;**92**:271–2.

57 Damaj G, Gressin R, Bouabdallah K *et al*. Results from a prospective, open-label, phase II trial of bendamustine in refractory or relapsed T-cell lymphomas: the BENTLY trial. *J Clin Oncol* 2013;**31**:104–10.

58 Pro B, Advani R, Brice P *et al*. Brentuximab vedotin (SGN-35) in patients with relapsed or refractory systemic anaplastic large-cell lymphoma: results of a phase II study. *J Clin Oncol* 2012;**30**:2190–6.

59 Horwitz SM, Advani RH, Bartlett NL *et al*. Objective responses in relapsed T-cell lymphomas with single-agent brentuximab vedotin. *Blood* 2014;**123**:3095–100.

60 Hamadani M, Awan FT, Elder P *et al*. Allogeneic hematopoietic stem cell transplantation for peripheral T cell lymphomas; evidence of graft-versus-T cell lymphoma effect. *Biol Blood Marrow Transplant* 2008;**14**:480–3.

61 Itonaga H, Tsushima H, Taguchi J *et al*. Treatment of relapsed adult T-cell leukemia/lymphoma after allogeneic hematopoietic stem cell transplantation: the Nagasaki Transplant Group experience. *Blood* 2013;**121**:219–25.

62 Gallamini A, Zaja F, Patti C *et al.* Alemtuzumab (Campath-1H) and CHOP chemotherapy as first-line treatment of peripheral T-cell lymphoma: results of a GITIL (Gruppo Italiano Terapie Innovative nei Linfomi) prospective multi-center trial. *Blood* 2007;**110**:2316–23.

63 O'Connor OA, Pro B, Pinter-Brown L *et al.* Pralatrexate in patients with relapsed or refractory peripheral T-cell lymphoma: results from the pivotal PROPEL study. *J Clin Oncol* 2011;**29**:1182–9.

64 Piekarz RL, Frye R, Prince HM *et al.* Phase 2 trial of romidepsin in patients with peripheral T-cell lymphoma. *Blood* 2011;**117**:5827–34.

65 Coiffier B, Pro B, Prince HM *et al.* Results from a pivotal, open-label, phase II study of romidepsin in relapsed or refractory peripheral T-cell lymphoma after prior systemic therapy. *J Clin Oncol* 2012;**30**:631–6.

66 Reddy P, Sun Y, Toubai T *et al.* Histone deacetylase inhibition modulates indoleamine 2,3-dioxygenase-dependent DC functions and regulates experimental graft-versus-host disease in mice. *J Clin Invest* 2008;**118**:2562–73.

67 Dueck G, Chua N, Prasad A *et al.* Interim report of a phase 2 clinical trial of lenalidomide for T-cell non-Hodgkin lymphoma. *Cancer* 2010;**116**:4541–8.

68 Morschhauser F, Fitoussi O, Haioun C *et al.* A phase 2, multicentre, single-arm, open-label study to evaluate the safety and efficacy of single-agent lenalidomide (Revlimid) in subjects with relapsed or refractory peripheral T-cell non-Hodgkin lymphoma: the EXPECT trial. *Eur J Cancer* 2013;**49**:2869–76.

69 Ishida T, Joh T, Uike N *et al.* Defucosylated anti-CCR4 monoclonal antibody (KW-0761) for relapsed adult T-cell leukemia-lymphoma: a multicenter phase II study. *J Clin Oncol* 2012;**30**:837–42.

70 Gambacorti Passerini C, Farina F, Stasia A *et al.* Crizotinib in advanced, chemoresistant anaplastic lymphoma kinase-positive lymphoma patients. *J Natl Cancer Inst* 2014;**106**:djt378.

CHAPTER 20

Transplantation in Burkitt and lymphoblastic lymphoma

Gregory A. Hale

Introduction

Burkitt and lymphoblastic non-Hodgkin lymphomas (NHLs) constitute two distinct groups of highly aggressive lymphoid neoplasms, each requiring aggressive induction chemotherapy that influences disease outcome [1–5]. Both these malignancies require intensive chemotherapy regimens with central nervous system (CNS)-directed therapy to prevent extramedullary relapse. Because of the relative infrequency of Burkitt lymphoma and lymphoblastic lymphoma in adults, the majority of published studies of transplantation in these diseases are markedly limited to pediatric reports, adult studies with small numbers of patients, or transplant reports of NHL patients with low-, intermediate-, and high-grade histologies, varied donor types, and conditioning regimens [6–11]. Presently there is no well-defined role for autologous or allogeneic HSCT in first remission in either malignancy, given the excellent outcomes reported with standard chemotherapy regimens. The majority of transplants for these disorders have been in patients with recurrent disease. Relapse remains the primary reason for treatment failure after autologous transplantation for both Burkitt and lymphoblastic NHL.

Allogeneic HSCT is most commonly studied in series of patients with all histologies of NHL and is rarely focused on Burkitt or lymphoblastic lymphoma [6–12]. Allogeneic HSCT finds its place in the treatment of those patients with relapsed or refractory disease for whom autologous stem cell transplant has failed or is not feasible. The issues of selecting the appropriate candidate, conditioning regimen, and timing of transplant remain topics of ongoing research. In general, allogeneic HSCT has several distinct advantages over autologous HSCT, including having a healthy stem cell source without the risk for tumor contamination, a lesser risk of treatment-related secondary hematopoietic malignancies, and a potential immunologic graft-versus-lymphoma (GVL) effect. The challenges of allogeneic HSCT include increased toxicities from the conditioning regimen, risk of infection from prolonged immunosuppression, and chance of graft-versus-host disease (GVHD); all these factors result in an increased risk of transplant-related mortality (TRM) compared with standard chemotherapy or autologous HSCT.

Burkitt lymphoma (Table 20.1)

Burkitt lymphoma is a high-grade malignancy that occurs more commonly in children, accounting for 30% of childhood lymphomas [13,14]. In adults, this malignancy is often associated with an underlying immunodeficiency and accounts for 2% of adult lymphomas [15–20]. In the Western hemisphere, the tumor most commonly occurs as bulky disease, originating in the abdomen, particularly the ileocecal region but may also involve other extranodal sites such as kidneys, ovaries, and breasts. In Africa the jaw and facial bones are commonly the primary site. Epstein–Barr virus (EBV) is often associated with endemic Burkitt lymphoma but less often in the Western hemisphere. The genetic origin of this disease is well known, arising from clonal rearrangements of the immunoglobulin heavy (*IGH*) and/or the immunoglobulin light (*IGL*) chain genes, associated

Clinical Guide to Transplantation in Lymphoma, First Edition. Edited by Bipin N. Savani and Mohamad Mohty.
© 2015 John Wiley & Sons, Ltd. Published 2015 by John Wiley & Sons, Ltd.

Table 20.1 Published studies of transplantation in Burkitt lymphoma.

Reference	Diseases	Type of HSCT (N)	Conditioning	TRM	PFS	OS	Comments
Maramattom et al. [27]	Burkitt	Auto (113)	MAC	4%	1-year 60%	1-year 62%	Patients transplanted in CR1 had 5-year OS 83% vs. 31% in non-CR1 patients
Maramattom et al. [27]	Burkitt	Allo (128)	10% RIC	20%	1-year 33% MRD; 24% URD	1-year 33% MRD; 25% URD	More chemotherapy-resistant advanced-stage disease
Gross et al. [33]	Pediatric; recurrent Burkitt	Auto (17)	MAC	1-year 14%	5-year 27%	NR	Similar outcomes with autologous or allogeneic HSCT
Gross et al. [33]	Pediatric; recurrent Burkitt	Allo (24)	MAC	1-year 17%	5-year 31%	NR	
Sweetenham et al. [25]	Burkitt; adults	Auto (117)	MAC	8.5%	3-year 54%	3-year 53%	3-year PFS 72% for CR1 Relapse PFS: chemotherapy sensitive 37% vs. chemotherapy resistant 7%
Gajewski et al. [42]	Burkitt	Auto (113)	MAC	5%	48%	5-year 54%	5-year PFS 78% in CR1 vs. 29% non-CR1
Gajewski et al. [42]	Burkitt	Allo (128)	MAC	26% MRD; 28% URD/MMRD	30% MRD; 22% URD/MMRD	5-year 32% MRD; 23% URD/MMRD	5-year PFS 50% in CR1 vs. 19% non-CR1
Krishnan et al. [18]	HIV + NHL, including Burkitt	Auto (6)	MAC	5%	85%	70% at 2.6 years	Low TRM and low infection risk
Belsalobre et al. [20]	HIV + NHL, including Burkitt	Auto (8)	MAC	7.5%	56%	61% at 2.5 years	Patients not in remission had decreased PFS
Diez-Martin et al. [19]	HIV + NHL, including Burkitt	Auto (3)	MAC	8%	58%	58% at 2.5 years	Nonsignificant increased risk of TRM in first year for HIV-positive patients

CR1, first remission; HSCT, hematopoietic stem cell transplant; MAC, myeloablative conditioning; MMRD, mismatched related donor; MRD, matched related donor; NHL, non-Hodgkin lymphoma; NR, not reported; OS, overall survival; PFS, progression-free survival; RIC, reduced-intensity conditioning; TRM, transplant-related mortality; URD, unrelated donor.

with the *CMYC* oncogene on chromosome 8, being translocated adjacent to *IGH* on chromosome 14 (most common) or *IGL* on chromosome 2 or 22 [21]. This malignancy is reported to be the most rapidly growing tumor, with doubling times approximating 24 hours, and is typically resistant to radiation therapy. Recently, aggressive multiagent chemotherapy regimens containing rituximab, alkylating agents, high-dose methotrexate, and cytarabine with aggressive CNS-directed prophylaxis have resulted in survival rates of 60–90%, being highest in pediatric patients and those with more limited-stage disease [22–26]. However, for patients with recurrent disease, allogeneic or autologous HSCT is necessary for long-term disease-free survival.

Autologous transplantation has been employed as both consolidation of first remission and as treatment for patients with relapsed disease. In an early study of autologous HSCT for Burkitt lymphoma, Sweetenham *et al.* [25] retrospectively analyzed patients reported to the European Society for Blood and Marrow Transplantation (EBMT), showing a 72% 3-year overall survival (OS) rate for patients in first remission (CR1). For patients in first remission at the time of transplantation, the survival rates are very similar to those who receive intensive chemotherapy regimens, with pediatric regimens reporting 73% 2-year survival when used in adult populations. With autologous HSCT as consolidation, the highest risk patients were reported to have a 59% 2-year survival rate, comparable to outcomes reported with intense chemotherapy regimens. For patients with relapsed disease, those with chemotherapy-sensitive disease had improved outcomes of 37% compared with 7% for those with chemotherapy-resistant disease.

The Center for International Blood and Marrow Transplant Research (CIBMTR) recently published their registry experience in 241 patients with Burkitt lymphoma transplanted between 1985 and 2007 [27]. Over this period there has been a significant decline in autologous HSCT for this disease, with only 19% performed after 2001. Survival rates were significantly higher for autograft recipients after 2000 compared to before 2000, suggesting improved survival rate with improved patient selection, better identification of patients likely to benefit from autologous HSCT, and improved supportive care [28]. Progression-free survival (PFS) at 5 years was 78% and 27% for those in first remission and those not in first remission, respectively. In this same series, those transplanted in second remission had a 5-year PFS of 44%, suggesting that autologous transplantation may

salvage patients with chemotherapy-sensitive disease. Autologous recipients were more likely to have had chemotherapy-sensitive disease, receive peripheral blood stem cell grafts, and be transplanted in first remission than allogeneic transplant recipients. The majority of deaths were from recurrent or progressive lymphoma. The authors concluded that autologous HSCT in first remission did not offer a survival advantage over present-day aggressive chemotherapy regimens, but could be used successfully to salvage patients with chemotherapy-sensitive disease.

Burkitt lymphoma is commonly seen as a malignancy in patients with HIV infection. Most studies demonstrate that HIV-positive patients with high- or intermediate-grade NHL can be cured with high-dose chemotherapy and autologous HSCT; however, disease recurrence rates are higher in patients with non-diffuse large B-cell lymphoma histologies [20]. Other investigators have demonstrated that HIV-positive and HIV-negative NHL patients undergoing autologous HSCT have similar outcomes [19]. Published studies suggest that HIV status should not be the sole factor used to preclude autologous HSCT for these patients, if otherwise indicated.

Future studies should aim to identify those patients in first remission who are destined to relapse, for whom autologous HSCT may be beneficial [25,27,29]. Certainly it appears that patients with chemotherapy-resistant Burkitt lymphoma are not likely to benefit from autologous HSCT, although autologous HSCT may salvage a significant proportion of patients who are able to achieve a second remission.

The data for the role of allogeneic HSCT for Burkitt lymphoma is quite scarce. The EBMT reported 101 patients who had undergone autologous or allogeneic HSCT for Burkitt lymphoma; patients in the two groups were carefully selected, being matched for known disease- and transplant-related risk factors [30]. In this retrospective registry study, eight Burkitt lymphoma patients were included in each cohort and there was no difference in relapse rate or OS rates in autologous or allogeneic transplant recipients for the Burkitt lymphoma patient group.

A single-institution publication of allogeneic HSCT for adult patients with chemotherapy-refractory aggressive NHL included 46 patients, 32 of whom had stable disease before transplant [12]. Three of them had Burkitt lymphoma, all with stable disease status prior to transplantation. The 5-year OS and PFS for Burkitt lymphoma patients were 33% and 33%, respectively. The authors concluded that patients with stable disease should not be excluded from allogeneic HSCT based solely on the presence of chemotherapy-insensitive disease.

In the CIBMTR registry publication, allogeneic HSCT resulted in PFS rates at 5 years of 50% and 19% for Burkitt lymphoma patients in first remission and those not in first remission, respectively [27]. Following National Comprehensive Cancer Network (NCCN) guidelines for a higher-risk subset of patients, allogeneic HSCT resulted in a 5-year PFS rate of 27%. Evidence of a GVL effect could not be determined in this study as no association was observed between survival and GVHD. The majority of deaths were from recurrent or progressive lymphoma.

Reduced-intensity conditioning (RIC) regimens are increasingly employed to treat lymphoma patients, particularly after autologous HSCT or in patients who are elderly or have comorbid conditions [6,31,32]. However, the kinetics of high-grade lymphomas makes these cells less susceptible targets for a GVL effect. In a Japanese study of RIC transplantation, patients with high-grade histology (including Burkitt lymphoma) had an increased relative risk of treatment failure when compared with patients with low- and intermediate-grade histologies [32].

In the largest publication of transplant experience in 182 pediatric lymphoma patients (90 autologous, 92 allogeneic), the CIBMTR reported no significant difference in the 5-year probabilities of OS, PFS, and relapse/progression for the 41 Burkitt lymphoma patients between autologous and allogeneic transplantation [33]. This trial only included patients less than 18 years of age with recurrent disease with no prior autologous HSCT. This was a retrospective study and the authors concluded that the rapid course of Burkitt lymphoma can make achieving disease control difficult, with short-lived responses that make transitioning to transplantation difficult.

Allogeneic transplantation has been successful in patients with recurrent Burkitt lymphoma, and can salvage chemotherapy-resistant patients. Its routine use in patients in first remission cannot be recommended at this time.

Lymphoblastic lymphoma (Table 20.2)

Lymphoblastic lymphoma accounts for approximately 2% of all cases of NHL and up to 30% of pediatric lymphomas [1,5,34]. It most commonly arises from precursor T lymphocytes and is frequently associated with extramedullary disease such as a mediastinal mass. Less commonly, this malignancy may be of B-cell origin. In either case, the disease is often associated with hepatosplenomegaly, a mediastinal mass, marked adenopathy, and marrow involvement. Morphologically, the disease is indistinguishable from acute lymphoblastic leukemia (ALL), with the primary difference being the percentage of malignant blasts in the marrow. This disease has a very aggressive clinical course and requires intensive ALL-like chemotherapy, with remission rates approaching 80% and up to 60% of patients having long-term survival, primarily pediatric patients and those with limited-stage disease [35–37].

Autologous HSCT has been used to consolidate initial remissions in an attempt to improve long-term disease-free survival, with both registries and single-institution publications demonstrating long-term survival rates of 50–80% [30,33,38–44]. One randomized study attempted to address the role of early autologous HSCT in first remission by randomizing patients who achieved a complete or partial remission after standard therapy to high-dose chemotherapy and autologous HSCT versus conventional chemotherapy consolidation and maintenance. Of the initial 119 patients enrolled, only 65 were eligible for randomization due to patient refusal, disease progression, toxicity, or a decision to undergo allogeneic HSCT. No significant difference in survival was observed between the nontransplant and the chemotherapy arms; however, these findings are difficult to interpret given the high number of patients who were not evaluable.

Allogeneic HSCT has been increasingly used in the setting of relapsed disease. In a study of the EBMT, investigators reported outcomes of 101 allogeneic HSCT recipients and compared them with those of 101 autologous HSCT recipients with a variety of NHL histologies [30]. Approximately half of patients had lymphoblastic lymphoma. PFS was similar between the two groups, with 49% for allogeneic HSCT and 46% for autologous HSCT. For those with lymphoblastic lymphoma, there was a statistically lower relapse rate in those undergoing allogeneic HSCT compared to those receiving autologous HSCT; however, OS was similar due to the higher TRM in the allogeneic group. Furthermore, there was a lower relapse rate among those with chronic GVHD, suggesting a GVL effect.

Published registry data for lymphoblastic lymphoma patients retrospectively compared 128 patients treated with autologous HSCT and 76 patients undergoing matched sibling donor HSCT [38]. At 5 years post

Table 20.2 Published studies of transplantation in lymphoblastic lymphoma.

Reference	Diseases	Type of HSCT (N)	Conditioning	TRM	DFS	OS	Comments
Gross et al. [33]	Pediatric; recurrent lymphoma	Auto	MAC	1-year 14%	4%	NR	
Gross et al. [33]	Pediatric; recurrent lymphoma	Allo	MAC	1-year 17%	40%	NR	Allogeneic HSCT had improved DFS vs. autologous (P < 0.01)
Chopra et al. [30]	NHL, approximately half lymphoblastic	Auto (101); 8 Burkit; 49 lymphoblastic	MAC	10%	46%		Lymphoblastic NHL patients had decreased relapse rate after allo-HSCT vs. auto-HSCT (48% vs. 24%)
Chopra et al. [30]	NHL, approximately half lymphoblastic	Allo (101); 8 Burkit; 49 lymphoblastic	MAC	24%	49%		Decreased relapse rate noted in cGVHD patients: 35% no cGVHD vs. 0% with cGVHD; 14/18 with cGVHD had lymphoblastic NHL
Levine et al. [38]	Adult lymphoblastic	Auto (128)	MAC	5-year 5%	5-year 39%	5-year 44%	
Levine et al. [38]	Adult lymphoblastic, MRD	Allo (76)	MAC	5-year 25%	5-year 36%	5-year 39%	Decreased relapse rates after allo-HSCT vs. auto-HSCT at 5 years (56% vs. 34%)
Sweetenham et al. [39]	Lymphoblastic NHL, adult	Auto 218); 105 in CR	MAC	14%	6-year 41%	6-year 42%	6-year OS for CR1 patients 63%
Sweetenham et al. [40]	Lymphoblastic, adult; auto vs. chemotherapy	Auto 31); chemotherapy (34)	MAC	NR	3-year 55% after auto vs. 24% after chemo	3-year 56% after auto vs. 45% after chemo	OS after auto-HSCT was not significantly better than chemotherapy

cGVHD, chronic graft-versus-host disease; CR1, first remission; DFS, disease-free survival; HSCT, hematopoietic stem cell transplant; MAC, myeloablative conditioning; MRD, matched related donor; NHL, non-Hodgkin lymphoma; NR, not reported; OS, overall survival; TRM, transplant-related mortality.

transplantation, the disease-free survival rate was similar in the two treatment arms, with 36% for allograft recipients and 39% for autologous recipients. Fewer relapses were observed after allogeneic HSCT. Irrespective of the type of transplant, patients transplanted after relapse and those with marrow involvement had inferior outcomes.

Investigators in a retrospective EBMT study concluded that high-dose treatment with autologous HSCT was an effective strategy for adults with lymphoblastic lymphoma even when the malignancy was resistant to conventional therapy [39]. However, this study was done in an era prior to the current aggressive induction used to treat this malignancy. With modern induction regimens, chemotherapy resistance is typically treated with allogeneic transplantation to utilize the GVL effect. In a registry study of 283 unrelated donor transplants for NHL employing myeloablative regimens reported to the CIBMTR, factors identified in multivariate analysis to be associated with a poor outcome included patients with high-grade histology (Burkitt or lymphoblastic NHL), poor performance status, advanced disease at HSCT, and refractory disease [8]. These findings confirm observations in other smaller trials and retrospective studies [45].

In the CIBMTR study of pediatric lymphoma, 53 patients had lymphoblastic lymphoma; 14 underwent autologous HSCT and 39 allogeneic HSCT [33]. In this trial of relapsed patients, event-free survival (EFS) was significantly higher for allograft recipients (40% vs. 4%, $P < 0.01$). For all subtypes, predictive factors for EFS were disease status at HSCT and the use of allogeneic donor for lymphoblastic lymphoma. There was no difference in outcome by donor type for any other histology. In this retrospective nonrandomized study of registry data the authors concluded that an allogeneic donor was preferred for lymphoblastic lymphoma.

With the inclusion of the nucleoside analog nelarabine in many upfront treatment regimens for T-cell malignancies, there are no published data on how this agent will alter outcomes in this population. Similar to its cousin medication clofarabine, now used as a component of regimens to treat B-cell precursor ALL, nelarabine may play a role in bridging patients to transplant.

Conclusion

In general, both adult and pediatric patients with NHL enjoy an excellent prognosis with the advent of more aggressive chemotherapy regimens, as the majority of these patients achieve durable remissions with these front-line therapies. Autologous HSCT has been demonstrated to result in prolonged remissions in Burkitt NHL patients in first remission or those with recurrent chemotherapy-sensitive disease. Nonetheless, allogeneic HSCT offers a potential option as salvage therapy for those with refractory and/or multiply-relapsed disease. In allogeneic HSCT for NHL, multiple recent studies have demonstrated better OS and PFS with RIC in the setting of HLA-matched donor stem cell grafts compared to myeloablative conditioning (MAC), in which the therapeutic benefit of dose intensification is frequently negated by the increased TRM. However, RIC regimens have not been proven effective in patients with high-grade histologies such as Burkitt or lymphoblastic NHL [31,45]. The reduced TRM with RIC justifies the use of allogeneic HSCT in patients with refractory but indolent subtypes of NHL. The greater GVL effect observed with some of the NHL subtypes in the clinical setting further augments the therapeutic potential of allogeneic HSCT.

Most newly diagnosed patients with Burkitt and lymphoblastic NHL will respond to conventional chemotherapy and most of them will experience long-term survival. Autologous HSCT may be beneficial in certain patients with Burkitt lymphoma in first remission but there are currently no criteria that identify those individuals. Data suggest that autologous transplant as part of initial therapy may benefit patients with high-risk features in first remission or those patients who have a slow response to chemotherapy. Patients with recurrent disease may benefit from autologous HSCT if they have chemotherapy-sensitive Burkitt lymphoma and are able to attain a second remission. Patients with recurrent disease or who are unable to undergo autologous HSCT due to marrow involvement may be candidates for allogeneic HSCT, realizing that TRM may be significant. Myeloablative regimens likely offer improved disease control compared to reduced-intensity regimens. For patients with chemotherapy-resistant or progressive disease, allogeneic transplantation or clinical trials can be considered.

Patients with lymphoblastic lymphoma appear to have better outcomes after allogeneic HSCT than after autologous HSCT. For those patients with refractory disease, allogeneic HSCT should be considered as salvage therapy. The decision to undergo allogeneic HSCT must account for patient performance, disease status, treatment history, comorbidities and, most importantly, personal wishes, as the TRM associated with any type of allogeneic HSCT is not minimal. RIC with related or unrelated HLA-matched donor stem cell graft provides an excellent outcome in the setting of refractory or multiply relapsed NHL and should be considered preferentially to MAC. With the improvements in supportive care and GVHD management, we should consider offering allogeneic HSCT earlier, such as after the first relapse, if a suitable donor is available. This strategy may further improve the outcome of allogeneic HSCT, with patients having better performance, less resistant disease, and less comorbidity. Future efforts should be directed to identifying those high-risk patients likely to fail at diagnosis for more aggressive consolidation. Autologous HSCT is currently used sparingly in Burkitt and lymphoblastic lymphoma, with allogeneic HSCT offering a putative GVL effect and some patients being cured of their disease, even those with chemotherapy-resistant lymphoma. Incorporation of new agents that optimize the immunologic GVL effect, or utilizing radio-immunotherapy and novel cellular therapies must be explored to improve survival rates [46–48].

References

1 The Non-Hodgkin's Lymphoma Classification Project. A clinical evaluation of the International Lymphoma Study Group classification of non-Hodgkin's lymphoma. *Blood* 1997;**89**:3909–18.

2 Sandlund JT, Pui CH, Zhou Y *et al.* Results of treatment of advanced-stage lymphoblastic lymphoma at St. Jude Children's Research Hospital from 1962 to 2002. *Ann Oncol* 2013;**24**: 2425–9.

3 Bouabdallah R, Xerri L, Dardou V J *et al.* Role of induction chemotherapy and bone marrow transplantation in adult lymphoblastic lymphoma: a report on 62 patients from a single center. *Ann Oncol* 1998;**9**:619–25.

4 Sandlund JT. The combination of monoclonal antibodies and conventional chemotherapy for children with malignant lymphoma: opportunities and challenges. *Pediatr Blood Cancer* 2009;**52**:150–2.

5 Hochberg J, Waxman IM, Kelly KM *et al.* Adolescent non-Hodgkin lymphoma and Hodgkin lymphoma: state of the science. *Br J Haematol* 2008;**144**: 24–40.

6 Hale GA, Shrestha S, Le-Rademacher J *et al.* Alternate donor hematopoietic cell transplantation (HCT) in non-Hodgkin lymphoma using lower intensity conditioning: a report from the CIBMTR. *Biol Blood Marrow Transplant* 2012;**18**: 1036–43.

7 Lazarus HM, Carreras J, Boudreau C *et al.* Influence of age and histology on outcome in adult non-Hodgkin's lymphoma patients undergoing autologous HCT: a report from the Center

for International Blood and Marrow Transplant Research (CIBMTR). *Biol Blood Marrow Transplant* 2008;**14**:1323–33.

8 van Besien K, Carreras J, Bierman PJ *et al.* Unrelated donor hematopoietic cell transplantation for non-Hodgkin lymphoma: long-term outcomes. *Biol Blood Marrow Transplant* 2009;**15**:554–63.

9 Devetten MP, Hari PN, Carreras J *et al.* Unrelated donor reduced intensity allogeneic hematopoietic stem cell transplant for relapsed and refractory Hodgkin lymphoma. *Biol Blood Marrow Transplant* 2009;**15**:109–17.

10 Schmitz N, Dreger P, Glass B, Sureda A. Allogeneic transplantation in lymphoma: current status. *Haematologica* 2007;**92**:1533–48.

11 Reddy NM, Oluwole O, Greer JP *et al.* Outcomes of autologous or allogeneic stem cell transplantation for non-Hodgkin lymphoma. *Exp Hematol* 2014;**42**:39–45.

12 Hamadani M, Benson DM Jr, Hofmeister CC *et al.* Allogeneic stem cell transplantation, for patients with relapsed chemo-refractory aggressive non-Hodgkin lymphoma. *Biol Blood Marrow Transplant* 2009;**15**:547–53.

13 Burkitt DP. Geographical distribution. In: Burkett DP, Wright DH, eds. *Burkett's Lymphoma*. Edinburgh: Churchill Livingstone, 1970:186.

14 Yano T, van Krieken JHJM, Magrath IT *et al.* Histogenetic correlations between subcategories of small noncleaved cell lymphoma. *Blood* 1992;**79**:1282–90.

15 Blum KA, Kozanski G, Byrd JC. Adult Burkitt leukemia and lumphoma. *Blood* 2004;**104**:3009–20.

16 Magrath I, Shiramizu B. Biology and treatment of small non-cleaved cell lymphoma. *Oncology* 1989;**3**:41–53.

17 Ballerini P, Gaidano G, Gong JZ *et al.* Multiple genetic lesions in AIDS-related non-Hodgkin's lymphoma. *Blood* 1993;**81**; 166–76.

18 Krishnan A, Molina, Zaia J *et al.* Durable remissions with autologous stem cell transplantation for high-risk HIV-associated lymphomas. *Blood* 2005;**105**: 874–8.

19 Diez-Martin JL, Balsalobre P, Re A *et al.* Comparable survival between HIV positive and HIV negative non-Hodgkin and Hodgkin lymphoma patients undergoing autologous peripheral blood stem cell transplantation. *Blood* 2009;**113**: 6011–14.

20 Balsalobre O, Diez-Martin JL, Re A *et al.* Autologous stem-cell transplantation in patients with HIV-related lymphoma. *J Clin Oncol* 2009;**27**:2192–8.

21 Poirel HA, Cairo MS, Heerema NA *et al.* Specific cytogenetic abnormalities are associated with a significantly inferior outcome in children and adolescents with mature B-cell non-Hodgkin's lymphoma: results of the FAB/LMB 96 international study. *Leukemia* 2009;**23**:323–31.

22 Sharkey RM, Press OW, Goldenberg DM. A re-examination of radioimmunotherapy in the treatment of non-Hodgkin lymphoma: prospects for dual-targeted antibody/radioantibody therapy. *Blood* 2009;**113**:3891–5.

23 Wollner N, Exelby PR, Liebermann PH. Non-Hodgkin's lymphoma in children: a progress report on the original patients treated with the LSA2L2 protocol. *Cancer* 1979;**44**:1990–9.

24 Magrath I, Adde M, Shad A *et al*. Adults and children with small non-cleaved-cell lymphoma have a similar excellent outcome when treated with the same chemotherapy regimen. *J Clin Oncol* 1996;**14**:925–34.

25 Sweetenham JW, Pearce R, Taghipour G, Blaise D, Gisselbrecht C, Goldstone AH. Adult Burkitt's and Burkitt-like non-Hodgkin's lymphoma: outcome for patients treated with high-dose therapy and autologous stem-cell transplantation in first remission or at relapse. Results from the European Group for Blood and Marrow Transplantation. *J Clin Oncol* 1996;**14**:2465–72.

26 Patte C, Phillip T, Radary C *et al*. High survival rate in advanced B-cell lymphomas and leukemias without CNS involvement with a short intensive polychemotherapy. *J Clin Oncol* 1991;**9**:123–32.

27 Maramattom LV, Hari PN, Burns LJ *et al*. Autologous and allogenic transplantation for Burkitt lymphoma outcomes and changes in utilization: a report from the Center for International Blood and Marrow Transplant Research. *Biol Blood Marrow Transplant* 2013;**19**:173–9.

28 McCarthy PL, Hahan T, Hassebroek A *et al*. Trends in use of and survival after autologous hematopoietic cell transplantation in North America, 1995–2005: significant improvement in survival of lymphoma and myeloma during a period of increasing recipient age. *Biol Blood Marrow Transplant* 2013;**19**:1116–23.

29 Jost LM, Jacky E, Dommann-Scherrer C *et al*. Short term weekly chemotherapy followed by high-dose therapy and autologous bone marrow transplantation for lymphoblastic and Burkitt's lymphoma in adult patients. *Ann Oncol* 1995;**6**:445–51.

30 Chopra R, Goldstone AH, Pearce R *et al*. Autologous versus allogeneic bone marrow transplantation for non-Hodgkin's lymphoma: a case-controlled analysis from the European Bone Marrow Transplant Group Registry data. *J Clin Oncol* 1992;**10**;1690–5.

31 Hamadani M, Saber W, Ahn KW *et al*. Impact of pretransplant conditioning regimens on outcomes of allogeneic transplantation for chemotherapy-unresponsive diffuse large B-cell lymphoma and grade-III follicular lymphoma. *Biol Blood Marrow Transplant* 2013;**19**:746–53.

32 Kusumi E, Kami M, Kanda Y *et al*. Reduced-intensity hematopoietic stem-cell transplantation for malignant lymphoma: a retrospective survey of 12 adult patients in Japan. *Bone Marrow Transplant* 2005;**36**:205–13.

33 Gross TG, Hale GA, He W *et al*. Hematopoietic stem cell transplantation for refractory and recurrent non-Hodgkin lymphoma in children and adolescents. *Biol Blood Marrow Transplant* 2010;**16**:223–30.

34 Slater DE, Mertelsmann R, Koziner B *et al*. Lymphoblastic lymphoma in adults. *J Clin Oncol* 1986;**4**:57–67.

35 Coustan-Smith E, Sandlund JT, Perkins SL *et al*. Minimal disseminated disease in childhood T-cell lymphoblastic lymphoma: a report from the Children's Oncology Group. *J Clin Oncol* 2009;**27**:3533–9.

36 Picozzi VJ, Coleman CN. Lymphoblastic lymphoma. *Semin Oncol* 1990;**17**:96–103.

37 Streuli RA, Kaneko Y, Variakojis D, Kinnealey A, Golomb HM, Rowley JD. Lymphoblastic lymphoma in adults. *Cancer* 1981;**47**:2510–16.

38 Levine JE, Harris RE, Loberiza FR *et al*. A comparison of allogeneic and autologous bone marrow transplantation for lymphoblastic lymphoma. *Blood* 2003;**101**:2476–82.

39 Sweetenham JW, Liberti G, Pearce R, Taghipour G, Santini G, Goldstone AH. High dose therapy and autologous bone marrow transplantation for adult patients with lymphoblastic lymphoma: results of the European Group for Bone Marrow Transplantation. *J Clin Oncol* 1994;**12**:1358–65.

40 Sweetenham JW, Santini G, Qian W *et al*. High-dose therapy and autologous stem-cell transplantation versus conventional-dose consolidation/maintenance therapy as postremission therapy for adult patients with lymphoblastic lymphoma: results of a randomized trial of the European Group for Blood and Marrow Transplantation and the United Kingdom Lymphoma Group. *J Clin Oncol* 2001;**19**:2927–36.

41 Verdonck LF, Dekker AW, De Gast GC, Lokhorst HM, Nieuwenhuis HK. Autologous bone marrow transplantation for adult poor risk lymphoblastic lymphoma in first remission. *J Clin Oncol* 1992;**10**;644–6.

42 Gajewski JL, Carreras J, Lazarus HM *et al*. The role of hematopoietic cell transplantation (SCT) for Burkitt lymphoma: a report from the Center for International Blood and Marrow Transplant Research (CIBMTR). *Blood (ASH Annual Meeting Abstracts)* 2010;**116**:Abstract 2390.

43 Milpied N, Ifrah N, Kuentz M *et al*. Bone marrow transplantation for adult poor prognosis lymphoblastic lymphoma in first complete remission. *Br J Haematol* 1989;**73**:82–7.

44 Santini G, Coser P, Chisesi T *et al*. Autologous bone marrow transplantation for advanced stage adult lymphoblastic lymphoma in first complete remission. *Ann Oncol* 1991;**2**(Suppl 2):181–5.

45 Robinson SP, Goldstone AH, Mackinnon S *et al*. Chemoresistant or aggressive lymphoma predicts for a poor outcome following reduced intensity allogeneic progenitor cell transplantation: an analysis from the Lymphoma Working Party of the European Group for Blood and Marrow Transplantation. *Blood* 2002;**100**:4310–16.

46 Ratanatharathorn V, Uberti J, Karanes C *et al*. Prospective comparative trial of autologous versus allogeneic transplantation in patients with non-Hodgkin's lymphoma. *Blood* 1994;**84**:1050–5.

47 Miles RR, Cairo MS, Satwani P *et al*. Immunophenotypic identification of possible therapeutic targets in paediatric non-Hodgkin lymphomas: a Children's Oncology Group report. *Br J Haematol* 2007;**138**:506–12.

48 Sharkey RM, Press OW, Goldenberg DM. A re-examination of radioimmunotherapy in the treatment of non-Hodgkin lymphoma: prospects for dual-targeted antibody/radioantibody therapy. *Blood* 2009;**113**:3891–5.

CHAPTER 21

Transplantation in adult T-cell leukemia/lymphoma

Ali Bazarbachi and Olivier Hermine

Introduction

Adult T-cell leukemia/lymphoma (ATL) is an aggressive lymphoid proliferation associated with the human lymphotropic virus type I (HTLV-I) [1,2]. The viral oncoprotein Tax plays a central role in T-cell transformation through deregulation of multiple cellular pathways [3]. ATL usually occurs in individuals from HTLV-I endemic regions, such as southern Japan, the Caribbean, Central and South America, inter-tropical Africa, Romania, and northern Iran [4–7]. HTLV-I causes transformation and clonal expansion of T cells, resulting in ATL in approximately 1–4% of the estimated 10–20 million infected hosts, with a mean latency period of more than 50 years [4,6,8]. It appears that early infection during childhood is associated with a higher risk of ATL development.

Clinical presentation and classification

The most recent World Health Organization lymphoma classification lists ATL as a peripheral T-cell lymphoma (PTCL) [9]. The diversity in clinical features and prognosis of patients with ATL has led to its subclassification into the following four subtypes (Shimoyama classification): smoldering, chronic and acute leukemic forms, and ATL lymphoma [10]. A borderline state between healthy carriers of HTLV-I and ATL patients has been described and named pre-ATL [11].

Acute and lymphoma subtypes

When ATL presents aggressively with massive enlargement of lymph nodes and visceral involvement, it is associated with or without a leukemic phase, referred to as "acute ATL" (60% of all cases) or "lymphomatous" ATL (20% of all cases), respectively [12]. In the acute variant, approximately 70% of patients will develop hypercalcemia. ATL patients are functionally immunocompromised and may develop a variety of opportunistic infections, including cytomegalovirus or *Pneumocystis carinii* pneumonias, malignant strongyloidiasis, disseminated cryptococcosis or toxoplasmosis, disseminated fungal infections, as well as bacterial abscesses and sepsis [12–14].

Smoldering and chronic subtypes

Smoldering ATL is characterized by skin or lung infiltration without any other visceral involvement, a low number of leukemic cells (1–5% abnormal peripheral blood lymphocytes), and a normal leukocyte count. In chronic ATL, a high leukocyte count is observed and this is associated with a tumor syndrome (lymphadenopathy and hepatosplenomegaly). However, there is no associated hypercalcemia, infiltration of the central nervous system (CNS), gastrointestinal tract or bones, and the lactate dehydrogenase (LDH) level is normal or only slightly increased (less than twice the upper limit of normal).

Diagnostic criteria

The diagnosis of ATL is based on a combination of characteristic clinical presentation, morphologic and immunophenotypic features of the malignant cells,

Clinical Guide to Transplantation in Lymphoma, First Edition. Edited by Bipin N. Savani and Mohamad Mohty.

along with confirmation of HTLV-I infection [11]. ATL tumor cells are detected in peripheral blood in cases of acute, chronic, or smoldering type with leukemic manifestations or from biopsy of involved organs in ATL lymphoma. At least 5% of circulating abnormal T lymphocytes is required to diagnose ATL in patients without histologically proven tumor lesions [10]. These tumor cells, also termed "flower cells" and considered pathognomonic of ATL, are malignant activated lymphocytes with convoluted nuclei, and basophilic cytoplasm [12] expressing CD2, CD4 and CD5, CD45RO, CD29, T-cell receptor αβ and are usually negative for CD7, CD8 and CD26 and show reduced CD3 expression. The lymphocytic activation markers HLA-DP, -DQ, -DR and IL-2Rα (CD25) are always present [12] whereas terminal deoxynucleotidyl transferase (TdT) is typically absent.

Treatment options

Treatment of ATL is usually dependent on the ATL subtype. Patients with aggressive forms (acute and lymphoma) have a very poor prognosis because of intrinsic chemoresistance, a large tumor burden, hypercalcemia and/or frequent infectious complications due to profound immunodeficiency (2,10,15–17).

Conventional chemotherapy

Multiple Japanese trials in aggressive ATL clearly demonstrated that although combinations of chemotherapy have improved the response rates, particularly in ATL lymphoma, they failed to achieve a significant impact on long-term survival. A Japanese Phase III study demonstrated that the LSG15 regimen is superior to biweekly CHOP (cyclophosphamide, doxorubicin, vincristine, and prednisone) in newly diagnosed acute, lymphoma, or unfavorable chronic ATL. The complete remission (CR) rate in the LSG15 and CHOP arms was 40% and 25%, respectively, while 3-year overall survival (OS) in the LSG15 and CHOP arms was 24% and 13%, respectively. However, the median survival of 13 months remains disappointing [18].

Watch and wait policy for indolent ATL

Patients with smoldering or chronic ATL subtypes have a better prognosis than the aggressive variants of ATL [10]. In a recent Brazilian study, in which patients with ATL were followed on an expectant policy for 14 years, the reported median survival of chronic and smoldering types was only 18 months and 58 months, respectively,

and the OS rates were less than 20% at 5 years in both types [19]. Another recent Japanese study with a longer follow-up period confirmed that indolent ATL had a poor prognosis: patients with smoldering ATL had an estimated 15-year survival rate of 12.7% with a median survival of 2.9 years, while patients with chronic ATL had an estimated 15-year survival rate of 14.7% with a median survival of 5.3 years [20]. Importantly, in this study, patients who received chemotherapy had a significantly lower survival as compared to patients treated on a watch and wait policy [20].

Antiviral therapy

An important advance in the treatment of ATL was initially reported in two preliminary Phase II studies with the combination of the antiretroviral agent zidovudine (AZT) and interferon alpha (IFN) [21–23]. The efficacy of this combination was then confirmed in multiple small series [24]. A worldwide meta-analysis including survival data on 238 patients with ATL treated between 1995 and 2008 [25] showed that first-line antiviral therapy (AVT) alone resulted in 5-year OS of 46% compared with 20% following chemotherapy alone. Patients with acute, chronic, and smoldering ATL obtained significant benefit from first-line AVT alone while chemotherapy alone was superior in lymphoma ATL. Achievement of CR following AVT alone in patients with acute ATL resulted in 82% 5-year OS. In chronic ATL, treatment with AVT was associated with 100% 5-year survival. Multivariate analysis confirmed that first-line AVT significantly improved OS of ATL patients.

Novel agents and monoclonal antibodies

Multiple preclinical or preliminary clinical studies have reported the efficacy of novel agents including arsenic trioxide either alone or combined with IFN [26–28], bortezomib [29], and monoclonal antibodies against CD25 (daclizumab) [30], CD52 (alemtuzumab) [31], CCR4 (KW-0761) [32] or CD30 (brentuximab vedotin). The most promising results are those reported with the combination of arsenic trioxide and IFN or with KW-0761.

Hematopoietic stem cell transplantation for ATL

A review of the published literature reveals that hematopoietic stem cell transplantation (HSCT) has been applied to a limited number of ATL patients, with all the reported series originating from one geographical location, Japan.

Autologous HSCT

High-dose chemotherapy and autologous (auto)-HSCT has been reported in only 16 ATL patients [33,34]. All patients relapsed or died from transplant-related mortality (TRM). Hence, this treatment strategy is not currently recommended.

Allogeneic HSCT

Retrospective studies have confirmed that allografting using either myeloablative conditioning (MAC) [35–37] or reduced-intensity conditioning (RIC) [38] is a feasible option for patients with ATL. Age and remission status at HSCT were identified as predictors of survival. A large retrospective study included 386 patients allografted between 1995 and 2005 using either MAC or RIC [39]. After a median follow-up of 41 months, the 3-year OS was 33%. Interestingly, donor HTLV-I seropositivity adversely affected disease-associated mortality, specifically for patients who received transplants from related donors.

Myeloablative conditioning

A large serie of 40 MAC allogeneic (allo)-HSCT performed for ATL in Japan between 1997 and 2002 has been reported [37]. The majority of donors were siblings, five of whom were mismatched, while eight unrelated donors were used. Although 12 of 40 (30%) had resistant disease before transplant, all evaluable cases entered CR after allo-HSCT but the median OS for all patients was only 9.6 months. The estimated 3-year OS and progression free survival (PFS), and relapse rate were 45.3%, 33.8%, and 39.3%, respectively. Interestingly, among 10 patients with ATL relapse, five patients achieved CR again, three of whom attained remission following reduction or cessation of immunosuppressive agents, which suggested a graft-versus-ATL effect. TRM was high at 41%. On multivariate analysis the use of a related donor significantly improved the relapse-free survival through a reduction in graft-versus-host disease (GVHD), while the occurrence of acute GVHD reduced OS with no benefit in reduction of relapse.

Reduced-intensity conditioning

Recently, interesting long-term results of 30 patients who received RIC HSCT demonstrated OS and PFS rates of 36% and 31%, respectively [40].

Related donors

A nationwide Japanese retrospective analysis reported 154 ATL patients who received allo-HSCT from matched related donors [39]. Despite 37% relapse after a median of around 2 months and a median OS of 9.8 months, long-term results were encouraging with 3-year OS of 41%. However, allo-HSCT from mismatched related donors remains experimental. Indeed, of 43 Japanese ATL patients who received this transplant modality, 51% relapsed at a median of 2 months with a median OS of 2.5 months and a 3-year OS of 24% [39].

Unrelated donors

A small ($N = 8$) Japanese retrospective analysis demonstrated the efficacy of MAC ($N = 5$) or RIC ($N = 3$) allo-HSCT using unrelated donors [41]. Six patients (75%) were transplanted in CR. Five of eight patients were alive and disease-free at median follow-up of 20 months after HSCT. Two early deaths were secondary to an encephalopathy of unknown etiology. A larger retrospective analysis of 33 patients with ATL who underwent HSCT from unrelated donors through the Japan Marrow Donor Program has been reported [42]. In this study only 13 patients (39%) were in CR at time of transplant. OS, PFS, and cumulative incidence of disease progression and progression-free mortality at 1 year after allo-HSCT were 49.5%, 49.2%, 18.6%, and 32.3%, respectively, indicating that allo-HSCT from unrelated donors appears to be efficacious in ATL but with significant TRM. Univariate analysis identified recipient age ($P = 0.022$) and nonremission at time of transplant ($P = 0.044$) as prognostic factors, whereas on multivariate analysis only recipient age was significant for OS ($P = 0.044$). GVHD was not significantly associated with survival. While grade II–IV acute GVHD occurred in 61% of patients, only 26% of long-term survivors developed chronic GVHD, and thus the possible association of GVHD with a graft-versus-ATL effect on OS could not be assessed. Previous reports have indicated that GVHD rates may be lower in Japanese compared to Western populations through reduced diversity of HLA genes [43]. The TRM in this study was high at 27%, explained in part by the high proportion of MAC transplants and the high median age.

Umbilical cord blood transplantation

A retrospective report from Japan on the use of RIC umbilical cord blood transplantation in 70 relatively elderly patients (median age 61 years), included 12

(17%) patients with ATL [44]. Overall nonrelapse mortality was high at 62%, and 2-year OS was 23%. Similar poor outcome was reported in 90 patients undergoing single umbilical cord blood transplantation with a 3-year OS of 17% [39].

Proviral load and follow-up of minimal residual disease

Several reports suggested that negative minimal residual disease (MRD) using HTLV-I proviral DNA following MAC or RIC allo-HSCT is associated with prolonged remission of ATL [45–48]. However, a secondary rise in HTLV-I proviral DNA or conversion from MRD negativity to MRD positivity may not necessarily indicate early ATL relapse. Indeed, MRD conversion may be related to *de novo* infection of donor lymphocytes. Hence, the significance of post-transplant monitoring of HTLV-I proviral DNA in ATL should be explored in prospective studies.

Donor lymphocyte infusion and evidence for graft-versus-ATL effect

The observation that some ATL relapses could be successfully managed with a reduction in immunosuppression suggests a graft-versus-leukemia effect [38,49,50]. Objective responses were reported in Nagasaki among ATL patients treated with donor lymphocyte infusion for relapse after allo-HSCT. Interestingly, these responses were durable, with three cases of long-term remission of more than 3 years [51]. A graft-versus-ATL effect is also suggested by the results of the national Japanese retrospective study [52].

EBMT report

A recent retrospective analysis of the European Society for Blood and Marrow Transplantation (EBMT) registry revealed 21 HTLV-I seropositive ATL patients, including seven acute and 12 lymphoma subtypes [53]. Four patients received auto-HSCT and rapidly died from ATL. Of 17 allo-HSCT patients (4 MAC, 13 RIC), six are still alive (four were in CR1 at HSCT). Eleven patients died within 2 years, eight from relapse/progression and three from transplant toxicity. Six of seven informative patients who lived more than 12 months had chronic GVHD. Overall, allo-HSCT but not auto-HSCT may salvage a subset of ATL patients, supporting the

existence of a graft-versus-ATL effect also in non-Japanese patients.

Recommendations for ATL therapy

Chronic and smoldering ATL

All patients with chronic and smoldering ATL should be treated, but not with chemotherapy. Outside clinical trials, the current standard therapy for chronic and smoldering ATL is combination therapy with AZT and IFN (Figure 21.1). However, this requires continuous therapy, since relapse always occurs when treatment is stopped. The recommended starting dose is AZT 900 mg/day (in three divided doses) and IFN (5–6 million IU/m^2 daily). Usually, after 1 month, AZT dose can be titrated down to 600 mg/day in two divided doses and IFN dose can be reduced to 3–5 million IU/day or alternatively 1.5 µg/kg of pegylated IFN weekly.

ATL lymphoma

Chemotherapy should be the preferred option for patients with ATL lymphoma. Recent results from the UK suggest that the combination of AVT with CHOP chemotherapy is superior to CHOP alone in patients with ATL lymphoma [55]. Finally, following recent encouraging results, allo-HSCT is recommended for young patients with ATL lymphoma and matched donor.

Acute ATL

Outside clinical trials, the current standard therapy for acute ATL is combination therapy with AZT and IFN (Figure 21.1) but it should be noted that only achievement of a CR is associated with a long-term response. Preliminary results indicate that patients with wild-type p53 are responders [56]. However, long-term disease control requires continuous therapy, since relapse is always noted when treatment is stopped. The recommended starting dose is AZT 900 mg/day (in three divided doses) and IFN (5–6 million IU/m^2 daily). Usually, after 1 or 2 months, AZT dose can be reduced to 600 mg/day in two divided doses and IFN dose can be reduced to 3–5 million IU/day. Allo-HSCT is recommended for young patients with acute ATL and matched donor in the absence of CR after AVT.

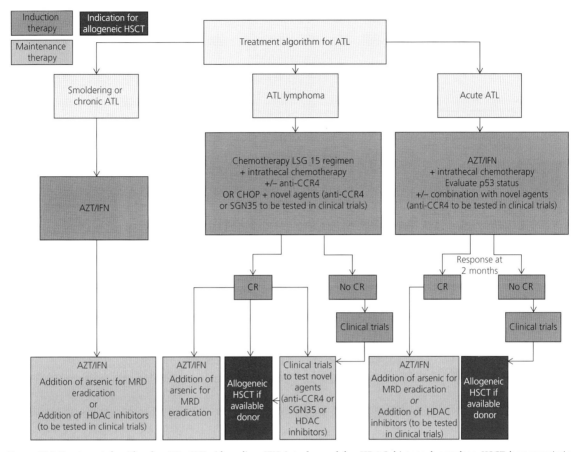

Figure 21.1 Treatment algorithm for ATL. AZT, zidovudine; IFN, interferon alpha; HDAC, histone deacetylase; HSCT, hematopoietic stem cell transplantation; MRD, minimal residual disease.

Supportive therapy in ATL

Hyercalcaemia should be managed with treatment of the disease, hydration, and bisphosphonate therapy. Trimethoprim–sulfamethoxazole, valacyclovir, and antifungal agents are recommended for the prophylaxis of *Pneumocystis jiroveci* pneumonia, viral and fungal infections [18]. Prophylaxis with anti-strongyloidiasis agents, such as ivermectin or albendazole, should be considered to avoid systemic infection in patients with a history of past and/or present exposure to the parasite. Intrathecal prophylaxis should be considered for patients with aggressive ATL even in the absence of clinical symptoms because more than half of relapses at new sites after chemotherapy are in the CNS.

Conclusion

Allo-HSCT using MAC or RIC should be considered in suitable patients. These include all newly diagnosed ATL lymphoma cases, acute ATL patients who fail to achieve CR with AVT, and relapsed ATL patients regardless of subtype. Importantly, HSCT should be planned early in the course of treatment because of the rapidly progressive nature of aggressive ATL and the potential difficulty in identifying a suitable donor, particularly for patients from ethnic minorities. Sibling donors should be tested initially, although outcome seems inferior with HTLV-I positive donors [39]. When matched related or unrelated donors cannot be identified, the use of alternative donor sources such as mismatched haploidentical sibling donors and umbilical cord blood transplantation remains experimental.

Case study

A 47-year-old female from the Dominican Republic with no significant past medical history presented with a 5-month history of asymptomatic cervical lymph nodes. Physical examination showed peripheral lymphadenopathies and splenomegaly. Computed tomography (CT) of chest, abdomen, and pelvis showed diffuse axillary, retroperitoneal, iliac, and inguinal lymph nodes and splenomegaly. Complete blood count showed lymphocytosis (white cell count 23,000 with 80% lymphocytes), normal hemoglobin and platelets. Blood smear showed atypical lymphocytes with basophilic cytoplasm and convoluted nuclei. Chemistry showed normal electrolytes, normal renal and liver function, and LDH at 1.8 upper normal level. Flow cytometry revealed expression of CD2, CD4, CD25, and HLA-DR whereas CD8 and CD7 were negative. HIV serology was negative. HTLV-I serology was positive. Diagnosis of adult T-cell leukemia/lymphoma, chronic subtype was made. What is the recommended management?

A Watch and wait.

B CHOP chemotherapy.

C Fludarabine-based chemotherapy.

D Combination of zidovudine and interferon alpha.

E Allogeneic HSCT.

Correct answer: D

Although chronic ATL is asymptomatic and labeled as indolent ATL, long-term prognosis is dismal if patients are managed on a watch-and-wait strategy or treated with chemotherapy. Conversely, the combination of zidovudine and interferon alpha is highly effective in indolent ATL, resulting in excellent long-term survival. There is no need for transplantation.

    The patient was treated with the combination of zidovudine and interferon alpha and achieved complete remission after 3 months. She was advised to continue treatment indefinitely. However, she stopped treatment on her own after 8 months of therapy and was lost to follow-up. One year later she presented with a 1-month history of dry cough, fatigue, weight loss, and epigastric pain. Routine blood tests revealed 70,000 circulating white cells (80% lymphocytes, most of them with atypical features), and severe hypercalcemia. CT of chest showed lung leukemic infiltrates. She still had excellent performance status. She was diagnosed with acute ATL subtype. She received symptomatic treatment for hypercalcemia and was restarted on zidovudine and interferon-alpha. Follow-up at 3 months and at 6 months showed only partial response. What is the recommended management?

A Continue zidovudine and interferon-alpha.

B Salvage chemotherapy.

C Salvage chemotherapy followed by autologous HSCT.

D Allogeneic HSCT.

Correct answer: D

Interruption of zidovudine and interferon-alpha always results in disease relapse. Acute ATL patients have a dismal prognosis. The combination of zidovudine and interferon-alpha results in response in two-thirds of the patients but in CR in only one-third of them. Only CR patients on zidovudine and interferon-alpha have an excellent long-term survival. Allogeneic HSCT is the only potentially curative modality and results in long-term survival in 35–40% of acute ATL patients. Chemotherapy and autologous HSCT are not effective in acute ATL and should not be proposed.

References

1 Uchiyama T, Yodoi J, Sagawa K, Takatsuki K, Uchino H. Adult T-cell leukemia: clinical and hematologic features of 16 cases. *Blood* 1977;50:481–92.

2 Bazarbachi A, Ghez D, Lepelletier Y *et al.* New therapeutic approaches for adult T-cell leukaemia. *Lancet Oncol* 2004; 5:664–72.

3 Matsuoka M, Jeang KT. Human T-cell leukaemia virus type 1 (HTLV-1) infectivity and cellular transformation. *Nat Rev Cancer* 2007;7:270–80.

4 Kaplan JE, Khabbaz RF. The epidemiology of human T-lymphotropic virus types I and II. *Rev Med Virol* 1993;3: 137–48.

5 Paun L, Ispas O, Del Mistro A, Chieco-Bianchi L. HTLV-I in Romania. *Eur J Haematol* 1994;52:117–18.

6 Höllsberg P, Hafler DA, Gessain A. Epidemiology of HTLV-1 and associated disease. In: Höllsberg P, Hafler DA, eds. *Human T-Cell Lymphotropic Virus Type 1*. Chichester: John Wiley & Sons, 1996:33–64.

7 Abbaszadegan MR, Gholamin M, Tabatabaee A, Farid R, Houshmand M, Abbaszadegan M. Prevalence of human

T-lymphotropic virus type 1 among blood donors from Mashhad, Iran. *J Clin Microbiol* 2003;41:2593–5.

8 Franchini G, Ambinder RF, Barry M. Viral disease in hematology. *Hematology Am Soc Hematol Educ Program* 2000;409–23.

9 Swerdlow SH, Campo E, Harris NL, Jaffe ES, Pileri SA, Stein H, Thiele J, Vardiman JW (eds) *World Health Organization Classification of Tumours of Haematopoietic and Lymphoid Tissues*, 4th edn. Lyon: IARC Press, 2008.

10 Shimoyama M. Diagnostic criteria and classification of clinical subtypes of adult T-cell leukaemia-lymphoma. A report from the Lymphoma Study Group (1984–87). *Br J Haematol* 1991;79:428–37.

11 Tsukasaki K, Hermine O, Bazarbachi A *et al*. Definition, prognostic factors, treatment, and response criteria of adult T-cell leukemia-lymphoma: a proposal from an international consensus meeting. *J Clin Oncol* 2009;27:453–9.

12 Takatsuki K, Yamaguchi K, Hattori T. Adult T-cell leukemia/lymphoma. In: Gallo RC, Wong-Staal F, eds. *Retrovirus Biology and Human Disease*. New York: Marcel Dekker, 1990:147–59.

13 Bunn PA Jr, Schechter GP, Jaffe E *et al*. Clinical course of retrovirus-associated adult T-cell lymphoma in the United States. *N Engl J Med* 1983;309:257–64.

14 Verdonck K, Gonzalez E, Van Dooren S, Vandamme AM, Vanham G, Gotuzzo E. Human T-lymphotropic virus 1: recent knowledge about an ancient infection. *Lancet Infect Dis* 2007;7:266–81.

15 Hermine O, Wattel E, Gessain A, Bazarbachi A. Adult T cell leukaemia: a review of established and new treatments. *BioDrugs* 1998;10:447–62.

16 Bazarbachi A, Hermine O. Treatment of adult T-cell leukaemia/lymphoma: current strategy and future perspectives. *Virus Res* 2001;78:79–92.

17 Tobinai K. Current management of adult T-cell leukemia/lymphoma. *Oncology (Williston Park)* 2009;23:1250–6.

18 Tsukasaki K, Utsunomiya A, Fukuda H *et al*. VCAP-AMP-VECP compared with biweekly CHOP for adult T cell leukemia-lymphoma: Japan Clinical Oncology Group Study JCOG9801. *J Clin Oncol* 2007;25:5458–64.

19 Bittencourt AL, da Gracas Vieira M, Brites CR, Farre L, Barbosa HS. Adult T-cell leukemia/lymphoma in Bahia, Brazil: analysis of prognostic factors in a group of 70 patients. *Am J Clin Pathol* 2007;128:875–82.

20 Takasaki Y, Iwanaga M, Imaizumi Y *et al*. Long-term study of indolent adult T-cell leukemia-lymphoma. *Blood* 2010; 115:4337–43.

21 Gill PS, Harrington W Jr, Kaplan MH *et al*. Treatment of adult T-cell leukemia-lymphoma with a combination of interferon alfa and zidovudine. *N Engl J Med* 1995;332: 1744–8.

22 Hermine O, Bouscary D, Gessain A *et al*. Brief report: treatment of adult T-cell leukemia-lymphoma with zidovudine and interferon alfa. *N Engl J Med* 1995;332: 1749–51.

23 Bazarbachi A, Hermine O. Treatment with a combination of zidovudine and alpha-interferon in naive and pretreated adult T-cell leukemia/lymphoma patients. *J Acquir Immune Defic Syndr Hum Retrovirol* 1996;13(Suppl 1):S186–90.

24 Hermine O, Allard I, Levy V, Arnulf B, Gessain A, Bazarbachi A. A prospective phase II clinical trial with the use of zidovudine and interferon-alpha in the acute and lymphoma forms of adult T-cell leukemia/lymphoma. *Hematol J* 2002;3:276–82.

25 Bazarbachi A, Plumelle Y, Carlos Ramos J *et al*. Meta-analysis on the use of zidovudine and interferon-alfa in adult T-cell leukemia/lymphoma showing improved survival in the leukemic subtypes. *J Clin Oncol* 2010;28:4177–83.

26 Hermine O, Dombret H, Poupon J *et al*. Phase II trial of arsenic trioxide and alpha interferon in patients with relapsed/refractory adult T-cell leukemia/lymphoma. *Hematol J* 2004;5:130–4.

27 Kchour G, Tarhini M, Kooshyar MM *et al*. Phase 2 study of the efficacy and safety of the combination of arsenic trioxide, interferon alpha, and zidovudine in newly diagnosed chronic adult T-cell leukemia/lymphoma (ATL). *Blood* 2009;113:6528–32.

28 El Hajj H, El-Sabban M, Hasegawa H *et al*. Therapy-induced selective loss of leukemia-initiating activity in murine adult T cell leukemia. *J Exp Med* 2010;207:2785–92.

29 Nasr R, El-Sabban ME, Karam JA *et al*. Efficacy and mechanism of action of the proteasome inhibitor PS-341 in T-cell lymphomas and HTLV-I associated adult T-cell leukemia/lymphoma. *Oncogene* 2005;24:419–30.

30 Ceesay MM, Matutes E, Taylor GP *et al*. Phase II study on combination therapy with CHOP-Zenapax for HTLV-I associated adult T-cell leukaemia/lymphoma (ATLL). *Leukemia Res* 2012;36:857–61.

31 Mone A, Puhalla S, Whitman S *et al*. Durable hematologic complete response and suppression of HTLV-1 viral load following alemtuzumab in zidovudine/IFN-α-refractory adult T-cell leukemia. *Blood* 2005;106:3380–2.

32 Yamamoto K, Utsunomiya A, Tobinai K *et al*. Phase I study of KW-0761, a defucosylated humanized anti-CCR4 antibody, in relapsed patients with adult T-cell leukemia-lymphoma and peripheral T-cell lymphoma. *J Clin Oncol* 2010;28:1591–8.

33 Tsukasaki K, Maeda T, Arimura K *et al*. Poor outcome of autologous stem cell transplantation for adult T cell leukemia/lymphoma: a case report and review of the literature. *Bone Marrow Transplant* 1999;23:87–9.

34 Phillips AA, Willim RD, Savage DG *et al*. A multi-institutional experience of autologous stem cell transplantation in North American patients with human T-cell lymphotropic virus type-1 adult T-cell leukemia/lymphoma suggests ineffective salvage of relapsed patients. *Leukemia Lymphoma* 2009;50:1039–42.

35 Utsunomiya A, Miyazaki Y, Takatsuka Y *et al*. Improved outcome of adult T cell leukemia/lymphoma with allogeneic hematopoietic stem cell transplantation. *Bone Marrow Transplant* 2001;27:15–20.

36 Kami M, Hamaki T, Miyakoshi S *et al*. Allogeneic haemato-poietic stem cell transplantation for the treatment of adult T-cell leukaemia/lymphoma. *Br J Haematol* 2003;120:304–9.

37 Fukushima T, Miyazaki Y, Honda S *et al*. Allogeneic hemato-poietic stem cell transplantation provides sustained long-term survival for patients with adult T-cell leukemia/lymphoma. *Leukemia* 2005;19:829–34.

38 Okamura J, Utsunomiya A, Tanosaki R *et al*. Allogeneic stem-cell transplantation with reduced conditioning inten-sity as a novel immunotherapy and antiviral therapy for adult T-cell leukemia/lymphoma. *Blood* 2005;105:4143–5.

39 Hishizawa M, Kanda J, Utsunomiya A *et al*. Transplantation of allogeneic hematopoietic stem cells for adult T-cell leu-kemia: a nationwide retrospective study. *Blood* 2010;116: 1369–76.

40 Uike N, Tanosaki R, Utsunomiya A, Choi I, Okamura J. Can allo-SCT with RIC cure ATLL? Long-term survivors with excellent PS and with heterogenous HTLV-1 proviral load level. *Retrovirology* 2011;8(Suppl 1):A33.

41 Nakase K, Hara M, Kozuka T, Tanimoto K, Nawa Y. Bone marrow transplantation from unrelated donors for patients with adult T-cell leukaemia/lymphoma. *Bone Marrow Transplant* 2006;37:41–4.

42 Kato K, Kanda Y, Eto T *et al*. Allogeneic bone marrow trans-plantation from unrelated human T-cell leukemia virus-I-negative donors for adult T-cell leukemia/lymphoma: retrospective analysis of data from the Japan Marrow Donor Program. *Biol Blood Marrow Transplant* 2007;13:90–9.

43 Morishima Y, Kodera Y, Hirabayashi N *et al*. Low incidence of acute GVHD in patients transplanted with marrow from HLA-A,B,DR-compatible unrelated donors among Japanese. *Bone Marrow Transplant* 1995;15:235–9.

44 Uchida N, Wake A, Takagi S *et al*. Umbilical cord blood trans-plantation after reduced-intensity conditioning for elderly patients with hematologic diseases. *Biol Blood Marrow Transplant* 2008;14:583–90.

45 Tajima K, Amakawa R, Uehira K *et al*. Adult T-cell leukemia successfully treated with allogeneic bone marrow transplan-tation. *Int J Hematol* 2000;71:290–3.

46 Abe Y, Yashiki S, Choi I *et al*. Eradication of virus-infected T-cells in a case of adult T-cell leukemia/lymphoma by non-myeloablative peripheral blood stem cell transplantation with conditioning consisting of low-dose total body irradia-tion and pentostatin. *Int J Hematol* 2002;76:91–3.

47 Ogata M, Ogata Y, Imamura T *et al*. Successful bone marrow transplantation from an unrelated donor in a patient with adult T cell leukemia. *Bone Marrow Transplant* 2002;30: 699–701.

48 Choi I, Tanosaki R, Uike N *et al*. Long-term outcomes after hematopoietic SCT for adult T-cell leukemia/lymphoma: results of prospective trials. *Bone Marrow Transplant* 2011; 46:116–18.

49 Harashima N, Kurihara K, Utsunomiya A *et al*. Graft-versus-Tax response in adult T-cell leukemia patients after hematopoietic stem cell transplantation. *Cancer Res* 2004; 64:391–9.

50 Shiratori S, Yasumoto A, Tanaka J *et al*. A retrospective anal-ysis of allogeneic hematopoietic stem cell transplantation for adult T cell leukemia/lymphoma (ATL): clinical impact of graft-versus-leukemia/lymphoma effect. *Biol Blood Marrow Transplant* 2008;14:817–23.

51 Itonaga H, Tsushima H, Taguchi J *et al*. Treatment of relapsed adult T-cell leukemia/lymphoma after allogeneic hemato-poietic stem cell transplantation: the Nagasaki Transplant Group experience. *Blood* 2013;121:219–25.

52 Ishida T, Hishizawa M, Kato K *et al*. Impact of graft-versus-host disease on allogeneic hematopoietic cell transplanta-tion for adult T cell leukemia-lymphoma focusing on preconditioning regimens: nationwide retrospective study. *Biol Blood Marrow Transplant* 2013;19:1731–9.

53 Bazarbachi A, Cwynarski K, Boumendil A *et al*. Outcome of patients with HTLV-1 associated adult T-cell leukemia/lym-phoma (ATL) who have undergone stem cell transplanta-tion: a retrospective study of the EBMT Lymphoma Working Party. *Blood (ASH Annual Meeting Abstracts)* 2013; 122:3398.

54 Yamada Y, Tomonaga M, Fukuda H *et al*. A new G-CSF-sup-ported combination chemotherapy, LSG15, for adult T-cell leukaemia-lymphoma: Japan Clinical Oncology Group Study 9303. *Br J Haematol* 2001;113:375–82.

55 Hodson A Montoto S, Mir N *et al*. Addition of anti-viral therapy to chemotherapy improves overall survival in acute and lymphomatous adult T-cell leukemia/lymphoma (ATLL). *Blood (ASH Annual Meeting Abstracts)* 2010;116; Abstract 3961.

56 Datta A, Bellon M, Sinha-Datta U *et al*. Persistent inhibition of telomerase reprograms adult T-cell leukemia to p53-dependent senescence. *Blood* 2006;108:1021–9.

CHAPTER 22

Hematopoietic cell transplantation for HIV-related lymphomas

Joseph C. Alvarnas

Origins and epidemiology of HIV/AIDS

A syndrome of immunodeficiency associated with atypical opportunistic infections and unusual malignancies was initially recognized in the United States in 1981 [1–3]. The acquired immunodeficiency syndrome (AIDS) was shortly thereafter recognized as a unique clinically entity and the Centers for Disease Control (CDC) definition of the disease achieved worldwide acceptance [4,5]. By 1984, investigators identified a retroviral infection, caused by two lentiviruses, as the underlying cause of AIDS. These viruses were respectively termed human immunodeficiency virus (HIV) 1 and 2 (Figure 22.1) [6,7]. Following entry into the body, HIV rapidly propagates throughout the lymphoid tissues. HIV enters host CD4+ T cells by binding to the CD4 surface receptor and, depending on its trophism, enters the cell through interaction with the CXC chemokine receptor 4 (CXCR4) (X4 trophic) or C-C chemokine receptor 5 (CCR5) (R5 trophic) [8]. Over time there is progressive depletion of naïve and memory CD4+ T cells that leads to a profoundly immunodeficient state [9].

As of 2012, the World Health Organization (WHO) estimates that more than 35 million people are living with HIV infection, including 17.1 million women and 3.3 million children less than 15 years of age [10,11]. Since the beginning of the epidemic, more than 25 million people have died from HIV infection [12]. In 2012 there were an estimated 2.3 million people who were newly infected with HIV, including 260,000 children less than 15 years of age [11]. Today more than half of all those infected with HIV are women and heterosexual transmission of the virus accounts for a majority of new infections worldwide [10,11].

Highly active antiretroviral therapy

Prior to the advent of highly active antiretroviral therapy (HAART) care of patients with HIV/AIDS was largely supportive [13]. In March 1987 the Food and Drug Administration (FDA) approved zidovudine (AZT) as the first anti-HIV antiretroviral [13,14]. The impact of single-agent antiretroviral therapy was limited; by 1993 there was evidence of HIV-1 resistance to zidovudine. Additional antiretrovirals were introduced in the following years, but the impact of these agents was modest at best [15,16]. By the end of 1995, over 513,000 cases of AIDS had been reported in the United States with 319,849 associated deaths [15].

At the 1996 XI International AIDS Conference in Vancouver, Canada, several groups reported on the profound effectiveness of novel combinations of antiretroviral agents [15,17,18]. HAART regimens resulted in marked suppression of HIV viral load, promoted recovery of CD4+ T-cell counts, and produced a profound decline in the rate of opportunistic infections [19–21]. By 1997, US AIDS deaths had declined by 42% [15,19,20]. WHO estimates that 700,000 deaths were averted in 2010 alone through the use of HAART [22].

Clinical Guide to Transplantation in Lymphoma, First Edition. Edited by Bipin N. Savani and Mohamad Mohty.

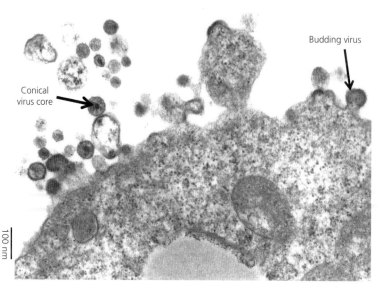

Figure 22.1 HIV-1 virion structures. Electron micrograph of CD4+ H9 T lymphocyte infected with HIV-1 strain IIIB (magnification 71,250×). Arrows indicate either a budding structure at the cell margin or a dense virus core of the nucelocapsid–RNA–protein structure. Photo-electron micrograph prepared at the City of Hope Electron Microscope Core by M. Miller PhD from tissue culture prepared by S. Li MD, Department of Virology, Beckman Research Institute of City of Hope.

In addition to reducing mortality, HAART also reduces transmission rates for HIV infection and decreases the risk of maternal–child transmission [19,22].

Cancer risk in patients with HIV/AIDS

Initial reports demonstrated that the risk of Kaposi sarcoma (KS) in AIDS was 2000-fold higher than in the general population [23]. There was also an increased risk of primary central nervous system lymphoma (PCNSL), particularly in patients with severely depleted immune systems [24,25]. The initial CDC definition of AIDS included KS and PCNSL as AIDS-defining diagnoses [5]. Based on the discovery of a 60–100 fold increased risk of non-Hodgkin lymphoma (NHL) in HIV-infected patients, the diagnostic criteria for AIDS were expanded to include all forms of NHL [25–27].

HIV-infected patients are also at higher risk for a number of non-AIDS-defining cancers [23,28–30]. The Swiss HIV Cohort study evaluated 7304 HIV-infected individuals who were followed for a total of 28,836 person-years. The investigators compared the cohort cancer incidence with that of the general population and calculated standardized incidence ratios (SIRs) for

the increased cancer risk. In addition to the AIDS-defining malignancies, SIRs were also increased for anal cancer (33.4), Hodgkin lymphoma (HL) (17.3), cervical cancer (8.0), liver cancer (7.0), and nonmelanoma skin cancers (3.2) [28].

Following the advent of HAART, the risk of AIDS-related lymphoma (ARL) has fallen by 50% [31,32]. The Swiss HIV Cohort study data demonstrate that risk ratios for development of ARL were much lower in individuals treated with HAART (24.2 vs. 99.3) [28]. Post HAART, ARL subtypes have also changed significantly, with a marked decline in PCNSL [28,32–34]. Interestingly, the risk of HL has not decreased post HAART [28,35].

NHL and HL in HIV-infected patients

Potential causes for ARL include chronic antigenic stimulation, profound loss of T-cell immunity, an abnormal cytokine milieu, and infection by oncogenic viruses [4,36–41]. There is a high rate of association with Epstein–Barr virus (EBV), with *in situ* hybridization studies demonstrating viral DNA present in 50% or more ARL samples [37,38]. Human herpesvirus

(HHV)-8 also plays a pathogenic role in the development of some subtypes of ARL, including primary effusion lymphoma (PEL) [36,42].

More than 95% of ARL is of B-cell derivation. The most common forms of ARL now include diffuse large B-cell lymphoma (DLBCL) (both centroblastic and immunoblastic variants) and Burkitt lymphoma (BL) [33,36,42,43]. Some forms of NHL are seen more frequently in patients with severely depleted immune systems, particularly PCNSL and plasmablastic lymphoma that typically occurs in patients with CD4$^+$ T-cell counts below 100/μL [24,25,36,42]. PEL represents less than 5% of ARL [32] and is unique because it is associated with coinfection by EBV and HHV-8 [42]. Peripheral T-cell lymphomas are quite rare and account for only 3.2% of ARL [36,44].

The WHO classification system recognizes three broad categories of HIV-associated lymphomas: those that also occur in immunocompetent patients; those that occur specifically in the setting of HIV infection; and those that also occur in other immunodeficiency states [36].

A majority of HIV-infected patients with HL have either the mixed cellularity or lymphocyte-depleted variants of the disease [35,36,45]. Evidence of EBV infection is found in 80–100% of patients with HIV-related HL [36].

Clinical presentation

Up to 80% of patients with ARL present with advanced-stage disease; 50% have gastrointestinal involvement and approximately 30% have bone marrow involvement at diagnosis. Up to 20% have evidence of CNS involvement at diagnosis. Patients with ARL are also more likely to have B symptoms (fevers, night sweats, weight loss >10% of body weight) at diagnosis [25,39]. HIV-infected patients diagnosed with HL are also more likely to present with more advanced-stage disease and up to 75% of patients present with B symptoms. Many have evidence of cytopenia and up to 60% have bone marrow involvement at diagnosis [35,45].

Prognosis and treatment of HIV-associated lymphoma

Prior to HAART, the prognosis for ARL was poor. In a series of 27 patients diagnosed with ARL prior to 1989, median survival was 0 months [37]. Initial attempts to deliver meaningful therapy to patients with ARL focused on the use of dose-attenuated regimens, such as low-dose m-BACOD (methotrexate, bleomycin, doxorubicin, cyclophosphamide, vincristine, dexamethasone) [46]. Following availability of HAART, there has been a shift toward use of standard-intensity regimens for patients with ARL and HL. This has resulted in significant improvements in patient outcomes. Gopol *et al.* [33] evaluated a cohort of patients with ARL who were diagnosed between 1996 and 2010. They reported 5-year overall survival (OS) rates that had risen to 61.6% for HL, 50.0% for BL, 44.1% for DLBCL, and 22.8% for PCNSL. The NHL International Prognostic Index (IPI) has demonstrated prognostic value in ARL [47,48]. The combination of CD4$^+$ T-cell counts at the time of lymphoma diagnosis and the IPI can be useful at predicting prognosis in ARL [39,49,50].

Survival rates for HIV-infected patients with NHL now clearly parallel those of non-HIV-infected patients [34]. The key to this progress has been ensuring effective control of HIV infection while managing this patient population [51]. CHOP (cyclophosphamide, doxorubicin, vincristine, prednisone) and rituximab (R)-CHOP are well tolerated by patients [52,53]. However, patients with CD4$^+$ T-cell counts below 50/μL receiving rituximab may have an increased risk of infection-related deaths [52].

Recent trials have demonstrated remarkable activity for infusional EPOCH-R (etoposide, prednisone, vincristine, cyclophosphamide, doxorubicin, rituximab) [31,41]. In a 2003 trial, 39 patients with ARL were treated with dose-adjusted EPOCH-R [54]; 31 had DLBCL and seven BL, while 26 patients had stage III/IV disease. HAART was suspended until the completion of chemotherapy. Patients were treated for six cycles. Complete response (CR) and partial response (PR) rates were 74% and 13%, respectively. At a median follow-up of 53 months, OS and progression-free survival (PFS) rates were 60% and 73%, respectively. Following resumption of HAART, patients achieved CD4$^+$ T-cell count recovery and control of viral load [54].

In a subsequent trial, 33 patients with AIDS-related DLCBL received a short course of EPOCH with double-dose rituximab (EPOCH-RR) [55]. Patients were treated with three to six cycles of therapy with treatment duration based on their response on imaging with fluorodeoxyglucose positron emission tomography (FDG-PET). Patients received a median of three cycles and 30 patients (91%) achieved a CR. At a median follow-up of 5 years, OS and PFS were 68% and 84%, respectively.

CHOP-like regimens are ineffective for patients with BL and are not recommended [41,56,57]. Post HAART, there has been a move toward treating BL patients with more intensive therapeutic regimens [58–60]. These include the hyper-CVAD regimen (cyclophosphamide, vincristine, doxorubicin, dexamethasone alternating with high-dose methotrexate/cytarabine) [59], CODOX-M/IVAC [60], and other dose-intensive regimens [58]. These intensive approaches produce 1-year PFS rates of up to 74.1% [60] but toxicity associated with some of these regimens may be limit their use [58].

EPOCH-RR appears to be both effective and well tolerated in HIV-infected patients with BL. Dunleavy *et al.* [61] published their experience using EPOCH-RR in 11 patients with AIDS-related BL. There were no treatment-related deaths and at a median follow-up of 73 months, OS was 100% with PFS of 90%.

In the HAART era, HL can be treated effectively with regimens such as ABVD (doxorubicin, bleomycin, vinblastine, dacarbazine), Stanford V, and BEACOPP (bleomycin, etoposide, doxorubicin, cyclophosphamide, vincristine, procarbazine, prednisone) with reasonable toxicity [62–64]. In a long-term update of outcomes for 62 patients who were treated with ABVD for advanced HL, the investigators found that at 9 years median follow-up, the 14-year probability of OS was estimated to be 65% [62]. These results rival those for non-HIV-infected patients.

Autologous hematopoietic cell transplantation for patients with AIDS-related lymphoma

The PARMA trial established autologous hematopoietic cell transplantation (HCT) as the standard of care for patients with chemotherapy-sensitive relapsed or refractory NHL [65]. Other groups have confirmed this finding and also demonstrated an essential role for autologous HCT for patients with relapsed and refractory HL [66]. Autologous HCT also now represents the standard of care for HIV-infected patients with relapsed and refractory NHL and HL who have controlled HIV infection.

Gabarre *et al.* [67] published the initial use of autologous HCT for a patient with ARL in 1996. The patient underwent autologous HCT in 1994 for chemotherapy-sensitive BL in second CR. His post-transplant course was complicated by a series of five opportunistic infections that culminated in his death. However, the patient remained in remission at the time of his death.

In 2000, this group published their expanded experience using autologous HCT for eight patients (including the previously reported patient) with HIV-related lymphoma, seven of whom were treated with HAART [68]. Median age at transplant was 39 years (range 27–53). The group included two patients with BL, two with immunoblastic lymphoma, and four with HL. All the patients mobilized adequately with a median hematopoietic progenitor cell (HPC) dose of CD34+ cells of 7.17×10^6/kg (range 4.5–17.6×10^6/kg). Five of the patients received total body irradiation (TBI)-containing preparative regimens; the remainder received chemotherapy alone. One patient died prior to engraftment; the remainder engrafted to neutrophils at a median of 12 days (range 9–18 days). All patients, except for the patient who underwent transplant prior to HAART, had undetectable HIV viral loads prior to transplant. Three patients experienced a post-HCT rise in their viral load. At the time of the publication, one patient had died of opportunistic infection (the index patient), three had died of progressive lymphoma, and four were alive and in CR at 4 to more than 15 months post HCT.

Beginning in 2000, the City of Hope group has published a series of reports demonstrating the feasibility, safety, and effectiveness of autologous HCT for patients with HIV-related lymphomas [69–72]. In 2005, they reported outcomes for 20 patients treated with autologous HCT for high-risk, relapsed, and refractory lymphoma [71]. Criteria for transplantation included the standard selection criteria for non-HIV-infected patients for autologous HCT, as well as the HIV-specific criteria of ongoing treatment with HAART, HIV viral load of less than 10,000 copies/mL, and no evidence of opportunistic infections for 1 year prior to HCT.

This group included four patients with IPI high-risk NHL who underwent HCT in first CR. Two patients underwent transplant for chemotherapy-sensitive relapsed HL. The remaining 14 patients underwent transplantation for chemotherapy-sensitive relapsed or refractory NHL. Median age was 44 years (range 11–68). At the time of transplant 17 patients had an undetectable viral load while the remaining three had viral loads ranging from 700 to 6500 copies/mL. Median CD4+ T-cell count at the time of transplant was 174/μL (range 30–500). A total of 17 patients underwent HCT using the CBV (carmustine, etoposide, cyclophosphamide) preparative regimen, while the remaining three were prepared with 12-Gy fractionated TBI, etoposide and cyclophosphamide. All patients successfully mobilized CD34+ cells; the group received a median CD34+ dose of 10.6×10^6/kg at the time of transplant. Median engraftment occurred at 11 days (range 9–23). One patient who was on zidovudine had evidence of delayed engraftment. There was one transplant-related death on day 22 post HCT due to the development of severe cardiomyopathy and renal failure. Post-transplant infectious complications included cytomegalovirus (CMV) viremia in two patients, CMV retinitis in one patient, and disseminated zoster in two patients. All responded to therapy. At a median follow-up of 31.8 months (range 5.5–70 months), OS for the group was 85% and PFS was 85%.

Eleven patients had interruptions of HAART due to gastrointestinal toxicities, while the remaining nine continued treatment throughout their transplant course. All patients experienced a nadir in their CD4+ T-cell counts that was maximal at 6 months post HCT, but all patients returned to their pretransplant CD4+ T-cell levels by 1 year post transplant. However, many patients experienced a rise in HIV viral levels post transplant, but 1 year after HCT 76% had undetectable viral loads. One patient had a persisting elevated viral load due to noncompliance with HAART regimen.

In 2003, Re *et al.* [73] reported their experience with autologous HCT for 16 HIV-infected patients with chemotherapy-sensitive relapsed or refractory lymphoma. All patients were responsive to treatment with HAART. Eight patients had NHL and eight had HL. Of the 16 patients, only 12 collected adequate CD34+ HPC grafts. One patient suffered disease progression prior to HPC collection. Two patients suffered progression of lymphoma after HPC collection and were not able to undergo transplant. Ten patients received high-dose therapy following the BEAM (BCNU, etoposide, ara-C, melphalan) preparative regimen. These patients achieved neutrophil engraftment at a median of 10 days (range 8–10 days). Of nine patients who were assessable for lymphoma response, seven achieved a CR and two patients achieved a PR. The estimated median survival for the entire patient group was 18 months and the projected 2-year OS was 39%. The investigators continued HAART through the entire treatment course. Only three patients required interruptions in HAART due to gastrointestinal toxicity. While the mean CD4+ T-cell counts dropped post

transplant, a recovery trend was seen by 6 months. No worsening in HIV infection was noted.

In 2004, Gabarre *et al.* [74] published a retrospective review of 14 HIV-infected patients who underwent autologous HCT. Six of the patients had relapsed or refractory HL; eight had relapsed NHL. The latter group included two patients with BL and one with PEL. Median age was 37 years (range 27–53). All patients received salvage chemotherapy prior to transplant; three patients had progressive disease and 11 responded (eight CR, three PR). All patients collected adequate HPC grafts with a median CD34+ cell yield of 5.8×10^6/kg (range $2.8–20 \times 10^6$/kg). Five patients were conditioned with BEAM; five received TBI and cyclophosphamide; two received TBI, cyclophosphamide, and thiotepa; one received TBI and melphalan; and one received busulfan, cytarabine, and melphalan. Seven patients died from relapsed lymphoma, one died from a secondary malignancy at 28 months post HCT, one patient died from AIDS-related complications at 16 months, and five remained alive at the time of the report. There was no loss of control over HIV infection following transplantation, although two patients experienced a spike in their viral loads following HAART interruption due to transplant-related gastrointestinal toxicity.

In a multicenter prospective trial published in 2005 by Serrano *et al.* [75], 14 patients with high-risk or relapsed HIV-related lymphoma underwent autologous HCT. The median patient age was 39.5 years (range 31–61). All patients were treated with HAART and had no opportunistic infections at the time of transplant. Three patients had HL and 11 had NHL (two anaplastic large cell, three BL or Burkitt-like, and six DLDCL). Ten patients had chemotherapy-sensitive relapsed or refractory lymphoma while four had high-risk NHL in first CR. All the patients collected HPC products successfully. Patients were prepared with either BEAM or BEAC (carmustine, etoposide, cytarabine, cyclophosphamide). Three patients died from disease progression prior to HCT. At a median of 30 months post HCT (range 7–36 months), the projected event-free survival (EFS) for the group was 65%. Of note, one of the patients in the group developed CMV infection following transplant.

In the AIDS Malignancy Consortium Study 020, the investigators prospectively studied autologous HPC in 27 patients with HIV-associated lymphoma [76]; 27 patients were enrolled in trial, but only 20 proceeded to HCT. Two patients failed to collect an adequate HPC dose, one developed cardiac toxicity, and four progressed prior to transplant. Patients were transplanted using the busulfan/cyclophosphamide preparative regimen. There was one transplant-related death due to venoocclusive disease of the liver. Neutrophil recovery was achieved at a median of 11 days (range 9–16 days). Nine of the patients demonstrated disease progression prior to day 100 following transplant. For the entire group, the median EFS was 23 weeks. As part of this trial, the investigators assessed CD4+ T-cell levels and HIV viral load during the peritransplant period and for 12 months afterward. Significant inter-patient variability was seen for both viral load and CD4+ T-cell counts. Some decrements in CD4+ T-cells counts were seen in the post-HCT period and some patients experienced spikes in their HIV viral load.

In 2009, Re *et al.* [77] published the results of an intention-to-treat study of 50 HAART-treated patients with HIV-related lymphoma. Median age was 39 years (range 28–59 years). The patients included 19 with HL and 31 with NHL. The patients had either relapsed or refractory disease. The patients received two to four cycles of salvage chemotherapy to test for responsiveness. Two of the patients died from therapy-related toxicity, 10 were chemotherapy resistant, and 38 chemotherapy sensitive. One patient withdrew from the study and 37 patients underwent HPC mobilization; six failed to mobilize. Of the 31 remaining patients, four developed disease progression. A total of 27 patients underwent high-dose therapy using the BEAM regimen. The patients engrafted at a median of 10 days (range 8–14). Post HCT, 24 patients achieved a CR and three had evidence of progressive disease. Of the 24 patients who achieved a CR, 21 remained in CR at the time of the study publication. Median survival for the entire patient cohort was 33 months. In the subgroup of 27 patients who underwent HCT, estimated PFS and OS were 75.9% and 74.6%, respectively, at a median of 44 months follow-up. Patients experienced nadir CD4+ T-cell counts at approximately 3 months post transplant with recovery by 6 months. Of 23 patients who had an undetectable viral load before HCT, eight developed a rise in the viral load after transplant, one of whom failed to suppress below the detectable level in the subsequent year. Five patients developed either CMV viremia or visceral disease post transplant.

In a retrospective review from the European Society for Blood and Marrow Transplantation (EBMT) Lymphoma

Working Party registry, 68 patients with HIV-related lymphoma who had undergone autologous HCT were analyzed [78]. Patients were treated at 20 different institutions with either the BEAM preparative regimen (65 patients) or TBI-containing regimens (three patients). These included 50 patients with NHL and 18 patients with HL. Of the patients, 16 were in first CR, 19 were in a second or greater CR, 25 were in PR, and eight patients had induction failures or chemotherapy-resistant disease. Median age was 41.3 years (range 29–62.5). Median time to neutrophil engraftment was 11 days (range 8–36). Four patients died from nonrelapse mortality, including one who died from multiorgan failure on day 15. At a median follow-up of 32 months, the 3-year estimated PFS and OS were 56% and 61%, respectively.

Two groups have now published case–control studies of autologous HCT for patients with HIV infection versus those without HIV infection that demonstrate comparable outcomes between the two groups. Krishnan *et al.* [72] compared 29 patients with HIV-related lymphoma with 29 HIV-negative controls who were matched for age, gender, time to transplant, transplant year, histology, number of prior regimens, disease status at transplant, and transplant preparative regimen. Figure 22.2 shows the results for OS by HIV status. The 2-year estimated disease-free survival (DFS) for the group of HIV-infected patients was 76% versus 56% for the control group ($P = 0.33$). Nonrelapse mortality was not statistically significant between groups (11% mortality in HIV-infected patients vs. 4% in the uninfected group; $P = 0.18$).

In a case–control study from the EBMT Lymphoma Working Party registry, investigators compared the results of autologous HCT for 53 patients with HIV-related lymphoma (35 with NHL and 18 with Hodgkin lymphoma) with 53 noninfected patients [79]. Patients were matched for age, histology, pretransplant treatment, disease status at transplant, preparative regimens, and post-HCT treatment. The only statistically significant differences between the patient groups were that the HIV-infected group had a higher proportion of male patients ($P = 0.05$) and a greater number of patients with the mixed cellularity subtype of HL ($P = 0.01$). The patient groups had similar rates of PFS, OS, and relapse rates.

The aggregate results from the trials cited in this section are detailed in Table 22.1. The trials reviewed here provide some important guidance regarding autologous HCT

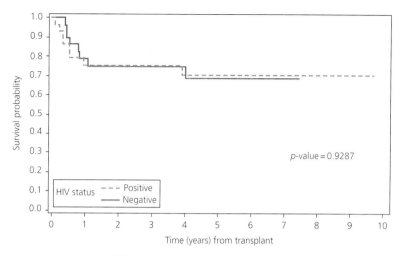

Figure 22.2 A case–control comparison of 20 HIV-infected and 20 HIV-uninfected patients who underwent autologous HCT for the treatment of relapsed or refractory lymphoma. Patients were matched for age, gender, date of transplant, histology, disease status at transplant, number of prior regimens, and preparative regimen. Overall survival between groups is not statistically significantly different. From Krishnan *et al.* [72]. Reproduced with permission of Elsevier.

Table 22.1 Overall patient survival for six published studies evaluating the impact of autologous hematopoietic cell transplantation in patients with HIV-associated NHL and HL. None of the trials were randomized.

Reference	Failed to mobilize (*N*)	Patients transplanted (*N*)	TRM (%)	Median follow-up (months)	Overall survival (%)
Krishnan *et al.* [71]	0	20	5	31.8	85
Spitzer *et al.* [76]	2	20	5	5.8	Median EFS 23 weeks
Re *et al.* [73]	4	10	0	18	39
Re *et al.* [77]	6	27*	0	44	74.6[†]
Serrano *et al.* [75]	0	11	0	32	73
Balsalobre *et al.* [78]	NA	68	7.5	32	61

*This was an intention-to-treat trial of patients with relapsed and refractory HIV-related lymphoma. Fifty patients were enrolled in the trial; only 27 underwent autologous HCT.
[†]For the entire group of 50 patients, median survival was 33 months. The overall survival result is reported only for the subset of 27 patients who underwent autologous HCT.
EFS, event-free survival; TRM, transplant-related mortality.

in HIV-infected patients. Patients who have uncontrolled or untreatable HIV infection are not appropriate candidates for transplantation. Zidovudine-containing HAART regimens may result in delayed engraftment or a failure to engraft. Patients should therefore be switched to an appropriate regimen that does not include zidovudine. In the post-transplant period, patients should receive appropriate prophylaxis for *Pneumocystis jiroveci* pneumonia and herpesviruses and should be monitored closely for evidence of CMV viremia by qPCR (quantitative real-time polymerase chain reaction) blood assay. In the event

of detection of viremia, patients should be treated preemptively with gancyclovir or another appropriate agent.

Mobilization, collection, and management of HPC products from HIV-infected patients

In the studies reviewed in the previous section, only a small number of HIV-infected patients have failed to mobilize adequate numbers of HPC. Re *et al.* [80] reviewed the outcomes for 155 HIV-infected patients who underwent autologous HPC mobilization at 10 different European centers. These included 120 patients with NHL and 35 with HL, 31% of whom were in CR. The majority (86%) of the patients underwent collection with chemotherapy followed by granulocyte colony-stimulating factor (G-CSF), while 14% underwent mobilization with G-CSF alone. A total of 113 patients achieved collection goals while 42 failed to mobilize adequately. Patients appeared to mobilize more efficiently with the combination of chemotherapy followed by G-CSF. In a multivariate analysis, refractory lymphoma ($P = 0.03$) and CD4$^+$ count less than 237/μL ($P = 0.009$) predicted failure to mobilize. For those patients who fail to mobilize adequately with the aforementioned measures, the use of plerixafor should be considered as an adjunct to chemotherapy and G-CSF [81].

Once hematopoietic stem cells are collected from HIV-infected patients, they may be subject to additional national, state, and local regulations during storage. The FDA requires (21CFR 1270 and 1271) that such products treated as nonconforming need to be marked with a biohazard sticker. At the City of Hope, these cells are cryopreserved in the vapor phase of liquid nitrogen in a separate quarantine cryofreezer that is used for storage of nonconforming products [82].

HIV infection and immunological recovery after transplant

A number of the studies detailed in this chapter demonstrate that patients may have spikes in HIV viral load post HCT [68,71,75,76]. The risk is higher for those patients who have interruptions in HAART. It is unclear what impact myeloablative therapy may have on the HIV viral reservoir; however, there is no evidence that autologous HCT can eradicate HIV infection. Even in those with undetectable viral loads, there is still evidence of residual HIV. Cillo *et al.* [83] evaluated 10 HAART-treated patients who underwent autologous HCT for HIV-related lymphoma who had HIV-1 RNA levels suppressed below 50 copies/mL using standard assays. Patient plasma samples were collected at a median of 686 days post transplant and were evaluated using qPCR with a single-copy sensitivity assay. In addition, peripheral blood mononuclear cells were analyzed for HIV-1 cDNA or 2-LTR circles (nonintegrated HIV cDNA).

Nine of the patients had detectable low-level plasma viremia and all had evidence of residual HIV DNA using the combined methods.

Patients with HIV infection appear to have post-transplant T-cell reconstitution comparable to that of non-infected patients. Even among noninfected patients there is ample evidence for qualitative abnormalities of T-cell reconstitution that persist up to 1 year following transplant [84]. While CD8$^+$ cells may recover numerically 2 months after HCT, CD4$^+$ T cells frequently fail to reach normal levels, even by 12 months, and recovery of naive CD4$^+$ T cells may be quite delayed [84]. Thymic maturation of T cells is an important component of immunologic reconstitution following autologous HCT [85]. During thymic maturation of T cells, excision of circular fragments of DNA occur during T-cell receptor gene rearrangements and may serve as markers of the rate of T-cell development. These are termed T-cell receptor excision circles (TRECs) and they may serve as markers of T-cell recovery following immunosuppressive or myeloablative therapy [86,87].

Simonelli *et al.* [88] prospectively assessed post-HCT immunologic recover in 24 HIV-infected and nine non-infected patients. Patients were evaluated by a flow cytometric T-cell subset analysis, TREC enumeration, and assessment of HIV viral RNA and DNA levels by qPCR. The two patient groups were comparable for histology, prior therapy, number of previous chemotherapeutic cycles, disease stage, and status at transplant. There was no difference in pre-HCT CD4$^+$ T cell, CD56$^+$ and CD19$^+$ cell counts between the groups; TREC levels were comparable as well. The groups only differed in that HIV-infected patients had higher CD8$^+$ cell counts prior to transplant ($P = 0.004$) and therefore had a lower CD4$^+$/CD8$^+$ ratio ($P < 0.001$). Both groups had a nadir in CD4$^+$ T-cell counts following HCT, with recovery continuing through 24 months post transplant, when the HIV-infected and noninfected groups reached 58% and 47% of their pretransplant values, respectively. TREC recovery was comparable between the two groups, with both groups achieving higher than baseline levels by 12 months. During transplant, 10 of the patients had interruptions in HAART due to transplant-related toxicity; eight experienced subsequent rebound viremia. At 24 months post HCT, HIV DNA levels appeared to be lower than those at baseline. Other investigators have found comparable levels of T-cell reconstitution post HCT in HIV-infected patients [89,90].

Allogeneic transplantation: the "Berlin patient" and a path toward a cure for HIV

In 1989, Holland *et al.* [91] published a case report describing a 41-year-old man with AIDS-related lymphoma who was treated with fully ablative allogeneic HCT. The preparative regimen consisted of TBI and cyclophosphamide. Prior to transplant, the patient was treated with high-dose zidovudine and it was continued post transplant. The patient engrafted by day 17 and demonstrated evidence of complete donor chimerism. Post-HCT qPCR analysis of peripheral blood was negative for HIV at day 32. Unfortunately, the patient died from progressive lymphoma on day 47. Postmortem analysis of samples of the patient's lymph nodes, bone marrow, brain, and lymphoma did not demonstrate evidence of HIV by either tissue culture or PCR.

A number of groups attempted to extend allogeneic HCT to HIV-infected patients throughout the pre-HAART era [92–94]. These attempts were largely unsuccessful, with the majority of patients dying in the year following transplant. There was little evidence of any impact on the underlying HIV infection [95]. In an analysis of 17 published case reports and trials describing the outcomes for allogeneic HCT for HIV-infected patients in the pre-HAART era, Hütter and Zaia [95] calculated that aggregate OS for these patients was less than 15%. In a review of Center for International Bone and Marrow Transplant Research (CIBMTR) registry data on HIV-infected patients who underwent allogeneic HCT pre HAART, Gupta *et al.* [96] found that at a median follow-up of 59 months only two of 14 patients remained alive.

HAART has made it possible to offer effective allogeneic transplantation to HIV-infected patients. In their review of 14 case reports and trials of allogeneic HCT for HIV-infected patients in the post-HAART era, Hütter and Zaia [95] reported an OS of approximately 50%. Three of these trials included patients who were underwent allogeneic HCT for treatment of NHL. In their CIBMTR dataset review of nine patients who underwent allogeneic transplant in the post-HAART era, Gupta *et al.* [96] reported that four of the nine patients remained alive at a median follow-up of 59 months.

Only a subset of those patients who have undergone allogeneic HCT in either the pre- or post-HAART eras have received their transplants for the management of

lymphoma. In the CIBMTR dataset, 10 of the 23 patients were treated for relapsed or refractory lymphoma, but the report does not describe disease-specific outcomes in this group [96]. In 1999, Campbell *et al.* [97] reported results for an HIV-infected patient who underwent syngeneic HCT for the treatment of relapsed chemotherapy-sensitive immunoblastic lymphoma. The patient received CBV conditioning and received mobilized HPC from his syngeneic brother. He received no immunosuppressive therapy following HCT. HAART was briefly interrupted 12 days post HCT due to toxicity. At the time of the report, the patient was 1 year post transplant and remained in CR, but his viral load at 13 months post HCT was still detectable (5000 copies/mL).

In 2002, Kang *et al.* [98] reported two patients who underwent nonmyeloablative allogeneic HCT for acute myelogenous leukemia (AML) and refractory HL. Both patients were treated with HAART at the time of transplant. The AML patient had a viral load of 494/mL while that of the patient with HL was undetectable. The preparative regimen consisted of fludarabine and cyclophosphamide. Graft-versus-host disease (GVHD) prophylaxis consisted of cyclosporine alone. The patient with AML received a gene-modified HPC graft while the HL patient received an unmanipulated graft. By day 96, both patients achieved 100% donor chimerism and both achieved a CR. Both patients developed grade II acute GVHD of the skin. Unfortunately, the patient with HL relapsed by day 180 post HCT and died within 1 year. The patient treated for AML demonstrated an undetectable HIV viral load post transplant and remained in remission at the time of the report.

Bryant and Milliken [99] published a case report of a patient who underwent allogeneic HCT for the treatment of HIV-related PEL. The patient initially underwent autologous HCT following BEAM for management of a chemotherapy-sensitive relapse. Based on his high risk for relapse, the investigators subsequently treated the patient with consolidative allogeneic HCT from an HLA-compatible sibling. The preparative regimen consisted of fludarabine and melphalan and GVHD prophylaxis consisted of tacrolimus, sirolimus, and mini-dose methotrexate. HAART was continued through the transplant and post-transplant period. Neutrophil engraftment occurred by day 17. The patient developed grade I acute GVHD of the skin that was managed with corticosteroids. The patient's HIV viral load remained undetectable throughout his course. At 31 months post HCT, the patient remained in CR.

The Ohio State University group published their experience using reduced-intensity allogeneic HCT for three HIV-infected patients, one with AML in second CR and two with ARL (BL and plasmablastic lymphoma) [100]. The conditioning included fludarabine and busulfan; the two lymphoma patients also received antithymocyte globulin (ATG). All the patients continued HAART uninterrupted throughout their transplant course. All patients achieved 100% lymphoid donor chimerism. One patient developed grade II acute GVHD and all the patients developed chronic GVHD (two extensive). At the time of publication, all three patients were alive, free of evidence of disease, and remained off all immunosuppressive therapy (range 368–802 days). At more than 1 year post HCT, only one patient had a detectable HIV viral load of 363/mL.

While early in the pre-HAART era some had naively hoped that allogeneic transplant might help eradicate HIV infection, these hopes had been largely dashed. However, the "Berlin patient" has upended our expectations about the potential to eradicate HIV through allogeneic HCT. By 1996, investigators had identified some individuals who, despite multiple high-risk exposures, remained free of evidence of HIV infection [8,9]. Further analysis demonstrated that these individuals shared a common homozygous variant of the CCR5 gene that included an internal 32-bp deletion that resulted in a truncated version of the CCR5 receptor protein [8]. This is referred to as the CCR5 Δ32 allele. It is found in up to 16% of people of northern European descent and is encountered far less frequently in individuals of Asian and African descent [101]. Approximately 1% of the white population is homozygous for this gene and it confers protection against infection by R5 trophic variants of HIV.

In 2009, Hütter *et al.* [102] reported long-term control of HIV infection in a patient following allogeneic HCT using a CCR5 Δ32 homozygous unrelated donor. The patient was a 40-year-old man with long-standing HIV infection who underwent allogeneic transplant for AML that relapsed 7 months following standard induction and consolidation therapy. At the time of AML diagnosis, the patient had a viral load that

was undetectable and the CD4 T-cell count was 415/μL. The patient received an allogeneic HCT from an unrelated donor who was CCR5 Δ32 homozygous. HAART was interrupted prior to transplant. The patient received a CD34$^+$ cell-selected graft. GVHD prophylaxis consisted of ATG, cyclosporine, and mycophenolate. The patient achieved engraftment on day 13. He developed grade I skin GVHD that responded to therapy. By 332 days post HCT the patient developed evidence of early relapse and was retreated with cytarabine and gemtuzumab. He subsequently received a second transplant from his original donor following 2-Gy TBI. At the time of the original report, the patient remained in remission and had an undetectable HIV viral load despite interruption of HAART at 20 months post HCT. The last detectable HIV viral load was noted on day 20 follow transplant. Evaluation of multiple tissues, including bone marrow, blood, and rectal mucosa demonstrated no evidence of HIV. The patient is now more than 6 years post HCT and has no evidence of recurrent HIV [103].

Investigators in Boston raised the question as to whether HIV could be eradicated following allogeneic HCT using donors who are not CCR5 Δ32 homozygous [104]. They treated two patients with HIV infection for relapsed HL and DLBCL, respectively. Both patients underwent allogeneic transplant and received HPC grafts from CCR5 wild-type donors. HAART was continued throughout the entire transplant course. Patients were evaluated for persistence of HIV using PCR quantification of HIV DNA and 2-LTR circles. While HIV was readily detected prior to transplant and up to 3 months post HCT, subsequent analysis up to 3.5 years post transplant did not demonstrate evidence of detectable HIV. The investigators raised the question as to whether the transplant procedure may have led to a sustained reduction in the HIV-1 reservoir. Unfortunately, both patients suffered detectable returns in HIV at 12 and 32 weeks, respectively, following cessation of HAART [105].

It is unclear whether allogeneic HCT with wild-type CCR5 donors can potentially affect the HIV reservoir. The triumph of the "Berlin patient" requires further validation as to whether this experience can be repeated or whether it can be replicated outside of the setting of a CCR5 Δ32 homozygous donor. Toward that end, the National Heart

Lung and Blood Institute and National Cancer Institute are sponsoring an ongoing trial of allogeneic transplantation for patients with advanced hematologic malignancies (clinicaltrials.gov, NCT01410344). Important secondary end points of this trial include evaluation of immunologic reconstitution of this patient population, the impact of transplant on the HIV viral reservoir, and long-term assessment of patient immunologic function. As part of this 15-patient trial, the investigators are searching for potential CCR5 Δ32 homozygous unrelated donors who might help to further validate the experience of Hütter and his colleagues.

Transplant as a platform for gene therapy

Allogeneic or autologous HCT may provide a platform for transplantation of gene-manipulated cells that could have the potential to impact HIV infection [106]. In 2001, Kang *et al.* [98] performed an allogeneic transplant in a patient with AML who received a gene-modified graft. The CD34+ cell graft was transduced with a transdominant *Rev* (TdRev) engineered to inhibit wild-type *Rev*. At 2 years post transplant, the patient demonstrated an undetectable HIV viral

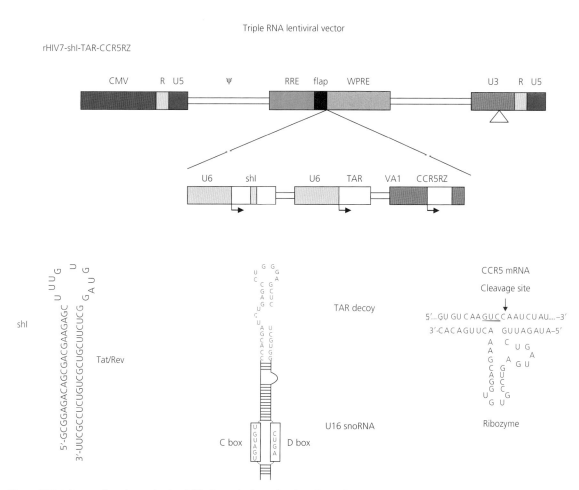

Figure 22.3 John Rossi, a pioneer in the field of RNA biology, developed a triple RNA construct targeting multiple cellular and viral molecules required for viral entry, replication, and maturation into mature virions. These small RNAs are driven from U6 and VA1 (PolIII) promoters and are thus expressed at high levels in recipient cells.

load and persistence of marked cells at a level of approximately 0.01%.

The City of Hope group performed autologous HCT in four patients with ARL using gene-modified HPC grafts [107]. The investigators performed CD34+ cell selection on the HPC products, then subsequently transfected them using a lentiviral vector that included three anti-HIV-directed RNA moieties. These included a *Tat/Rev* short hairpin RNA (shRNA), a *TAR* decoy, and a CCR5 ribozyme used in an attempt to render a functional knockout of CCR5 expression (Figure 22.3). Patients received both gene-manipulated and unmanipulated grafts. At a median follow-up of 18 months all patients remained in complete remission and two of the patients demonstrated quantifiable levels of gene marking (between 0.04 and 0.12%); the other two demonstrated unquantifiable but detectable levels of gene marking [107]. A number of groups have proposed alternative HCT-based gene therapeutic approaches for HIV-infected patients [98,106,108,109]. There are a significant number of technical barriers that need to be overcome before cure of HIV infection can be attempted using a gene therapy-based approach.

Conclusion

Over the past three decades there have been extraordinary strides in the care of patients suffering from HIV-related malignancies. HIV infection is associated with a profound degree of immunologic depletion that markedly increases the risk of lymphoma, yet compromises our ability to deliver effective care to this patient population. The advent and widespread availability of HAART has completely altered the prognosis for patients with ARL by making intensive therapeutic approaches both safe and effective. Outcomes for autologous HCT are equivalent between HIV-infected and noninfected patients with NHL and HL. We are in the process of verifying that allogeneic transplantation also represents the standard of care for HIV-infected patients with advanced hematologic malignancies. In the process, we continue to explore transplant-based therapeutic approaches, including gene-based therapeutics, that may hold the promise of a path toward the eradication of HIV infection.

References

1 Centers for Disease Control. *Pneumocystis* pneumonia – Los Angeles. *MMWR* 1981;**30**:1–3.

2 Centers for Disease Control. Kaposi sarcoma and *Pneumocystis* pneumonia among homosexual men – New York City and California. *MMWR* 1981;**30**:305–8.

3 Centers for Disease Control. Current trends update on acquired immunodeficiency syndrome (AIDS) – United States. *MMWR* 1982;**31**:507–8.

4 Fauci AS. The syndrome of Kaposi's sarcoma and opportunistic infections: an epidemiologically restricted disorder of immunoregulation. *Ann Intern Med* 1982;**96**:777–9.

5 World Health Organization. Acquired immunodeficiency syndrome: an assessment of the present situation in the world. Memorandum from a WHO meeting. *Bull WHO* 1984;**62**:419–32.

6 Gallo RC, Salahuddin SZ, Popovic M *et al.* Frequent detection and isolation of cytopathic retroviruses (HTLV-III) from patients with AIDS and at-risk for AIDS. *Science* 1984;**224**:500–3.

7 Wain-Hobson S, Vartanian JP, Henry M *et al.* LAV revisited: origins of the early HIV-1 isolates from the Institut Pasteur. *Science* 1991;**252**:961–5.

8 Liu R, Paxton WA, Choe S *et al.* Homozygous defect in HIV-1 coreceptor accounts for resistance of some multiply-exposed individuals to HIV-1 infection. *Cell* 1996;**86**:367–77.

9 Fauci A, Pantaleo G, Stanley S, Weissman D. Immunopathogenic mechanisms of HIV infection. *Ann Intern Med* 1996;**124**:654–63.

10 Henry J. Kaiser Family Foundation. The global HIV/AIDS epidemic, 2013. Available at http://kff.org/global-health-policy/fact-sheet/the-global-hivaids-epidemic/ (accessed April 10, 2014).

11 World Health Organization. UNAIDS core epidemiology slides, 2013. Available at http://www.unaids.org/en/media/unaids/contentassets/documents/epidemiology/2013/gr2013/201309_epi_core_en.pdf (accessed April 10, 2014).

12 Merson MH, O'Malley J, Serwada J, Apisuk C. The history and challenge of HIV prevention. *Lancet* 2008;**372**:475–88.

13 US Food and Drug Administration. HIV/AIDS historical time line 1981–1990. Available at http://www.fda.gov/ForConsumers/ByAudience/ForPatientAdvocates/HIVandAIDSActivities/ucm151074.htm (accessed April 10, 2014).

14 Fischl MA, Richman DD, Grieco MH *et al.* The efficacy of azidothymidine (AZT) in the treatment of patients with AIDS and AIDS-related complex. *N Engl J Med* 1987;**317**:185–91.

15 amfAR. Thirty years of HIV/AIDS: snapshots of an epidemic. Available at http://www.amfar.org/thirty-years-of-hiv/aids-snapshots-of-an-epidemic/ (accessed April 20, 2014).

16 Hammer SM, Katzenstein DA, Hughes MD *et al.* A trial comparing nucleoside monotherapy with combination therapy in HIV-infected adults with CD4 counts from 200 to 500 per cubic microliter. *N Engl J Med* 1996;**335**:1081–90.

17 Mellors JW, Rinaldo CR, Gupta P, White RM, Todd JA, Kingsley LA. Prognosis in HIV-1 infection predicted by the quantity of virus in plasma. *Science* 1996;**272**:1167–70.

18 O'Brien WA, Hartigan PM, Daar ES, Simberkoff MS, Hamilton JD. Changes in plasma HIV RNA and CD4+ lymphocyte counts predict both response to antiretroviral therapy and therapeutic failure. *Ann Intern Med* 1997;**126**:939–45.

19 Fauci AS. The AIDS epidemic: considerations for the 21st century. *N Engl J Med* 1999;**341**:1046–50.

20 Palella F, Delaney KM, Moorman AC *et al*. Declining morbidity and mortality among patients with advanced human immunodeficiency virus infection. *N Engl J Med* 1998;**338**:853–60.

21 Thompson MA, Aberg JA, Hoy JF *et al*. Antiretroviral treatment of adult HIV infection: 2012 recommendations of the international antiviral society, USA panel. *JAMA* 2012;**308**:387–402.

22 Fauci AS, Folkers GK. Toward an AIDS-free generation. *JAMA* 2012;**308**:343–4.

23 Schulz TF, Boshoff CH, Weiss RA. HIV infection and neoplasia. *Lancet* 1996;**348**:587–91.

24 Jiddane M, Nicoli F, Bergvall U, Vincentelli F, Hassoun J, Salamon G. Intracranial malignant lymphoma. Report of 30 cases and review of literature. *J Neurosurg* 1986;**65**:592–9.

25 Levine AM. Acquired immunodeficiency syndrome-related lymphoma. *Blood* 1992;**80**:8–20.

26 Centers for Disease Control. Revision of the CDC surveillance case definition for acquired immunodeficiency syndrome. *MMWR* 1987;**31**:1S–15S.

27 Centers for Disease Control. 1993 revised classification for HIV infection and expanded surveillance case definition for AIDS among adolescents and adults. *MMWR* 1992;**41**:961–2.

28 Clifford GM, Polesel J, Rickenbach M *et al*. Cancer risk in the Swiss HIV cohort study: associations with immunodeficiency, smoking, and highly active antiretroviral therapy. *J Natl Cancer Inst* 2005;**97**:425–32.

29 Cooksley CD, Hwang LY, Waller DK, Ford CE. HIV-related malignancies: community-based study using linkage of cancer registry and HIV registry data. *Int J STD AIDS* 1999;**10**:795–802.

30 Yanik EL, Napravnik S, Cole SR *et al*. Incidence and timing of cancer in HIV-infected individuals following initiation of combination antiretroviral therapy. *Clin Infect Dis* 2013;**57**:756–64.

31 Little RF, Dunleavy K. Update on the treatment of HIV-associated hematologic malignancies. *Hematology Am Soc Hematol Educ Program* 2013;382–8.

32 Kaplan LD. HIV-associated lymphoma. *Best Pract Res Clin Haematol* 2012;**25**:101–17.

33 Gopol S, Patel MR, Yanik EL *et al*. Temporal trends in presentation and survival for HIV-associated lymphoma in the antiretroviral therapy era. *J Natl Cancer Inst* 2013;**105**:1221–9.

34 Dunleavy K, Wilson W. Implications of the shifting pathobiology of AIDS-related lymphoma. *J Natl Cancer Inst* 2013;**105**:1170–1.

35 Martis N, Mounier N. Hodgkin lymphoma in patients with HIV infection: a review. *Curr Hematol Malig Rep* 2012;**7**:228–34.

36 Swerdlow SH, Campo E, Harris NL, Jaffe ES, Pileri SA, Stein H, Thiele J, Vardiman JW (eds) *World Health Organization Classification of Tumours of Haematopoietic and Lymphoid Tissues*, 4th edn. Lyon: IARC Press, 2008.

37 Hamilton-Dutoit SJ, Pallesen G, Franzmann MB *et al*. AIDS-related lymphoma: histopathology, immunophenotype, and association with Epstein–Barr virus as demonstrated by *in situ* nucleic acid hybridization. *Am J Pathol* 1991;**138**:149–63.

38 Shibata D, Weiss LM, Hernandez AM, Nathwani BN, Bernstein L, Levine AM. Epstein–Barr virus-associated non-Hodgkin's lymphoma in patients infected with the human immunodeficiency virus. *Blood* 1993;**81**:2102–9.

39 Vishnu P, Aboulafia DM. AIDS-related non-Hodgkin's lymphoma in the era of highly active antiretroviral therapy. *Adv Hematol* 2012; Article ID 485943.

40 Breen EC, Hussein SK, Magpantay L *et al*. B-cell stimulatory cytokines and markers of immune activation are elevated several years prior to diagnosis of systemic AIDS-associated non-Hodgkin B-cell lymphoma. *Cancer Epidemiol Biomarkers Prev* 2011;**20**:1303–14.

41 Dunleavy K, Wilson WH. How I treat HIV-associated lymphoma. *Blood* 2012;**119**:3245–55.

42 Cheung MC, Pantanowitz L, Dezube BJ. AIDS-related malignancies: emerging challenges in the era of highly active antiretroviral therapy. *Oncologist* 2005;**10**:412–26.

43 Sparano JA. Human immunodeficiency virus associated lymphoma. *Curr Opin Oncol* 2003;**15**:372–8.

44 Shiels MS, Pfeiffer RM, Gail MH *et al*. Proportions of Kaposi sarcoma, selected non-Hodgkin lymphomas and cervical cancer in the United States occurring in persons with AIDS, 1980–2007. *JAMA* 2011;**305**:1450–9.

45 Levine AM. Management of AIDS-related lymphoma. *Curr Opin Oncol* 2008;**20**:522–8.

46 Kaplan LD, Straus DJ, Testa MA *et al*. Low dose compared with standard-dose m-BACOD chemotherapy for non-Hodgkin's lymphoma associated with human immunodeficiency virus infection. *N Engl J Med* 1997;**336**:1641–8.

47 The International Non-Hodgkin's-Lymphoma Prognostic Factors Project. A predictive model for aggressive non-Hodgkin's lymphoma. *N Engl J Med* 1993;**329**:987–94.

48 Rossi G, Donisi A, Casari S, Re A, Cadeo G, Carosi G. The International Prognostic Index can be used as a guide to treatment decisions regarding patients with human immunodeficiency virus-related systemic non-Hodgkin lymphoma. *Cancer* 1999;**86**:2391–7.

49 Behler CM, Kaplan LD. Advances in the management of HIV-related non-Hodgkin lymphoma. *Curr Opin Oncol* 2006;**18**:437–43.

50 Mounier N, Spina M, Gabarre M *et al*. AIDS-related non-Hodgkin lymphoma: final analysis of 485 patients

treated with risk-adapted intensive chemotherapy. *Blood* 2006;**107**:3832–40.

51 Kaplan LD, Lee JY, Ambinder RF *et al*. Rituximab does not improve clinical outcome in a randomized phase 3 trial of CHOP with or without rituximab in patients with HIV-associated non-Hodgkin lymphoma: AIDS-Malignancies Consortium trial 010. *Blood* 2005;**106**:1538–43.

52 Boué F, Gabarre J, Gisselbrecht C *et al*. Phase II trials of CHOP plus rituximab in patients with HIV-associated non-Hodgkin's lymphoma. *J Clin Oncol* 2006;**24**:4123–8.

53 Little RF, Pittaluga S, Grant N *et al*. Highly effective treatment of acquired immunodeficiency syndrome-related lymphoma with dose-adjusted EPOCH: impact of antiretroviral suspension and tumor biology. *Blood* 2003;**101**:4653–9.

54 Dunleavy K, Little RF, Pittaluga S *et al*. The role of tumor histogenesis, FDG-PET, and short-course EPOCH with dose-dense rituximab (SC-EPOCH-RR) in HIV-associated diffuse large B-cell lymphoma. *Blood* 2010;**115**:3017–24.

55 Xicoy B, Ribera JM, Miralles P *et al*. Comparison of CHOP treatment with specific short-intensive chemotherapy in AIDS-related Burkitt's lymphoma or leukemia. *Med Clin (Barc)* 2011;**136**:323–8.

56 Lim ST, Karim R, Nathwani BN, Tulpule A, Espina B, Levine AM. AIDS-related Burkitt's lymphoma versus diffuse large cell lymphoma in the pre-highly active antiretroviral therapy (HAART) and HAART eras: significant differences in survival with standard chemotherapy. *J Clin Oncol* 2005;**23**:4430–8.

57 Xicoy B, Ribera JM, Müller M *et al*. Dose-intensive chemotherapy including rituximab is highly effective but toxic in human immunodeficiency virus-infected patients with Burkitt lymphoma/leukemia: parallel study of 81 patients. *Leukemia Lymphoma* 2014;**55**:2341–8.

58 Cortes J, Thomas D, Rios A *et al*. Hyperfractionated cyclophosphamide, vincristine, doxorubicin, and dexamethasone and highly active antiretroviral therapy for patients with acquired-immunodeficiency syndrome-related Burkitt lymphoma/leukemia. *Cancer* 2002;**94**:1492–9.

59 Noy A, Kaplan L, Lee JY. A modified dose-intensive CODOX-M/IVAC for HIV-associated Burkitt lymphoma and atypical Burkitt lymphoma (BL) demonstrates high cure rates and low toxicity: prospective multicenter trial of the AIDS Malignancy Consortium (AMC 048). *Blood* 2013;**122**:639.

60 Dunleavy K, Pittaluga S, Shovlin M *et al*. Low-intensity therapy in adults with Burkitt's lymphoma. *N Engl J Med* 2013;**369**:1915–25.

61 Xicoy B, Miralles P, Morgades M, Rubio R, Valencia ME, Ribera JM. Long-term follow up of patients with human immunodeficiency virus infection and advanced stage Hodgkin's lymphoma treated with doxorubicin, bleomycin, vinblastine, dacarbazine. *Haematologica* 2013;**98**:e85.

62 Spina M, Gabare J, Rossi G *et al*. Stanford V regimen and concomitant HAART in 59 patients with Hodgkin disease and HIV infection. *Blood* 2002;**100**:1984–8.

63 Hartmann P, Rehwald U, Salzberger B *et al*. BEACOPP therapeutic regimen for patients with Hodgkin's disease and HIV infection. *Ann Oncol* 2003;**14**:1562–9.

64 Philip T, Guglielmi C, Hagenbeek A *et al*. Autologous bone marrow transplantation as compared with salvage chemotherapy in relapses of chemotherapy-sensitive non-Hodgkin's lymphoma. *N Engl J Med* 1995;**333**:1540–5.

65 Nademanee A, O'Donnell MR, Snyder DS *et al*. High-dose chemotherapy with or without total body irradiation followed by autologous bone marrow and/or peripheral blood stem cell transplantation for patients with relapsed and refractory Hodgkin's disease: results in 85 patients with analysis of prognostic factors. *Blood* 1995;**85**:1381–90.

66 Gabarre J, Leblond V, Sutton L *et al*. Autologous bone marrow transplantation in relapsed HIV-related non-Hodgkin's lymphoma. *Bone Marrow Transplant* 1996;**18**:1195–7.

67 Gabarre J, Azar N, Autran B, Katlama C, Leblond V. High-dose therapy and autologous haematopoietic stem-cell transplantation for HIV-1-associated lymphoma. *Lancet* 2000;**355**:1071–2.

68 Molina A, Krishnan AY, Nademanee A *et al*. High dose therapy and autologous stem cell transplantation for human immunodeficiency virus-associated non-Hodgkin lymphoma in the era of highly active antiretroviral therapy. *Cancer* 2000;**89**:680–9.

69 Krishnan A, Molina A, Zaia J *et al*. Autologous stem cell transplantation for HIV-associated lymphoma. *Blood* 2001;**98**:3857–9.

70 Krishnan A, Molina A, Zaia J *et al*. Durable remissions with autologous stem cell transplantation for high-risk HIV-associated lymphomas. *Blood* 2005;**105**:874–8.

71 Krishnan A, Palmer JP, Zaia JA, Tsai NC, Alvarnas M, Forman SJ. HIV status does not affect the outcome of autologous stem cell transplantation (ASCT) for non-Hodgkin lymphoma (NHL). *Biol Blood Marrow Transplant* 2010;**16**:1302–8.

72 Re A, Cattaneo C, Michieli M *et al*. High-dose therapy and autologous peripheral-blood stem-cell transplantation as salvage treatment for HIV-associated lymphoma in patients receiving highly active antiretroviral therapy. *J Clin Oncol* 2003;**21**:4423–7.

73 Gabarre J, Marcelin AG, Azar N *et al*. High-dose therapy plus autologous hematopoietic stem cell transplantation for human immunodeficiency virus (HIV)-related lymphoma: results and impact on HIV disease. *Haematologica* 2004;**89**:1100–8.

74 Serrano D, Carrión R, Balsalobre P *et al*. HIV-associated lymphoma successfully treated with peripheral blood stem cell transplantation. *Exp Hematol* 2005;**33**:487–94.

75 Spitzer TR, Ambinder RF, Lee JY *et al.* Dose-reduced busulfan, cyclophosphamide, and autologous stem cell transplantation for human immunodeficiency virus-associated lymphoma: AIDS Malignancy Consortium study 020. *Biol Blood Marrow Transplant* 2008;**14**:59–66.

76 Re A, Michieli M, Casari S *et al.* High-dose therapy and autologous peripheral blood stem cell transplantation as salvage treatment for AIDS-related lymphoma: long-term results of the Italian Cooperative Group of AIDS and Tumors (GICAT) study with analysis of prognostic factors. *Blood* 2009;**114**:1306–13.

77 Balsalobre P, Díez-Martín JL, Re A *et al.* Autologous stem-cell transplantation in patients with HIV-related lymphoma. *J Clin Oncol* 2009;**27**:2192–8.

78 Díez-Martín JL, Balsalobre P, Re A *et al.* Comparable survival between HIV+ and HIV– non-Hodgkin and Hodgkin lymphoma patients undergoing autologous peripheral blood stem cell transplantation. *Blood* 2009;**113**:6011–14.

79 Re A, Cattaneo C, Skert C *et al.* Stem cell mobilization in HIV seropositive patients with lymphoma. *Haematologica* 2013;**98**:1762–8.

80 Attolico I, Pavone V, Ostuni AN *et al.* Plerixafor added to chemotherapy plus G-CSF is safe and allows adequate PBSC collection in predicted poor mobilizer patients with multiple myeloma or lymphoma. *Biol Blood Marrow Transplant* 2012;**18**:241–9.

81 Wang S. HIV-infected stem cell storage. E-mail to Joseph Alvarnas, May 2, 2010.

82 Cillo AR, Krishnan A, Mitsuyasu RT *et al.* Plasma viremia and cellular HIV-1 DNA persist despite autologous hematopoietic stem cell transplantation for HIV-related lymphoma. *J Acquir Immune Defic Syndr* 2013;**63**:438–41.

83 te Boeckhorst PAW, Lamers CHJ, Schipperus MR *et al.* T-lymphocyte reconstitution following rigorously T-cell depleted versus unmodified autologous stem cell transplants. *Bone Marrow Transplant* 2006;**37**:763–77.

84 Haynes BF, Markert ML, Sempowski D, Patel DD, Hale LP. The role of the thymus in immune reconstitution in aging, bone marrow transplantation, and HIV-1 infection. *Annu Rev Immunol* 2000;**18**:529–60.

85 Douek DC. The contribution of the thymus to immune reconstitution after hematopoietic stem-cell transplantation. *Cytotherapy* 2002;**4**:425–6.

86 Pratesi C, Simonelli C, Zanussi S *et al.* Recent thymic emigrants in lymphoma patients with and without human immunodeficiency virus infection candidates for autologous peripheral stem cell transplants. *Clin Exp Immunol* 2007;**151**:101–9.

87 Simonelli C, Zanussi S, Pratesi C *et al.* Immune recovery after autologous stem cell transplantation is not different for HIV-infected versus HIV-uninfected patients with relapsed or refractory lymphoma. *Clin Infect Dis* 2010;**50**: 1672–9.

88 Benicchi T, Ghidini C, Re A *et al.* T-cell immune reconstitution after hematopoietic stem cell transplantation for HIV-associated lymphoma. *Transplantation* 2005;**80**:673–82.

89 Resino S, Pérez A, Seoane E *et al.* Immune reconstitution after autologous peripheral blood stem cell transplantation in HIV-infected patients: might be better than expected? *AIDS Res Hum Retroviruses* 2007;**23**:543–8.

90 Holland HK, Sara R, Donnenberg AD *et al.* Allogeneic bone marrow transplantation, zidovudine, and human immunodeficiency virus type-1 (HIV-1) infection: studies in a patient with non-Hodgkin lymphoma. *Ann Intern Med* 1989;**111**:973–81.

91 Torlontano G, Di Bartolomeo P, Di Girolamo G *et al.* AIDS-related complex treated by antiviral drugs and allogeneic bone marrow transplantation following conditioning protocol with busulfan, cyclophosphamide and cyclosporin. *Haematologica* 1992;**77**:287–90.

92 Giri N, Vowels MR, Ziegler JB. Failure of allogeneic bone marrow transplantation to benefit HIV infection. *J Paediatr Child Health* 1992;**28**:331–3.

93 Contu L, La Nasa G, Arras M *et al.* Allogeneic bone marrow transplantation combined with multiple anti-HIV-1 treatment in a case of AIDS. *Bone Marrow Transplant* 1993;**12**:669–71.

94 Hütter G, Zaia JA. Allogeneic haematopoietic stem cell transplantation in patients with human immunodeficiency virus: the experiences of more than 25 years. *Clin Exp Immunol* 2011;**163**:284–95.

95 Gupta V, Tomblyn M, Pedersen TL *et al.* Allogeneic hematopoietic cell transplantation in HIV-positive patients with hematological disorders: a report from the Center for International Blood and Marrow Transplant Research (CIBMTR). *Biol Blood Marrow Transplant* 2009;**15**:864–71.

96 Campbell P, Iland H, Gibson J, Joshua D. Syngeneic stem cell transplantation for HIV-related lymphoma. *Br J Haematol* 1999;**105**:795–8.

97 Kang EM, de Witte M, Malech H *et al.* Nonmyeloablative conditioning followed by transplantation of genetically modified HLA-matched peripheral blood progenitor cells for hematologic malignancies in patients with acquired immunodeficiency syndrome. *Blood* 2002;**99**:698–701.

98 Bryant A, Milliken S. Successful reduced-intensity conditioning allogeneic HSCT for HIV-related primary effusion lymphoma. *Biol Blood Marrow Transplant* 2008;**14**:601–2.

99 Hamadani M, Devine S. Reduced-intensity conditioning allogeneic stem cell transplantation in HIV patients with hematologic malignancies: yes, we can. *Blood* 2009;**114**:2564–6.

100 November J, Galvani AP, Slatkin M. The geographic spread of the CCR5 Δ32 HIV-resistance allele. *PLOS Biol* 2005;**3**(11):e339.

101 Hütter G, Nowak D, Mossner M *et al.* Long-term control of HIV by *CCR5* Delta32/Delta32 stem-cell transplantation. *N Engl J Med* 2009;**360**:692–8.

102 Allers K, Hütter G, Hofmann J *et al.* Evidence for the cure of HIV infection by *CCR5Δ32/Δ32* stem cell transplantation. *Blood* 2011;**117**:2791–9.

103 Henrich TJ, Hu X, Li JZ *et al.* Long-term reductions in peripheral blood HIV type 1 reservoirs following reduced-intensity conditioning allogeneic stem cell transplantation. *J Infect Dis* 2013;**207**:1694–702.

104 Sanchez R, Wills S, Young S. HIV returns in two patients after bone marrow transplant. CNN Health: Breaking News, December 9, 2013. Retrieved from http://www.cnn.com/2013/12/07/health/hiv-patients/

105 Younan P, Kowalski J, Kiem HP. Genetically modified hematopoietic stem cell transplantation for HIV-1 infected patients: can we achieve a cure? *Mol Ther* 2014;**22**:257–64.

106 DiGiusto DL, Krishnan A, Li L *et al.* RNA-based gene therapy for HIV with lentiviral vector-modified CD34(+) cells in patients undergoing transplantation for AIDS-related lymphoma. *Sci Transl Med* 2010;**2**(36):36ra43.

107 Kiem HP, Jerome KR, Deeks SG, McCune JM. Hematopoietic stem cell-based gene therapy for HIV disease. *Cell Stem Cell* 2012;**10**:137–47.

108 Chung J, Scherer LJ, Gu A *et al.* Optimized lentiviral vectors for HIV gene therapy: multiplexed expression of small RNAs and inclusion of MGMT^P140K drug resistance gene. *Mol Ther* 2014;**22**:952–63.

Addendum

The Blood and Marrow Transplant Clinical Trials Network (BMT CTN)/AIDS Malignancy Consortium (AMC) 0803/071 trial is a prospective trial of autologous hematopoietic cell transplantation for patients with persistent and relapsed NHL and HL. In total, 40 patients underwent transplant using the BEAM preparative regimen. The patients were managed with a consistent approach to HAART. The use of zidovudine was prohibited due to its myelosuppressive effects. Antiretrovirals were held during the preparative regimen and were resumed 7 days post transplant or following complete resolution of significant transplant-related gastrointestinal toxicities. At a median follow-up of 24 months, the 1-year estimated OS and PFS were 86.6% and 82.3%, respectively. Transplant-related mortality for the group was 5.2%. The trial group was compared with 151 non-HIV-infected patients who were matched for age, performance status, diagnosis, disease response at the time of transplant, and performance status. These comparison patients were identified using the CIBMTR data registry. OS and PFS were not statistically significantly different between the HIV-infected patients treated on trial and the CIBMTR comparison group. In light of these data and given the body of evidence supporting the use of autologous transplant for patients with persisting and relapsed HIV-related lymphoma (HRL), transplant should be viewed as the standard of care for patients with chemotherapy-sensitive HRL who otherwise meet standard transplant criteria (http://www.bloodjournal.org/content/124/21/674?sso-checked=true).

CHAPTER 23

Stem cell transplantation for mycosis fungoides/Sézary syndrome

Eric D. Jacobsen

Epidemiology and clinical presentation

Mycosis fungoides (MF) and Sézary syndrome (SS) are the most common subtypes of cutaneous T-cell lymphoma (CTCL). MF and SS are more common in men and in the white population [1]. MF is characterized by skin patches or plaques that can be confused with common dermatologic conditions such as psoriasis or eczema. Lymph node and visceral involvement typically occur after a long interval of isolated cutaneous involvement but can be present at diagnosis. Apparent lymph node involvement by computed tomography (CT) or positron emission tomography (PET) frequently represents reactive (dermatopathic) changes and suspected lymph node involvement should be confirmed by biopsy. Peripheral T-cell lymphoma (PTCL) can frequently involve the skin and can be difficult to distinguish from MF with nodal involvement in patients who present initially with both nodal and cutaneous involvement.

The most common, and disabling, symptom of MF/SS is pruritus. Alopecia and nail hypertrophy are also common. Patients with CTCL are endogenously immunosuppressed so concomitant infections, particulary cutaneous superinfection with Gram-positive organisms such as *Staphylococcus aureus*, are very common.

Pathology

MF is typified by an epidermotrophic infiltrate of atypical lymphocytes classically manifesting as Pautrier's microabscesses (intraepidermal lymphocyte aggregates)

[2]. Establishing T-cell clonality by polymerase chain reaction (PCR) can support the diagnosis though a clonal infiltrate cannot be identified in all cases. Similarly, clonal T-cell infiltrates can occur in nonmalignant skin conditions, such as psoriasis. To further confuse the picture, MF can have an inflammatory prophase during which the classic histologic findings or clonal T-cell population are not manifest and often serial skin biopsies over many years are necessary to establish the diagnosis [3]. SS is characterized by generalized erythroderma and a circulating population of abnormal mononuclear cells with a grooved (cerebriform) nucleus. The cell of origin is generally a CD4-positive skin-homing T cell or central memory T cell that expresses CD3, cutaneous lymphocyte antigen (CLA), CCR4, and CCR7. The vast majority of cases are CD26 negative and loss of CD7 is also extremely common. Loss of other mature T-cell markers such as CD2 and CD5 is common but not as common as loss of CD7 or CD26. MF and SS probably represent a spectrum of the same disease, with no significant histologic differences between the two [4]. SS may evolve out of preexisting MF or may present as *de novo* disease. MF can transform to a more aggressive process frequently characterized by CD30 expression [5].

Staging

The staging of MF integrates the pattern and extent of cutaneous involvement with the presence or absence of lymph node, peripheral blood, and/or visceral involvement. Differing degrees of nodal involvement

Clinical Guide to Transplantation in Lymphoma, First Edition. Edited by Bipin N. Savani and Mohamad Mohty.
© 2015 John Wiley & Sons, Ltd. Published 2015 by John Wiley & Sons, Ltd.

Table 23.1 International Society for Cutaneous Lymphomas/ European Organization for Research and Treatment of Cancer (ISCL/EORTC) classification of mycosis fungoides and Sézary syndrome.

	T	N	M	B
I	1	0	0	0,1
IB	2	0	0	0,1
II	1,2	1,2	0	0,1
IIB	3	0–2	0	0,1
IIIA	4	0–2	0	0
IIIB	4	0–2	0	1
IV				
IVA1	1–4	0–2	0	2
IVA2	1–4	3	0	0–2
IVB	1–4	0–3	1	0–2

Source: Olsen *et al.* [27]. Reproduced with permission of American Society of Hematology.

and peripheral blood involvement further affect the staging system (Tables 23.1 and 23.2). Seventy percent of patients present with early-stage disease (IA–IIA) while 30% present with advanced-stage disease (IIB–IVB). In one large series the median overall survival (OS) for all diagnosed patients was 24 years, although disease-specific survival had not been reached. Only 8% of patients died of disease [6]. The 5-year OS for SS is only 11% [7].

Nontransplant therapies

A detailed description of the treatment of MF/SS is beyond the scope of this chapter. However, some general principles can be noted. Patients with early-stage disease (IA–IIA) are typically managed with skin-directed therapies such as moderate- to high-potency topical corticosteroids, topical nitrogen mustard, topical retinoids, and/or external beam or electron beam radiotherapy. Phototherapy with either narrow or broad-band ultraviolet (UV)B radiation or a combination of psoralen and UVA radiation (PUVA) is also used. Patients who present with stage IA infrequently require systemic chemotherapy over the course of their illness.

Systemic chemotherapy is often necessary in advanced-stage disease (IIB–IV). The use of combination chemotherapy regimens has not been shown to be superior to sequential single-agent treatments. The most commonly

Table 23.2 International Society for Cutaneous Lymphomas/ European Organization for Research and Treatment of Cancer (ISCL/EORTC) revision to the classification of mycosis fungoides and Sézary syndrome.

TNMB stages	
Skin	
T_1	Limited patches, papules, and/or plaques covering <10% of the skin surface. May further stratify into T_{1a} (patch only) vs. T_{1b} (plaque ± patch)
T_2	Patches, papules or plaques covering ≥10% of the skin surface. May further stratify into T_{2a} (patch only) vs. T_{2b} (plaque ± patch)
T_3	One or more tumors (≥1 cm diameter)
T_4	Confluence of erythema covering ≥80% body surface area
Node	
N_0	No clinically abnormal peripheral lymph nodes; biopsy not required
N_1	Clinically abnormal peripheral lymph nodes; histopathology Dutch grade 1 or NCI LN_{0-2}
N_{1a}	Clone negative
N_{1b}	Clone positive
N_2	Clinically abnormal peripheral lymph nodes; histopathology Dutch grade 2 or NCI LN_3
N_{2a}	Clone negative
N_{2b}	Clone positive
N_3	Clinically abnormal peripheral lymph nodes; histopathology Dutch grades 3–4 or NCI LN_4; clone positive or negative
N_x	Clinically abnormal peripheral lymph nodes; no histologic confirmation
Visceral	
M_0	No visceral organ involvement
M_1	Visceral involvement (must have pathology confirmation and organ involved should be specified)
Blood	
B_0	Absence of significant blood involvement: ≤5% of peripheral blood lymphocytes are atypical (Sézary) cells
B_{0a}	Clone negative
B_{0b}	Clone positive
B_1	Low blood tumor burden: >5% of peripheral blood lymphocytes are atypical (Sézary) cells but does not meet the criteria of B_2
B_{1a}	Clone negative
B_{1b}	Clone positive
B_2	High blood tumor burden: ≥1000/μL Sézary cells with positive clone

utilized initial systemic therapy in MF is bexarotene. The overall response rate is 45–55% [8]. Other agents approved by the Food and Drug Administration (FDA) to treat recurrent MF are the histone deacetylase inhibitors vorinostat and romidepsin [9,10]. Interferon-alpha is also a commonly utilized therapy in MF, frequently in combination with PUVA.

Traditional cytotoxics used to treat MF include oral methotrexate, alkylating agents, nucleoside analogs, gemcitabine, and liposomal doxorubicin, though none are formally approved for this indication. Pralatrexate appears to be active in the disease, though it is used at lower doses than when utilized in PTCL [11]. Finally, the anti-CD52 antibody alemtuzumab and the antibody–drug conjugate brentuximab vedotin have demonstrated promising activity [12,13]. Unfortunately, none of these therapies cures MF/SS and most patients experience frequent relapses over the course of their illness.

Autologous stem cell transplantation

Autologous stem cell transplantation is utilized routinely in PTCL. However, several trials in CTCL have failed to demonstrate a benefit to autologous stem cell transplantation [14–16]. Patients rarely achieve complete remission (CR) and relapses are universal. Thus, autologous transplantation is not generally utilized in CTCL.

Allogeneic stem cell transplantation

The utility of allogeneic stem cell transplantation (allo-SCT) in CTCL was first reported in several small case series. The presence of a graft-versus-lymphoma (GVL) effect was confirmed when patients who exhibited recurrence after allo-SCT subsequently responded to withdrawal of immune suppression and/or donor lymphocyte infusion (DLI) [17]. A meta-analysis confirmed that allogeneic transplant improved event-free survival (EFS) and OS compared to autologous transplant [18]. Although no prospective trials of allo-SCT have been published, restrospective series demonstrated 2-year progression-free survival (PFS) of 31–53% and 2-year OS of 57–79% [19,20]. Long-term data from the Center for International Blood and Marrow Transplant Research (CIBMTR) have demonstrated that remissions after allo-SCT are durable, with 5-year PFS of 17% and 5-year OS of 32% [21]. The European Society for Blood and Marrow Transplantation (EBMT) data demonstrated 5- and 7-year PFS of 32% and 30%, respectively, and 5- and 7-year OS of 46% and 44%, respectively [23]. The plateau in the survival curves suggests that this subgroup of patients is cured of the disease. The major studies of allo-SCT in MF/SS are listed in Table 23.3 [22,23].

Table 23.3 Selected studies of allogeneic peripheral blood stem cell transplantation in mycosis fungoides/Sézary syndrome.

Study	Patients	Conditioning	PFS	OS	NRM	Acute GVHD (grade II–IV)	Chronic GVHD
Duarte et al. [22]	60	RIC 44 MAC 16	34%*	53%*	22%	28%	48%[†]
Lechowicz et al. [21]	129	RIC 83 MAC 46	17%[‡]	41% (RIC)* 31% (MAC)*	19%	41%	43%[†]
de Masson et al. [20]	37	RIC 25 MAC 12	31%[†]	57%[†]	16%	49%	44%[†]
Wu et al. [18]	20	RIC 11 MAC 9	60% (EFS)[‡]	23%[‡]	20%	75%[§]	75%[¶]
Duvic et al. [19]	19	RIC 19	53%[†]	79%[†]	12%	28%	67%[¶]
Molina et al. [26]	8	RIC 4 MAC 4		6/8 patients alive and in CR at time of report	25%	50%[‖]	88%[¶]

*At 3 years.
[†]At 2 years.
[‡]At 5 years.
[§]Grades I–III.
[¶]Timing not reported.
[‖]Exact grading not recorded in all cases.
CR, complete remission; GVHD, graft-versus-host disease; MAC, myeloablative conditioning; NRM, nonrelapse mortality; OS, overall survival; PFS, progression-free survival; RIC, reduced-intensity conditioning.

Indications for allogeneic stem cell transplantation

Allo-SCT is not indicated in early-stage disease (IA–IIA) unless patients have relapsed after, or progressed on, a number of systemic and skin-directed therapies. The same is typically true of stage IIB–III disease, although transplant is more likely to become a necessity in this setting. In most series examining allo-SCT in MF, patients had failed skin-directed therapies in addition to four or more systemic therapies. However, this must be counterbalanced with the fact that allo-SCT is likely most efficacious when utilized while a patient is in CR or at least a very good partial remission (PR) and therefore patients should be considered for allo-SCT prior to exhausting available treatment options [24].

The prognosis of stage IVA or IVB disease, SS, and transformed MF is poor and allo-SCT should be considered early in those settings. Although some studies have suggested that disease stage does not impact the outcome of allo-SCT, the EBMT series did demonstrate a higher risk of relapse and lower PFS with advanced-stage disease [21]. Most published series of allo-SCT in MF/SS have included a preponderance of patients under age 60, but it is reasonable to consider allo-SCT in patients in their early to mid seventies so long as they have a good performance status and do not have substantial comorbidities.

Donor selection and stem cell source

Matched related donors (MRDs) are preferred over matched unrelated donors (MUDs), with improved PFS (hazard ratio 2.17) and OS (hazard ratio 4.81) and a trend toward decreased nonrelapse mortality (NRM) using MRD [21]. If no MRD is available, the outcomes with a well-matched unrelated donor are still favorable and transplantation should still be pursued since other series have not demonstrated any difference in outcome between use of MRD and MUD [20,22]. There are limited data for haploidentical or umbilical cord blood transplantation in MF/SS and such procedures should only be considered in the context of a clinical trial or the situation where a MRD or MUD is not available.

Comparisons of outcome between peripheral blood stem cell and bone marrow transplantation have not demonstrated a difference in graft-versus-host disease (GVHD), PFS, OS, or NRM by stem cell source [20–23]. However, these data must be interpreted with caution given the small numbers of patients involved. The majority of experience is with peripheral blood stem cells and in general this is favored, although bone marrow is acceptable if institutional, physician, or donor preference dictates.

Regardless of the stem cell source, T-cell depletion is not recommended outside the context of a well-designed clinical trial. Although T-cell depletion can decrease the incidence of GVHD, it may result in a threefold increase in the risk of relapse [21].

Conditioning regimen

The first factor in selecting a conditioning regimen is deciding between reduced-intensity/nonmyeloablative conditioning (RIC) versus myeloablative conditioning (MAC). A CIBMTR study compared MAC to RIC and showed no difference in OS or NRM; 1-year and 3-year OS were 56% and 41% for RIC and 51% and 31% for MAC, while NRM at 1 year was 19% and at 5 years was 22% and did not differ with the type of conditioning [22]. These data were corroborated by a French series demonstrating no difference in survival by intensity of conditioning [20].

However, an EBMT study demonstrated that MAC resulted in higher NRM and decreased OS compared to RIC, with hazard ratios of 4.5 and 2.99 respectively [21]. Thus, RIC is preferred since other series have shown no difference in outcomes by conditioning intensity and no series has demonstrated inferior outcomes with RIC.

There are no data defining the optimal conditioning for RIC. Most experience is with fludarabine-based regimens in combination with busulfan or alkylating agents (melphalan or cyclophosphamide). The choice of conditioning regimen at present is based on institutional or physician preference. In one series, the incorporation of antithymocyte globulin (ATG) did reduce NRM but at the cost of decreased PFS [20]. Based on these data, ATG should not be incorporated into the conditioning regimen unless donor and recipient characteristics predict a high risk of GVHD.

The utility of incorporating radiotherapy into the conditioning regimen is also unclear. Total body irradiation (TBI) at doses of 10–12 Gy does not clearly improve outcome and may be associated with increased skin toxicity and GVHD [20]. Data from autologous transplantation regimens that incorporate TBI also demonstrate near universal recurrence, reinforcing that TBI even in combination with ablative chemotherapy is not sufficient to cure MF/SS [14–16].

One intriguing approach is the incorporation of total body skin electron beam radiation (TBSEB). Duvic *et al.* [19] published a series of patients with advanced CTCL undergoing allo-SCT, 15 of whom underwent TBSEB to 36 Gy, administered over 8 weeks, 1–2 months prior to transplant. The study reported an impressive 58% CR rate and a median OS that has not yet been reached, though median follow-up was less than 2 years. The authors hypothesized that TBSEB not only offered tumor debulking but may also decrease recipient skin antigen-presenting cells (APCs). Since CD4+ T cells (from which MF is derived) proliferate in response to class II HLA-restricted antigen presentation, reducing skin APCs may remove the stimulus for malignant T-cell proliferation and regrowth. The incidence of GVHD in this trial was comparable to that in other series, although a separate meta-analysis suggested that the risk of GVHD may be higher with TBSEB. Although best done in the context of a clinical trial, incorporation of TBSEB before transplant is reasonable in patients with persistent cutaneous disease prior to transplantation. Given the possibility of an increased risk of GVHD, TBSEB should be restricted to matched related or well-matched unrelated donors until further data are available.

GVHD prophylaxis

Cutaneous GVHD may be more prevalent following allo-SCT for MF/SS than in other diseases, perhaps due to the plethora of skin-directed therapies, including UV therapy and radiation, that patients receive and the altered immunologic milieu in the skin induced by the disease itself. The overall incidence of grade II–IV acute GVHD ranges from 28 to 49%, with up to 60% of patients developing cutaneous acute GVHD of any grade. The incidence of chronic GVHD ranges from 33% at 1 year to 48% at 2 years [19–22]. The optimal GVHD prophylaxis regimen is unclear. ATG prior to transplant may decrease PFS and should be restricted to clinical trials or patients at high risk of GVHD. Most published series have utilized cyclosporine- or tacrolimus-based GVHD regimens in combination with methotrexate or mycophenolate mofetil. A report of lower recurrence rates with sirolimus-based prophylaxis in lymphoma is intriguing but has not been demonstrated definitively in MF/SS [25]. In the absence of emerging data, GVHD prophylaxis is generally based on physician/institutional preference and side-effect profile. As in other settings, corticosteroids are a mainstay of treatment should GVHD develop.

One important caveat is that recurrent CTCL can mimic cutaneous GVHD and vice versa. Also, patients with CTCL have a high risk of cutaneous infections before and after transplant given the inherent breakdown of skin barriers by the disease itself and prior skin-directed therapies. Co-management with a dermatologist with experience in CTCL is critical and biopsy of carefully selected skin sites is mandatory to distinguish GVHD from infection and/or recurrent CTCL.

Recurrence of CTCL often arises within months and almost always within a year of allo-SCT [19]. Therefore, regardless of the immunosuppressive regimen chosen, tapering of immunosuppression should occur as quickly as possible (preferably as soon as 90 days) after allo-SCT to maximize GVL effect while maintaining careful vigilance for the development of GVHD.

Post-transplant infectious prophylaxis

Post-transplant prophylaxis following allo-SCT for MF/SS is comparable to any other disease state post allo-SCT and is discussed elsewhere in this book. As mentioned previously, patients with MF/SS are susceptible to cutaneous infection. Similarly, they are susceptible to nonmelanoma skin cancers due to prior UV therapy or radiotherapy. Thus close follow-up with a dermatologist experienced in the management of CTCL is extremely important.

Monitoring for recurrence

Most recurrences arise within 1 year of transplant. The skin is the most common site of recurrence and skin examination is the most important part of surveillance. Patients should have a complete skin examination at least every 3 months for the first 2 years after transplant barring any interval signs of recurrence or GVHD. In the absence of recurrence the frequency of skin examinations can be decreased to every 6 months, with annual examination sufficing starting at year seven.

Radiographic surveillance plays a lesser role in MF/SS than in aggressive lymphomas. A post-transplant PET/CT or CT of the chest, abdomen, and pelvis is suggested at approximately day 100 post transplant if there was nodal or visceral involvement prior to transplant. If there is no evidence of recurrence on the day-100 scan, CT of the chest, abdomen, and pelvis every 6 months for 18–24 months is reasonable barring any clinical evidence of recurrence. Routine radiographic surveillance is not necessary beyond 24 months post transplant.

If there was bone marrow involvement before transplant, a repeat bone marrow biopsy is suggested at approximately day 100. If that study does not demonstrate involvement with lymphoma, routine bone marrow biopsies are not necessary unless there are clinical indicators of bone marrow recurrence such as worsening cytopenias. Peripheral blood flow cytometry (PBFC) is suggested for patients with SS or patients with MF with circulating disease. A reasonable schedule is day 30, day 100, and 6 months post transplant and then every 6 months until 24 months post transplant. Annual PBFC is reasonable thereafter. There are no studies demonstrating when PBFC is no longer necessary but it is reasonable to discontinue routine monitoring at year seven.

Management of relapse

Relapse remains a common problem after allo-SCT for MF/SS. However, patients can experience long-term survival after recurrence. In an analysis of long-term outcomes from the EBMT, 8 of 27 patients with recurrent disease were alive at a median of 8 years of follow-up [23]. Patients can experience subsequent remission after withdrawal of immunosuppression and/or DLI. For patients who do not respond to tapering of immunosuppression or patients with GVHD who cannot undergo tapering of immunosuppression, additional systemic therapy or skin-directed therapies are warranted. The selection of agents is similar to selection of agents before transplant and is based on prior agents received and comorbidities. Agents that were effective before transplant can be revisited if prior response duration was greater than 6 months. Novel agents in development include PI3 kinase inhibitors, monoclonal antibodies, and aurora kinase inhibitors and participation in clinical trials should always be encouraged.

Summary and recommendations

Allo-SCT is infrequently utilized in MF given the generally indolent nature of the disease. However, a small subgroup of patients with advanced-stage disease or multiple recurrences are candidates and allo-SCT can provide long-term disease control or even cure. Relapse and NRM from GVHD and infection remain major concerns.

The optimal timing of transplant is unclear. Although some studies have not demonstrated a correlation between disease stage, remission status or time since diagnosis and outcome, several reasonable conclusions can be reached. Patients with early-stage disease generally have an extremely long median survival and allo-SCT should only be considered in the context of a particularly aggressive disease course. Patients with advanced-stage (IVA or IVB) or transformed MF or SS have a median survival of only a few years so utilization of early allo-SCT even after only a few or even one course of systemic therapy is reasonable.

From existing data in CTCL and extrapolation from data for allo-SCT in more common diseases, we can surmise that patients should optimally have chemosensitive disease (preferably PR or CR) prior to allo-SCT, particularly since most recurrences arise within a few months of transplant. RIC is preferred over MAC and MRD is preferred over MUD or alternative donor sources. The utility of radiotherapy as part of conditioning is unclear but TBSEB prior to transplant is reasonable in patients with incomplete disease clearance from the skin. GVHD and infectious prophylaxis should follow institutional and society guidelines. All patients should be managed in conjunction with a dermatologist experienced with allo-SCT and CTCL.

References

1 Barton PT, Davesa SS, Anderson WF, Toro JR, Cutaneous lymphoma incidence patterns in the United States: a population based study of 3884 cases. *Blood* 2009;**113**:5064–73.

2 Kempf W, Kazakov DV, Kerl K, Cutaneous lymphomas: an update. Part 1: T-cell and natural killer/T-cell lymphomas and related conditions. *Am J Dermatopathol* 2014;**36**:105–23.

3 Zhang B, Beck AH, Taube JM *et al*. Combined used of PCR-based TCRG and TCRB clonality tests on paraffin-embedded skin tissue in the differential diagnosis of mycosis fungoides and inflammatory dermatoses. *J Mol Diagn* 2010;**12**:320–7.

4 Willemze R, Hodak E, Zinzani PL *et al*. Primary cutaneous lymphomas: ESMO clinical practice guidelines for diagnosis, treatment, and follow-up. *Ann Oncol* 2013;**24**(Suppl 6): vi149–54.

5 Hermann JL, Hughey LC. Recognizing large cell transformation of mycosis fungoides. *J Am Acad Dermatol* 2012;**67**:665–72.

6 Talpur R, Singh L, Davlat S *et al*. Long-term outcomes of 1,263 patients with mycosis fungoides and Sezary syndrome from 1982 to 2009. *Clin Cancer Res* 2012;**18**:5051–60.

7 Kim YH, Hoppe RT. Mycosis fungoides and the Sezary syndrome. *Semin Oncol* 1999;**26**:276–89.

8 Abbott RA, Whittaker SJ, Morris SL *et al*. Bexarotene therapy for mycosis fungoides and Sezary syndrome. *Br J Dermatol* 2009;**160**:1299–307.

9 Whittaker SJ, Demierre MF, Kim EJ *et al.* Final results from a multicenter, international, pivotal study of romidpesin in refractory cutaneous T cell lymphoma. *J Clin Oncol* 2010;**28**: 4485–91.

10 Olsen EA, Kim YH, Kuzel TM *et al.* Phase IIb multicenter trial of vorinostat in patients with persistent, progressive, or treatment-refractory cutaneous T-cell lymphoma. *J Clin Oncol* 2007;**25**:3109–15.

11 Horwitz SM, Kim YH, Foss F *et al.* Identification of an active, well-tolerated dose of pralatrexate in patients with relapsed or refractory cutaneous T cell lymphoma. *Blood* 2012;**119**: 4115–22.

12 de Masson A, Guitera P, Brice P *et al.* Long-term efficacy and safety of alemtuzumab in advanced primary cutaneous T-cell lymphomas. *Br J Dermatol* 2014;**170**:720–4.

13 Saintes C, Saint-Jean M, Renaut JJ, Dréno B, Quéreux G. Dramatic efficacy of brentuximab vedotin in 2 patients with epidermotrophic cutaneous T-cell lymphomas after treatment failure despite variable CD30 expression. *Br J Dermatol* 2014; doi: 10.1111/bjd.13337.

14 Bigler RD, Crilley P, Micaily B *et al.* Autologous bone marrow transplantation for advanced stage mycosis fungoides. *Bone Marrow Transplant* 1991;**7**:133–7.

15 Duarte RF, Schmitz N, Servitje O, Sureda A. Haematopoietic stem cell transplantation for patients with primary cutaneous T-cell lymphoma. *Bone Marrow Transplant* 2008;**41**:597–604.

16 Olavarria E, Childe F, Woolford A *et al.* T-cell depletion and autologous stem cell transplantation in the management of tumour stage mycosis fungoides with peripheral blood involvement. *Br J Haematol* 2001;**114**:624–31.

17 Soligo D, Ibaticic A, Berti E *et al.* Treatment of advanced mycosis fungoides by allogeneic stem-cell transplantation with a nonmyeloablative regimen. *Bone Marrow Transplant* 2003;**31**:663–6.

18 Wu PA, Kim YH, Lavori PW, Hoppe RT, Stockerl-Goldstein KE. A meta-analysis of patients receiving allogeneic or autologous hematopoietic stem cell transplant in mycosis fungoides and Sezary syndrome. *Biol Blood Marrow Transplant* 2009;**15**:982–90.

19 Duvic M, Donato M, Dabaja B *et al.* Total skin electron beam and non-myeloablative allogeneic hematopoietic stem-cell transplantation in advanced mycosis fungoides and Sezary syndrome. *J Clin Oncol* 2010;**28**:2365–72.

20 de Masson A, Beylot-Barry M, Bouaziz JD *et al.* Allogeneic stem cell transplantation for advanced cutaneous T-cell lymphomas: a study from the French Society of Bone Marrow Transplantation and French Study Group on Cutaneous Lymphomas. *Haematologica* 2014;**99**:527–34.

21 Lechowicz MJ, Lazarus HM, Carreras J *et al.* Allogeneic hematopoietic cell transplantation for mycosis fungoides and Sezary syndrome. *Bone Marrow Transplant* 2014;**49**:1360–5.

22 Duarte RF, Canals C, Onida F *et al.* Allogeneic hematopoietic cell transplantation for patients with mycosis fungoides and Sezary syndrome: a retrospective analysis of the Lymphoma Working Party of the European Group for Blood and Marrow Transplantation. *J Clin Oncol* 2010;**28**:4492–9.

23 Duarte RF, Boumendil A, Onida F *et al.* Long-term outcome of allogeneic hematopoietic cell transplantation for patients with mycosis fungoides and Sezary syndrome: a European Society for Blood and Marrow Transplantation Lymphoma Working Party extended analysis. *J Clin Oncol* 2014;**32**:1–2.

24 Jacobsen ED, Kim HT, Ho VT *et al.* A large single-center experience with allogeneic stem cell transplantation for peripheral T-cell non-Hodgkin lymphoma and advanced mycosis fungoides/Sézary syndrome. *Ann Oncol* 2011;**22**: 1608–13.

25 Armand P, Gannamaneni S, Kim HT *et al.* Improved survival in lymphoma patients receiving sirolimus for graft-versus-host disease prophylaxis after hematopoietic stem-cell transplantation with reduced-intensity conditioning. *J Clin Oncol* 2008;**26**:5767–74.

26 Molina A, Zain J, Arber DA *et al.* Durable clinical, cytogenetic, and molecular remissions after allogeneic hematopoietic cell transplantation for refractory Sezary syndrome and mycosis fungoides. *J Clin Oncol* 2005;**23**:6163–71.

27 Olsen E, Vonderheid E, Pimpinelli N *et al.* Revisions to the staging and classification of mycosis fungoides and Sézary syndrome: a proposal of the International Society for Cutaneous Lymphomas (ISCL) and the cutaneous lymphoma task force of the European Organization of Research and Treatment of Cancer (EORTC). *Blood* 2007;**110**: 1713–22.

CHAPTER 24

Role of transplantation in lymphoplasmacytic lymphoma

Silvia Montoto and Charalampia Kyriakou

Onbehalf of the Lymphoma Working Party-EBMT

Definition and diagnosis: Waldenström macroglobulinemia and lymphoplasmacytic lymphoma

The relationship between Waldenström macroglobulinemia (WM) and lymphoplasmacytic lymphoma (LPL) is frequently a source of confusion and object of controversy. Jan Gosta Waldenström described for the first time the entity that carries his name in 1944 in two patients with enlarged lymphadenopathy, plasma cell infiltration in the bone marrow, and hyperviscosity symptoms due to an abnormal monoclonal paraprotein in the blood [1]. In the past, the term "Waldenström macroglobulinemia" has been used as a synonym of hyperviscosity syndrome caused by the presence of a monoclonal paraprotein of IgM subtype, regardless of the underlying pathologic substrate. More recently, WM has been defined as a lymphoproliferative disorder characterized by the presence of an IgM paraprotein in the setting of LPL infiltration in the bone marrow [2]. The latest classification of the World Health Organization (WHO) published in 2008 defines LPL as a neoplasm of small B lymphocytes, plasmacytoid lymphocytes, and plasma cells usually infiltrating the bone marrow, with or without lymph node involvement; thus, the presence of a monoclonal component, which can be of IgM or of another subtype, is not a requisite for the diagnosis of LPL [3]. The recently described somatic mutation MYD-88 L265P is present in 90% of cases with WM/LPL [4] and thus can be used as a marker of WM/LPL in its frequently difficult differential diagnosis from other lymphoproliferative disorders such as marginal zone lymphoma [5].

Epidemiology

WM/LPL is a rare lymphoproliferative disorder that represents 1–2% of all non-Hodgkin lymphomas. The incidence in the white population in Western countries is 0.3–0.4 per 100,000 inhabitants, whereas it seems to be lower in the non-white population. The median age at diagnosis is over 70 years and there is a male predominance [6]. Having either a personal or family history of autoimmune, inflammatory and infective disorders such as autoimmune hemolytic anemia and Sjögren syndrome is associated with an increased risk of WM/LPL. Along the same lines, a family history of WM/LPL has been associated with an increased risk of WM/LPL [7].

Clinical characteristics at diagnosis and criteria for treatment

Patients can present symptoms due to (i) the IgM paraprotein, (ii) cytopenias, or (iii) tumor burden. Hyperviscosity syndrome is detected in around 30% of patients. There is not a linear relationship between the size of the monoclonal component and the presence of hyperviscosity symptoms, but the latter are more common in patients with an M-band of 40 g/L or more.

Clinical Guide to Transplantation in Lymphoma, First Edition. Edited by Bipin N. Savani and Mohamad Mohty.
© 2015 John Wiley & Sons, Ltd. Published 2015 by John Wiley & Sons, Ltd.

Other symptoms directly caused by the IgM paraprotein are amyloidosis, peripheral neuropathy, cold agglutinin disease, and acquired von Willebrand disease, but these are significantly less common than hyperviscosity syndrome. Bone marrow infiltration can cause cytopenias: 40% of the patients present with anemia at diagnosis, whereas leukopenia and thrombocytopenia are much less common. The presence of B symptoms is observed in around one-quarter of patients. Some patients are diagnosed following investigations of peripheral lymphadenopahy. The presence of bulky disease is rare, but 20% of the patients present lymphadenopathy at diagnosis and splenomegaly can be detected in a similar percentage of patients. However, a considerable proportion of patients, up to one-third, are asymptomatic at presentation, the disease frequently being diagnosed during the course of investigations of a small monoclonal component detected in a routine blood test.

As in other indolent lymphomas, the advanced age at diagnosis, the fact that a significant proportion of patients are asymptomatic at presentation, and the lack of a curative treatment in a disease with an indolent course and prolonged survival makes expectant management the standard treatment at diagnosis, and the decision to start treatment should be based on the presence of clear signs and symptoms. In general, treatment is dictated by the presence of hyperviscosity symptoms or cytopenias. A high monoclonal component does not constitute per se an indication to start therapy, but these patients should be closely monitored for symptoms of hyperviscosity and initiation of treatment if the M-band is rapidly rising. The recommendations of the Second International Workshop on Waldenström macroglobulinemia include cytopenias, constitutional symptoms, symptomatic hyperviscosity or other symptoms directly attributable to the monoclonal component, and symptomatic lymphadenopathy or organomegaly as the criteria for immediate treatment [8].

Prognostic factors

As mentioned, patients newly diagnosed with WM/LPL enjoy a prolonged survival, the median overall survival (OS) being longer than 7 years in a recent series [9]. A number of studies have analyzed the clinical characteristics that are associated with a poor outcome. Not surprisingly, older age is among the most

Table 24.1 International Prognostic Scoring System for Waldenström macroglobulinemia.

Risk group	Risk factors*	Percentage of patients	Median overall survival (months)
Low	0–1 (except age)	27%	143
Intermediate	Age or 2	38%	99
High	3 or more	35%	44

*Age >65 years; hemoglobin <11.5 g/dL; platelet count <100 × 10^9/L; β_2-microglobulin >3 mg/L; IgM >7.0 g/dL.

important factors associated with a poor outcome. Other clinical features such as anemia, raised β_2-microglobulin, and low albuminemia have also been associated with a shortened survival. The International Prognostic Scoring System for Waldenström macroglobulinemia (ISSWM) has recently been described, based on data from 587 symptomatic patients with WM and includes age, hemoglobin, platelet count, β_2-microglobulin, and IgM level [9]. One of the strengths of the ISSWM is that it distributes patients in three risk groups that are well balanced in terms of the proportion of patients in each group. Patients in the low-risk group (young patients with zero to one adverse factor) have a median OS of 143 months, whereas it is 99 months for patients in the intermediate-risk group (two adverse factors or age >65 years), and 44 months for patients in the high-risk group (more than three factors) (Table 24.1).

Novel agents

The development of new agents has revolutionized the management of patients with indolent lymphomas and LPL is not an exception in this sense. Although not new, and despite the fact that LPL was not included in the original studies, rituximab is now fully incorporated in the management of patients with LPL. Along the same lines, bendamustine and bortezomib are nowadays included as treatment options for first-line therapy. More recently, research has led to the development of drugs that target the B-cell receptor such as ibrutinib, which has shown excellent promising results in monotherapy and is currently being tested in combination with other drugs. Other targeted drugs that inhibit different pathways such as the PI3 kinase inhibitor idelalisib are also under investigation.

It is against this background of an indolent disease, frequently diagnosed in elderly asymptomatic patients, with a plethora of new drugs with very promising results on the horizon, that the role of HSCT will be discussed.

Initial management: any role for HSCT?

As mentioned, a significant proportion of patients present asymptomatically and do not require treatment at diagnosis. In contrast with follicular lymphoma, there are no randomized studies comparing this approach with immediate therapy, and hence data on the median time to treatment are scarce. As LPL is a rare disease, very few randomized studies have been performed in this population and data have to be extrapolated from studies in indolent lymphomas or extracted from subgroup analysis. Both alkylating agents and purine analogs are still included among the treatment options for first-line therapy [2,10], although the results of a randomized study comparing chlorambucil and fludarabine showed that fludarabine results in a better outcome in terms of progression-free survival (PFS) and response duration [11]. The efficacy of fludarabine is unfortunately accompanied by a significantly higher hematologic toxicity, which makes it inappropriate in elderly patients and those who are potential candidates for an autologous stem cell transplant (ASCT). Anthracyclines are rarely used as part of the initial treatment given the old age at presentation, and this was further reinforced by a randomized trial comparing bendamustine/rituximab and R-CHOP which demonstrated that the former results in a significantly better outcome with much less toxicity, also in the small group of patients with WM/LPL [12]. Some Phase II studies have investigated the incorporation of novel agents such as bortezomib as part of first-line therapy. Thus, the combination of bortezomib, dexamethasone, and rituximab (BDR) resulted in an overall response rate (RR) of 85% with a median PFS of 42 months [13]. The recommendations of the Fourth International Workshop on Waldenström macroglobulinemia included combinations of alkylating agents, purine analogs and rituximab as the potential first-line treatment options, the choice among them driven by age and comorbidities, clinical presentation, and potential

for ASCT [14]. Table 24.2 shows the results obtained with conventional chemotherapy as first-line treatment.

The data on ASCT as part of first-line therapy are very limited, as this procedure is generally not recommended in this setting given the relatively good prognosis and advanced age of the patients. Data from small studies support the feasibility of such an approach [15,16] (Table 24.3). In the largest study on ASCT in WM/LPL published to date from the Lymphoma Working Party of the European Society for Blood and Marrow Transplantation (LWP-EBMT) [17], 69 patients (44%) were transplanted in first response. The 5-year PFS in this subgroup was 52%, with a 5-year OS of 77% (Table 24.3). These results are better than those achieved with conventional chemotherapy in patients with high-risk disease according to the ISSWM and suggest that it might be worth exploring HSCT as consolidation of first response in this high-risk population.

For obvious reasons, data on allogeneic transplant to consolidate first response are even more limited. Anecdotal case reports have been published suggesting the existence of a graft-versus-lymphoma (GVL) effect [18]. The LWP-EBMT study, the largest study published on allogeneic transplant in WM/LPL, included six patients (7%) who were transplanted after one line of chemotherapy, but no data on the outcome of this subgroup are provided [19]. Along the same lines, in the Center for International Blood and Marrow Transplant Research (CIBMTR) registry study, 19% of the patients were transplanted following one line of treatment but their outcome was not reported separately [20].

Management at relapse: when, if at all, is the right time for HSCT?

As in other indolent lymphomas, treatment options at relapse include the same drugs/regimens that can be used as first-line treatment, provided the patient has not received them. Table 24.2 shows the results of conventional treatment in patients with relapsed WM/LPL, with RRs ranging from 62 to 83% and a median PFS of around 1.5 years [21–23]. As mentioned already, new drugs are showing very promising results. Most of the data come, for obvious reasons, from Phase II trials in patients with relapsed lymphoma (Table 24.2). Advani *et al.* [24] reported on 56 patients with relapsed indolent lymphoma who received salvage ibrutinib. In this study,

Table 24.2 Conventional treatment and novel agents for WM/LPL.

Series	Drugs	N	RR (%)	Median PFS (months)	OS
Initial therapy					
Leblond et al. (2013) [11]	Chlorambucil	202*	39	27 months	62% (at 5 years)
Leblond et al. (2013) [11]	Fludarabine	203*	48	36 months	69% (at 5 years)
Rummel et al. (2013) [12]	Bendamustine/rituximab	261†	93	70 months	NR
Dimopoulos et al. (2013) [13]	Bortezomib/dexamethasone/rituximab	59	68	42 months	82% (at 3 years)
Relapse					
Ghobrial et al. (2010) [21]	Bortezomib/rituximab	37	62	16 months	94% (at 1 year)
Treon et al. (2011) [22]	Bendamustine/rituximab	30	83	Median TTP, 13 months	—
Tedeschi et al. (2012) [23]	Fludarabine/cyclophosphamide/rituximab	40	80	NR (median follow-up, 51 months)	—
Advani et al. (2012) [24]	Ibrutinib	56‡	54	14 months	—
Gopal et al. (2014) [25]	Idelalisib	125§	57	11 months	Median OS, 20 months

*Including 184 and 187 patients with WM/LPL.
†Including 22 patients with WM/LPL.
‡Including four patients with WM/LPL.
§Including 10 patients with WM/LPL.
NR, not reached; OS, overall survival; PFS, progression-free survival; RR, response rate; TTP, time to progression.

Table 24.3 Autologous stem cell transplantation in WM/LPL.

Series	N	Median follow-up (months)	PFS	OS
Initial therapy				
Dreger et al. (2007) [15]	12	69	Median PFS, 69 months	100% (at 69 months)
Caravita et al. (2009) [16]	5	66	100% (at 66 months)	—
Kyriakou et al. (2010) [17]	69	54	52% (at 5 years)	77% (at 5 years)
Relapse				
Anagnostopoulos et al. (2006) [20]	10	63	65% (at 3 years)	70% (at 3 years)
Gilleece et al. (2008) [26]	9	44	DFS, 43% (at 4 years)	73% (at 4 years)
Kyriakou et al. (2010) [17]	158	50	40% (at 5 years)	69% (at 5 years)

DFS, disease-free survival; OS, overall survival; PFS, progression-free survival.

the RR among four patients with WM/LPL was 75%. Data recently published on idelalisib, the PI3Kδ inhibitor, in patients with indolent lymphoma are also very promising, with RR of 57% and median PFS of 11 months in a highly refractory population [25].

A few small studies have reported on the outcome of patients with relapsed WM/LPL following ASCT, with PFS ranging from 65% at 3 years [20] to 43% at 4 years [26] (Table 24.3). Patients included in these series were heavily pretreated [27] and in some cases, as in the CIBMTR study, a significant proportion presented with chemoresistant disease at the time of

ASCT [20]. The largest registry study published is the LWP-EBMT study, which included 158 patients [17] (Table 24.3). In this study, one-third of the patients had received three or more lines of chemotherapy prior to ASCT and 54% had high-risk disease at diagnosis according to the ISSWM. The nonrelapse mortality (NRM) at 5 years was 6%, and after a median follow-up of longer than 4 years the relapse rate at 5 years was 54%. The number of prior chemotherapy lines and being transplanted with chemoresistant disease were the most important predictors of outcome. These data suggest that ASCT

Table 24.4 Allogeneic transplantation in WM/LPL.

Series	N	Median follow-up (months)	NRM	PFS	OS
Anagnostopoulos et al. (2006) [20]	MAC 21 RIC 5	75	40% (at 3 years)	31% (at 3 years)	46% (at 3 years)
Garnier et al. (2010) [28]	MAC 12 RIC 13	63	25% (at 1 year)	58% (at 5 years)	67% (at 5 years)
Kyriakou et al. (2010) [19]	MAC 37 RIC 49	63 44	33% (at 3 years) 23% (at 3 years)	56% (at 5 years) 49% (at 5 years)	62% (at 5 years) 64% (at 5 years)

MAC, myeloablative conditioning; NRM, nonrelapse mortality; OS, overall survival; PFS, progression-free survival; RIC, reduced-intensity conditioning.

is an excellent option to prolong response duration, but it does not result in cure of LPL.

Earlier series on allogeneic transplant in patients with WM/LPL included mostly patients who received a myeloablative conditioning (MAC) regimen and this resulted in a high NRM of around 40% [20,26,27]. In more recent series, a higher proportion of patients who received a reduced-intensity conditioning (RIC) transplant are included, and this translates into a lower NRM (Table 24.4). Thus, in the French registry study, 13 of 25 patients included had an RIC transplant, and the 1-year NRM for the whole series was 25% [28]. Of note, whereas one could assume that RIC allogeneic transplants are rarely performed as the first transplant but are more frequently performed in patients relapsing after an autologous transplant, a relatively small proportion of patients received RIC allogeneic transplant following ASCT failure (23% in Garnier et al. series [28] and 12% in Kyriakou et al study [19]). In 2010, the LWP-EBMT reported on 86 patients who had an allogeneic transplant for WM/LPL during the period 1998–2005 [19]. Around 60% of the patients received an RIC transplant and, as in the majority of studies published, donors were HLA-identical siblings in around 80% of the cases. The patients included represented a heavily pretreated population, with two-thirds of them having received three or more prior treatment lines. No differences were observed in this study in the outcome of patients according to the type of conditioning regimen received, but patients in the RIC group had more advanced disease and were significantly older. Of note, in this study an association between the development of chronic graft-versus-host disease and a lower risk of progression was observed and a significant proportion of patients who received donor lymphocyte infusions achieved a response, supporting the existence of a GVL effect.

Conclusions

Defining the role of HSCT in a disease such as WM/LPL, characterized by advanced age at presentation, an indolent course, and a long survival, represents a difficult challenge. Evidence-based data to support the appropriate timing for HSCT are scarce, given the low incidence of this disease and hence most of the available data come from registry studies. Against this background, the recently described ISSWM provides a powerful tool to select a high-risk population with a poor prognosis when treated with conventional therapy that might benefit from HSCT. Registry data suggest that both ASCT and allogeneic transplant result in better outcomes than conventional treatment in high-risk patients. Efforts should be made to identify young patients with high-risk disease and encourage their early referral for consideration of HSCT.

References

1 Waldenstrom JG. Incipient myelomatosis or "essential" hyperglobulinemia with fibrinogenopenia: a new syndrome? *Acta Med Scand* 1944;**117**:216–47.

2 Owen RG, Pratt G, Auer RL *et al.* Guidelines on the diagnosis and management of Waldenstrom macroglobulinaemia. *Br J Haematol* 2014;**165**:316–33.

3 Swerdlow SH, Berger F, Pileri SA, Harris NL, Jaffe ES, Stein H. Lymphoplasmacytic lymphoma. In: Swerdlow SH, Campo E, Harris NL, Jaffe ES, Pileri SA, Stein H, Thiele J, Vardiman JW, eds.

World Health Organization Classification of Tumours of Haematopoietic and Lymphoid Tissues, 4th edn. Lyon: IARC Press, 2008.

4 Treon SP, Xu L, Yang G *et al*. MYD88 L265P somatic mutation in Waldenstrom's macroglobulinemia. *N Engl J Med* 2012;**367**:826–33.

5 Xu L, Hunter ZR, Yang G *et al*. MYD88 L265P in Waldenstrom macroglobulinemia, immunoglobulin M monoclonal gammopathy, and other B-cell lymphoproliferative disorders using conventional and quantitative allele-specific polymerase chain reaction. *Blood* 2013;**121**:2051–8.

6 Phekoo KJ, Jack RH, Davies E, Moller H, Schey SA. The incidence and survival of Waldenstrom's macroglobulinaemia in South East England. *Leuk Res* 2008;**32**:55–9.

7 Kristinsson SY, Goldin LR, Turesson I, Bjorkholm M, Landgren O. Familial aggregation of lymphoplasmacytic lymphoma/Waldenstrom macroglobulinemia with solid tumors and myeloid malignancies. *Acta Haematol* 2012;**127**:173–7.

8 Kyle RA, Treon SP, Alexanian R et al. Prognostic markers and criteria to initiate therapy in Waldenstrom's macroglobulinemia: consensus panel recommendations from the Second International Workshop on Waldenstrom's Macroglobulinemia. *Semin Oncol* 2003;**30**:116–20.

9 Morel P, Duhamel A, Gobbi P *et al*. International prognostic scoring system for Waldenstrom macroglobulinemia. *Blood* 2009;**113**:4163–70.

10 Anderson KC, Alsina M, Bensinger W *et al*. Waldenstrom's macroglobulinemia/lymphoplasmacytic lymphoma, version 2.2013. *J Natl Compr Canc Netw* 2012;**10**:1211–19.

11 Leblond V, Johnson S, Chevret S *et al*. Results of a randomized trial of chlorambucil versus fludarabine for patients with untreated Waldenstrom macroglobulinemia, marginal zone lymphoma, or lymphoplasmacytic lymphoma. *J Clin Oncol* 2013;**31**:301–7.

12 Rummel MJ, Niederle N, Maschmeyer G *et al*. Bendamustine plus rituximab versus CHOP plus rituximab as first-line treatment for patients with indolent and mantle-cell lymphomas: an open-label, multicentre, randomised, phase 3 non-inferiority trial. *Lancet* 2013;**381**:1203–10.

13 Dimopoulos MA, Garcia-Sanz R, Gavriatopoulou M *et al*. Primary therapy of Waldenstrom macroglobulinemia (WM) with weekly bortezomib, low-dose dexamethasone, and rituximab (BDR): long-term results of a phase 2 study of the European Myeloma Network (EMN). *Blood* 2013;**122**:3276–82.

14 Dimopoulos MA, Gertz MA, Kastritis E *et al*. Update on treatment recommendations from the Fourth International Workshop on Waldenstrom's Macroglobulinemia. *J Clin Oncol* 2009;**27**:120–6.

15 Dreger P, Schmitz N. Autologous stem cell transplantation as part of first-line treatment of Waldenstrom's macroglobulinemia. *Biol Blood Marrow Transplant* 2007;**13**:623–4.

16 Caravita T, Siniscalchi A, Tendas A *et al*. High-dose therapy with autologous PBSC transplantation in the front-line treatment of Waldenstrom's macroglobulinemia. *Bone Marrow Transplant* 2009;**43**:587–8.

17 Kyriakou C, Canals C, Sibon D *et al*. High-dose therapy and autologous stem-cell transplantation in Waldenstrom macroglobulinemia: the Lymphoma Working Party of the European Group for Blood and Marrow Transplantation. *J Clin Oncol* 2010;**28**:2227–32.

18 Meniane JC, El-Cheikh J, Faucher C *et al*. Long-term graft-versus-Waldenstrom macroglobulinemia effect following reduced intensity conditioning allogeneic stem cell transplantation. *Bone Marrow Transplant* 2007;**40**:175–7.

19 Kyriakou C, Canals C, Cornelissen JJ *et al*. Allogeneic stem-cell transplantation in patients with Waldenstrom macroglobulinemia: report from the Lymphoma Working Party of the European Group for Blood and Marrow Transplantation. *J Clin Oncol* 2010;**28**:4926–34.

20 Anagnostopoulos A, Hari PN, Perez WS *et al*. Autologous or allogeneic stem cell transplantation in patients with Waldenstrom's macroglobulinemia. *Biol Blood Marrow Transplant* 2006;**12**:845–54.

21 Ghobrial IM, Hong F, Padmanabhan S *et al*. Phase II trial of weekly bortezomib in combination with rituximab in relapsed or relapsed and refractory Waldenstrom macroglobulinemia. *J Clin Oncol* 2010;**28**:1422–8.

22 Treon SP, Hanzis C, Tripsas C *et al*. Bendamustine therapy in patients with relapsed or refractory Waldenstrom's macroglobulinemia. *Clin Lymphoma Myeloma Leuk* 2011;**11**:133–5.

23 Tedeschi A, Benevolo G, Varettoni M *et al*. Fludarabine plus cyclophosphamide and rituximab in Waldenstrom macroglobulinemia: an effective but myelosuppressive regimen to be offered to patients with advanced disease. *Cancer* 2012;**118**:434–43.

24 Advani RH, Buggy JJ, Sharman JP *et al*. Bruton tyrosine kinase inhibitor ibrutinib (PCI-32765) has significant activity in patients with relapsed/refractory B-cell malignancies. *J Clin Oncol* 2012;**31**:88–94.

25 Gopal AK, Kahl BS, de Vos S *et al*. PI3Kdelta inhibition by idelalisib in patients with relapsed indolent lymphoma. *N Engl J Med* 2014;**370**:1008–18.

26 Gilleece MH, Pearce R, Linch DC *et al*. The outcome of haemopoietic stem cell transplantation in the treatment of lymphoplasmacytic lymphoma in the UK: a British Society Bone Marrow Transplantation study. *Hematology* 2008;**13**:119–27.

27 Tournilhac O, Leblond V, Tabrizi R *et al*. Transplantation in Waldenstrom's macroglobulinemia: the French experience. *Semin Oncol* 2003;**30**:291–6.

28 Garnier A, Robin M, Larosa F *et al*. Allogeneic hematopoietic stem cell transplantation allows long-term complete remission and curability in high-risk Waldenstrom's macroglobulinemia. Results of a retrospective analysis of the Societe Francaise de Greffe de Moelle et de Therapie Cellulaire. *Haematologica* 2010;**95**:950–5.

CHAPTER 25

Transplantation outcome in primary mediastinal large B-cell lymphoma

Amanda F. Cashen

Introduction

Primary mediastinal large B-cell lymphoma (PMBL) is a subtype of diffuse large B-cell lymphoma (DLBCL) that is listed as a distinct entity in the World Health Organization (WHO) classification. PMBL typically occurs in young adults, with a modest female predominance. Most patients present with a bulky mediastinal mass, which can cause superior vena cava syndrome or invade into adjacent thoracic structures. Involvement outside the chest is uncommon at the time of diagnosis, and bone marrow involvement is rare [1]. On the other hand, extranodal disease is frequently seen in relapsed PMBL.

PMBL derives from thymic B cells, probably in late germinal-center differentiation [2–4]. The tumors are marked by sclerosis in the surrounding stroma, and immunohistochemical staining demonstrates expression of B-cell markers, including CD20, CD19, and CD22, as well as weak expression of CD30. Common chromosome abnormalities in PMBL include gains in 2p, leading to overexpression of cREL, and gains in 9p, associated with janus kinase (JAK)-2 overexpression [5]. Gene expression profiling studies have established significant overlap in the pattern of genes overexpressed in both PMBL and Hodgkin lymphoma, in contrast to DLBCL [3]. Similar to Hodgkin lymphoma, the nuclear factor (NF)-κB survival pathway and the JAK-STAT (janus kinase/signal transducer and activator of transcription) pathway are activated and provide a survival advantage in PBML [2,6].

First-line therapy of PMBL

PMBL has been treated with a variety of standard-intensity and dose-dense regimens derived from the management of DLBCL. Historically, most patients have also been treated with mediastinal radiation, although the necessity of radiation is debated. Retrospective studies comparing CHOP (cyclophosphamide, adriamycin, vincrinstine, prednisone) or CHOP-like regimens with the dose-intense regimens VACOP-B and MACOP-B (etoposide or methotrexate, adriamycin, cyclophosphamide, vincristine, prednisone, bleomycin) suggest superiority of the latter regimens [7–10], although no prospective randomized data are available. Overall survival (OS) at 3 years or more following CHOP or CHOP-like regimens has ranged from 44 to 71%, compared with 71–87% following VACOP-B or MACOP-B [8–16]. In the largest retrospective series of patients treated in the pre-rituximab era, 10-year progression-free survival (PFS) and OS were 35% and 44% for patients treated with CHOP ($N = 105$) compared to 67% and 71% for patients treated with MACOP-B and other third-generation regimens ($N = 277$) [7]. Most relapses occur quickly, so that progressive disease more than 2 years after therapy is rare.

Addition of rituximab to CHOP may match the efficacy of the third-generation regimens, with retrospective studies reporting PFS of 74–88% and long-term OS exceeding 80% when patients with PMBL are treated with R-CHOP [9,10,16–19]. On the other hand, addition of rituximab to third-generation regimens does not clearly improve their efficacy [10,20]. Although no

Clinical Guide to Transplantation in Lymphoma, First Edition. Edited by Bipin N. Savani and Mohamad Mohty.
© 2015 John Wiley & Sons, Ltd. Published 2015 by John Wiley & Sons, Ltd.

Table 25.1 Upfront high-dose chemotherapy/ASCT in PMBL.

Study	N	Eligibility for ASCT	Radiation	PFS	OS
Rodríguez et al. [25]	71	Retrospective, any response to induction chemotherapy	53%	81% (4 year)	84% (4 year)
Zinzani et al. [7]	44	Enrolled in prospective study	Yes	78% (10 year)	77% (10 year)
Hamlin et al. [14]	17	Enrolled in prospective study	Yes	60% (10 year)	78% (10 year)
Cairoli et al. [34]	15	Retrospective, high intermed or high IPI score	Yes	93% (3 year)	NR
Sehn et al. [28]	12	Retrospective, first CR or PR	NR	83% (5 year)	NR

ASCT, autologous stem cell transplantation; CR, complete remission; NR, not reported; OS, overall survival; PFS, progression-free survival; PR, partial remission.

randomized study has been undertaken specifically in PMBL patients, an analysis of the subset of 87 PBML cases treated in the Mabthera International Trial, which assigned young, newly diagnosed DLBCL patients to treatment with CHOP-like therapy with or without rituximab, found that addition of rituximab decreased the rate of disease progression from 24% to 2.5% in the PBML patients, so that event-free survival (EFS) was 78 versus 52% ($P = 0.012$) with and without rituximab [17].

Other dose-intense regimens that incorporate rituximab have also demonstrated excellent outcomes in PMBL. In the dose-adjusted EPOCH-R regimen, infusional doxorubicin, etoposide, and vincristine are combined with bolus cyclophosphamide, prednisone, and rituximab, and the doses delivered with each cycle are adjusted to maximize therapeutic intensity. No consolidative radiation is given. In a subset analysis of PMBL patients treated within a larger DLBCL study, DA-EPOCH, without rituximab, provided EFS of 67% and OS of 78% [21]. In a Phase II study, 51 patients with PBML were treated with DA-EPOCH plus rituximab and, after a median follow-up of 5 years, EFS and OS were 93% and 97%, respectively [22]. Another dose-dense regimen, combining R-CHOP and consolidative ICE (ifosfamide, carboplatin, etoposide), provided PFS of 78% and OS of 88% in 54 patients with PMBL, with no radiation delivered to responding patients [23,24].

Prognostic factors in PMBL and the role of consolidative autologous stem cell transplant

Randomized trials have demonstrated improved outcomes in high-risk DLBCL patients treated with autologous stem cell transplantation (ASCT) in first remission.

These results prompted the exploration of ASCT in consolidating response in patients with PBML who were considered at high risk of relapse. The available reports include small numbers of patients treated with variable pretransplant chemotherapy, transplant conditioning regimens, and radiation strategies (Table 25.1). Despite the limitations of the data, it is reasonable to conclude that ASCT can provide durable disease control and excellent long-term survival when incorporated into the upfront therapy of patients with PMBL. However, no data have established the superiority of consolidative ASCT over induction chemotherapy alone.

It is unlikely that upfront ASCT could improve on the outcomes achieved with current immunochemotherapy approaches, given that fewer than 20% of patients fail therapy with R-CHOP, R-VACOP-B, or DA-EPOCH-R. Identifying the patients who are at high risk of treatment failure, and who might benefit from consolidative ASCT, has proven difficult. The International Prognostic Index and other accepted risk factors in DLBCL have inconsistent prognostic value in PMBL [10,13,20,25]. Functional imaging with ^{18}F-fluorodeoxyglucose positron emission tomography (FDG-PET) has also failed to identify patients who may benefit from additional therapy. FDG-PET has a low positive predictive value in PMBL, whether performed during the course of therapy [10,23,26] or at the end of therapy [22,27], suggesting that residual masses, even if FDG avid, are more likely to represent fibrosis and inflammation than disease. In the absence of prospective data demonstrating benefit of ASCT in first remission of PMBL, transplant is best reserved for those patients who have biopsy-proven residual lymphoma at the end of induction chemotherapy or who relapse after initial response.

Treatment of relapsed or refractory PMBL

The management of relapsed or refractory PMBL mirrors that undertaken for relapsed DLBCL: salvage chemotherapy followed by ASCT for patients with chemosensitive disease. However, the response to salvage chemotherapy in PMBL is low, and outcomes for patients with relapsed or refractory PMBL have been poor, as reported in retrospective series [11]. For example, in one series, response to salvage chemotherapy was 38% among 23 patients with relapsed or refractory PMBL [28], and in another only 4 of 27 patients (15%) treated with salvage chemotherapy survived [18]. Salvage chemotherapy options for PMBL are the same as those used for DLBCL, and there is no evidence to support one regimen over another [29,30]. The CD30-targeted antibody–drug conjugate brentuximab vedotin is one novel approach to the treatment of relapsed PMBL, given the common albeit low-level expression of CD30 on the malignant B cells. However, among the PBML subset of a larger Phase II study, the overall response rate was only 17% [31].

Autologous stem cell transplant for relapsed PMBL

The limiting factor in the use of ASCT for patients with relapsed PMBL is the chemorefractory nature of the lymphoma, so that many patients are never eligible for ASCT. In a Memorial Sloan-Kettering retrospective series [14], 64 PMBL patients relapsed after front-line chemotherapy and only 36 (56%) had subsequent ASCT. OS among the transplanted patients was 54%. The same group reported that among 54 PMBL patients treated with dose-intense chemotherapy, 11 failed upfront dose-intense chemotherapy and five of them were successfully salvaged with therapy that included ASCT [23].

Among the patients who do respond to salvage chemotherapy, ASCT can provide long-term disease control similar to that achieved in DLBCL. Kuruvilla *et al.* [32] evaluated 37 patients with relapsed/refractory PMBL who were treated with standard platinum-based salvage chemotherapy regimens between 1995 and 2004 and compared their outcomes with a cohort of DLBCL patients treated during the same period. Fewer than 10% of patients in their cohort received rituximab. Patients who responded to salvage therapy with a partial remission or better received subsequent high-dose chemotherapy and ASCT. Among the PMBL patients, the response to salvage chemotherapy was remarkably low (25%), so that only 22% of patients underwent ASCT. The 2-year PFS was 15% for the PMBL cohort, which was statistically significantly worse than for the DLBCL patients (34%, $P = 0.018$). However, PMBL patients who did undergo ASCT had PFS and OS of 57% and 67%, respectively, which was not different from the results for the DLBCL patients.

The M.D. Anderson Cancer Center group also retrospectively compared ASCT outcomes in PMBL and DLBCL patients [33]. Among the 31 patients with PMBL, 14 had induction failure, 11 were in chemosensitive relapse, and six had chemorefractory relapse. Disease-free survival (DFS) and OS were 55% and 56% for the PMBL patients, compared to 32% and 35% for the 50 patients with DLBCL ($P = 0.07$ for DFS; $P = 0.05$ for OS). The study concluded that PMBL may be more sensitive to high-dose chemotherapy than DLBCL, but it is hard to support this conclusion given the high failure rate to pre-transplant salvage chemotherapy.

Selin *et al.* [28] reported the outcome of 35 patients who underwent ASCT prior to 1995 (12 first response, 12 primary refractory, 11 relapsed). For the entire cohort, 5-year PFS after ASCT was 57%. Chemosensitivity and disease status at the time of transplant were significantly associated with PFS. PFS was 83%, 58%, and 27% for patients transplanted in first response, primary refractory, and relapse, respectively, while 5-year PFS was 75% in patients with chemosensitive disease at the time of transplant versus 33% who had less than partial remission prior to transplant. Although these results suggest that a portion of patients with primary refractory disease can be salvaged with additional chemotherapy followed by ASCT, not all the primary refractory patients in this series had functional imaging and/or biopsy. Some of them may have had residual fibrotic masses that were incorrectly classified as active lymphoma.

Allogeneic stem cell transplant

Information about allogeneic stem cell transplant in the management of PMBL is relegated to case reports. This modality could be approached as for other aggressive lymphomas, with allogeneic transplant considered for patients who fail multiple lines of therapy and/or who relapse after prior ASCT.

Conclusions

Most patients diagnosed with PMBL will enjoy long-term DFS after treatment with immunochemotherapy, so that additional therapy with stem cell transplant is not indicated. Unfortunately, for the minority of PMBL patients who do fail first-line therapy, the response to salvage chemotherapy is low. Patients who have chemosensitive relapsed disease should proceed with consolidative ASCT, as the outcomes after transplant are comparable to those achieved when ASCT is used to treat DLBCL.

Case study

A 28-year-old woman presents with cough, chest pain, and shortness of breath. Chest X-ray reveals a large mediastinal mass. Chest CT confirms a 12-cm mediastinal mass, associated with pleural extension and a pleural effusion. Biopsy is performed via mediastinoscopy, and pathology reveals sclerosis and an infiltration of large cells that are positive for CD20, CD19, and CD30, consistent with primary mediastinal B-cell lymphoma. She is treated with six cycles of R-CHOP. At the end of therapy, FDG-PET shows resolution of the pleural effusion, but a 4-cm mediastinal mass remains, with a focus of FDG uptake. The residual mass is biopsied, and pathology demonstrates persistent lymphoma. She is treated with a platinum-based salvage regimen, with a negative FDG-PET scan at the end of three cycles. She then undergoes high-dose chemotherapy with BEAM, followed by ASCT. She is alive and disease-free 2 years post transplant.

References

1 Cazals-Hatem D, Lepage E, Brice P *et al*. A clinicopathologic study of 141 cases compared with 916 nonmediastinal large B-cell lymphomas, a GELA (Groupe d'Etude des Lymphomes de l'Adulte) study. *Am J Surg Pathol* 1996;**20**:877–88.

2 Savage KJ, Monti S, Kutok JL *et al*. The molecular signature of mediastinal large B-cell lymphoma differs from that of other diffuse large B-cell lymphomas and shares features with classical Hodgkin lymphoma. *Blood* 2003;**102**:3871–9.

3 Rosenwald A, Wright G, Leroy K *et al*. Molecular diagnosis of primary mediastinal B cell lymphoma identifies a clinically favorable subgroup of diffuse large B cell lymphoma related to Hodgkin lymphoma. *J Exp Med* 2003;**198**:851–62.

4 Pileri S, Gaidano G, Zinzani P *et al*. Primary mediastinal B-cell lymphoma: high frequency of BCL-6 mutations and consistent expression of the transcription factors OCT-2, BOB.1, and PU.1 in the absence of immunoglobulins. *Am J Pathol* 2003;**162**:243–53.

5 Joos S, Otano-Joos M, Ziegler S *et al*. Primary mediastinal (thymic) B-cell lymphoma is characterized by gains of chromosomal material including 9p and amplification of the REL gene. *Blood* 1996;**87**:1571–8.

6 Steidl C, Gascoyne RD. The molecular pathogenesis of primary mediastinal large B-cell lymphoma. *Blood* 2011;**118**: 2659–69.

7 Zinzani P, Martelli M, Bertini M *et al*. Induction chemotherapy strategies for primary mediastinal large B-cell lymphoma with sclerosis: a retrospective multinational study on 426 previously untreated patients. *Haematologica* 2002; **87**:1258–64.

8 Todeschini G, Secchi S, Morra E *et al*. Primary mediastinal large B-cell lymphoma (PMLBCL): long-term results from a retrospective multicentre Italian experience in 138 patients treated with CHOP or MACOP-B//VACOP-B. *Br J Cancer* 2004;**90**:372–6.

9 Savage KJ, Al-Rajhi N, Voss N *et al*. Favorable outcome of primary mediastinal large B-cell lymphoma in a single institution: the British Columbia experience. *Ann Oncol* 2006;**17**: 123–30.

10 Avigdor A, Sirotkin T, Kedmi M *et al*. The impact of R-VACOP-B and interim FDG-PET/CT on outcome in primary mediastinal large B cell lymphoma. *Ann Hematol* 2014;**93**:1297–304.

11 Lazzarino M, Orlandi E, Paulli M *et al*. Treatment outcome and prognostic factors for primary mediastinal (thymic) B-cell lymphoma: a multicenter study of 106 patients. *J Clin Oncol* 1997;**15**:1646–53.

12 Abou-Elella AA, Weisenburger DD, Vose JM *et al*. Primary mediastinal large B-cell lymphoma: a clinicopathologic study of 43 patients from the Nebraska Lymphoma Study Group. *J Clin Oncol* 1999;**17**:784.

13 Zinzani P, Martelli M, Bertini M *et al*. Induction chemotherapy strategies for primary mediastinal large B-cell lymphoma with sclerosis: a retrospective multinational study on 426 previously untreated patients. *Haematologica* 2002;**87**:1258–64.

14 Hamlin PA, Portlock CS, Straus DJ *et al*. Primary mediastinal large B-cell lymphoma: optimal therapy and prognostic factor analysis in 141 consecutive patients treated at memorial Sloan Kettering from 1980 to 1999. *Br J Haematol* 2005;**130**:691–9.

15 Mazzarotto R, Boso C, Vianello F *et al*. Primary mediastinal large B-cell lymphoma: results of intensive chemotherapy regimens (MACOP-B/VACOP-B) plus involved

field radiotherapy on 53 patients. A single institution experience. *Int J Radiat Oncol Biol Phys* 2007;**68**:823–9.

16 Tai WM, Quah D, Peng Yap S *et al*. Primary mediastinal large B-cell lymphoma: optimal therapy and prognostic factors in 41 consecutive Asian patients. *Leukemia Lymphoma* 2011;**52**:604–12.

17 Rieger M, Österborg A, Pettengell R *et al*. Primary mediastinal B-cell lymphoma treated with CHOP-like chemotherapy with or without rituximab: results of the Mabthera International Trial Group study. *Ann Oncol* 2011;**22**:664–70.

18 Xu L-M, Fang H, Wang W-H *et al*. Prognostic significance of rituximab and radiotherapy for patients with primary mediastinal large B-cell lymphoma receiving doxorubicin-containing chemotherapy. *Leukemia Lymphoma* 2013;**54**:1684–90.

19 Savage KJ, Yenson PR, Shenkier T *et al*. The outcome of primary mediastinal large B-cell lymphoma (PMBCL) in the R-CHOP treatment era.*Blood (ASH Annual Meeting Abstracts)* 2012;**120**:Abstract 303.

20 Zinzani P, Stefoni V, Finolezzi E *et al*. Rituximab combined with MACOP-B or VACOP-B and radiation therapy in primary mediastinal large B-cell lymphoma: a retrospective study. *Clin Lymphoma Myeloma* 2009;**9**:381–5.

21 Wilson WH, Grossbard ML, Pittaluga S *et al*. Dose-adjusted EPOCH chemotherapy for untreated large B-cell lymphomas: a pharmacodynamic approach with high efficacy. *Blood* 2002;**99**:2685–93.

22 Dunleavy K, Pittaluga S, Maeda LS *et al*. Dose-adjusted EPOCH-rituximab therapy in primary mediastinal B-cell lymphoma. *N Engl J Med* 2013;**368**:1408–16.

23 Moskowitz C, Hamlin PA Jr, Maragulia J, Meikle J, Zelenetz AD. Sequential dose-dense RCHOP followed by ICE consolidation (MSKCC protocol 01-142) without radiotherapy for patients with primary mediastinal large B cell lymphoma. *Blood (ASH Annual Meeting Abstracts)* 2010;**116**:Abstract 420.

24 Moskowitz CH, Schöder H, Teruya-Feldstein J *et al*. Risk-adapted dose-dense immunochemotherapy determined by interim FDG-PET in advanced-stage diffuse large B-cell lymphoma. *J Clin Oncol* 2010;**28**:1896–903.

25 Rodríguez J, Conde E, Gutiérrez A *et al*. Primary mediastinal large cell lymphoma (PMBL): frontline treatment with autologous stem cell transplantation (ASCT). The GEL-TAMO experience. *Hematol Oncol* 2008;**26**:171–8.

26 Moskowitz C, Hamlin PA, Horwitz SM *et al*. Phase II trial of dose-dense R-CHOP followed by risk-adapted consolidation with either ICE or ICE and ASCT, based upon the results of biopsy confirmed abnormal interim restaging PET scan, improves outcome in patients with advanced stage DLBCL. *Blood (ASH Annual Meeting Abstracts)* 2006;**108**:Abstract 532.

27 Ceriani L, Zucca E, Zinzani PL *et al*. Role of positron emission tomography (PET/CT) in primary mediastinal large B cell lymphoma (PMLBCL): preliminary results of an international Phase II trial (IELSG-26 Study) conducted on behalf of the International Extranodal Lymphoma Study Group (IELSG), the Fondazione Italiana Linfomi (FIL) and the UK NCRI Lymphoma Group. *Blood (ASH Annual Meeting Abstracts)* 2012;**120**:Abstract 1566.

28 Sehn LH, Antin JH, Shulman LN *et al*. Primary diffuse large B-cell lymphoma of the mediastinum: outcome following high-dose chemotherapy and autologous hematopoietic cell transplantation. *Blood* 1998;**91**:717–23.

29 Gisselbrecht C, Glass B, Mounier N *et al*. Salvage regimens with autologous transplantation for relapsed large B-cell lymphoma in the rituximab era. *J Clin Oncol* 2010;**28**:4184–90.

30 Matasar MJ, Czuczman MS, Rodriguez MA *et al*. Ofatumumab in combination with ICE or DHAP chemotherapy in relapsed or refractory intermediate grade B-cell lymphoma. *Blood* 2013;**122**:499–506.

31 Bartlett NL, Sharman JP, Oki Y *et al*. A Phase 2 study of brentuximab vedotin in patients with relapsed or refractory CD30-positive non-Hodgkin lymphomas: interim results in patients with DLBCL and other B-cell lymphomas. *Blood (ASH Annual Meeting Abstracts)* 2013;**122**:848.

32 Kuruvilla J, Pintilie M, Tsang R, Nagy T, Keating A, Crump M. Salvage chemotherapy and autologous stem cell transplantation are inferior for relapsed or refractory primary mediastinal large B-cell lymphoma compared with diffuse large B-cell lymphoma. *Leukemia Lymphoma* 2008;**49**:1329–36.

33 Popat U, Przepiork D, Champlin R *et al*. High-dose chemotherapy for relapsed and refractory diffuse large B-cell lymphoma: mediastinal localization predicts for a favorable outcome. *J Clin Oncol* 1998;**16**:63–9

34 Cairoli R, Grillo G, Tedeschi A *et al*. Efficacy of an early intensification treatment integrating chemotherapy, autologous stem cell transplantation and radiotherapy for poor risk primary mediastinal large B cell lymphoma with sclerosis. *Bone Marrow Transplant* 2002;**29**:473–7.

CHAPTER 26

Management of post-transplant lymphoproliferative disorders

Jan Styczynski and Per Ljungman

Introduction

Post-transplant lymphoproliferative disorders (PTLD) can be broadly defined as a heterogeneous group of lymphoproliferative diseases occurring in the setting of either hematopoietic stem cell transplantation (HSCT) or solid organ transplantation (SOT). PTLD is due to the uncontrolled neoplastic proliferation of plasmacytic or lymphoid cells, and is often life-threatening. It can occur at any age and after all types of transplants, although PTLD occurring after autologous transplantation is very rare. Recipients of allogeneic HSCT are at particular risk for developing PTLD [1,2].

Since the first report over 40 years ago, PTLD has remained one of the most severe complications associated with transplantation. Before the current methods of therapy with drugs that inhibit Epstein–Barr virus (EBV) were introduced, the mortality from PTLD was very high. Before 2000, an attributable mortality for PTLD of 84.6% after HSCT was reported [2].

Epidemiology

EBV is the predominant cause of PTLD in both adults and children. While both primary EBV infection and reactivation can trigger PTLD, the risk is higher after a primary infection and this is considered a major risk factor in transplant patients. Since the EBV seropositivity rate increases with age and 90% of adults worldwide are infected with EBV, adults have a lower risk of developing EBV-related PTLD (EBV-PTLD) than children, who are more likely to develop a primary EBV infection [3].

EBV-PTLD usually presents early after transplant, with the highest rates occurring within the first year. However, late PTLD can occur up to 10 years after SOT. While EBV still remains the major cause, a significant proportion of late PTLD in SOT patients (21–38%) may be EBV-negative and non-B cell. These tend to present more than 5 years after transplant and carry a worse prognosis [3,4].

In a recent European Society for Blood and Marrow Transplantation (EBMT) study, the overall incidence of PTLD after allogeneic HSCT was 3.2%, varying from 1.2% in matched family donor to 11.2% in mismatched unrelated donor recipients [5]. Overall, the frequency of PTLD after alternative donor (mismatched family donor or unrelated donor) allogeneic (allo)-HSCT was 4.7%, while PTLD frequency after cord blood transplantation was 4.1% [5].

The lower incidence of PTLD following matched family donor HSCT is probably due to a more rapid reconstitution of EBV-specific cytotoxic T lymphocyte (CTL) activity [2,6,7]. On the other hand, the increased risk in unrelated donor HSCT is likely due to delayed EBV CTL recovery in these patients [2,6,7]. Furthermore, a human leukocyte antigen (HLA) disparity may induce chronic B-cell stimulation and proliferation, which could predispose a patient to develop PTLD.

Risk factors for PTLD

Risk factors related to the HSCT setting can be divided into the following categories: (i) donor-related factors (unrelated or mismatched donor, unrelated cord

Clinical Guide to Transplantation in Lymphoma, First Edition. Edited by Bipin N. Savani and Mohamad Mohty.

blood, older recipient age, older donor age); (ii) the preparative regimen (total body irradiation, T-cell depletion, and especially the use of anti-T-cell monoclonal antibodies); and (iii) severe graft-versus-host disease (GVHD) [8–12]. The major risk factors for PTLD include an unrelated or mismatched HSCT, T-cell depletion (*in vivo* or *in vitro*), EBV serologic mismatch between donor and recipient, and cord blood HSCT. Minor risk factors include primary EBV infection, splenectomy, and chronic GVHD. The risk of PTLD increases with the number of risk factors. Allo-HSCT with at least one of the major risk factors is regarded as a high-risk transplant for PTLD development. A high incidence of PTLD in both pediatric and adult patients following reduced-intensity conditioning (RIC) regimens using antithymocyte globulin (ATG) or alemtuzumab has also been reported [13,14]. This likely reflects both the delayed recovery of EBV-specific immunity after such transplants and the persistence of recipient-derived B cells.

Pathogenesis

The pathogenesis of PTLD is a result of EBV-induced transformation of B cells in the setting of impaired anti-EBV cellular immunity due to iatrogenic immunosuppression and resulting in an outgrowth of EBV-infected B cells. GVHD prevention strategies that indiscriminately remove T cells from the graft increase the risk of PTLD [15]. PTLD is also associated with T-cell dysfunction such as poor response to interleukin (IL)-7 stimulation [16].

PTLDs reflect a wide spectrum of histologically diverse lymphoproliferative disorders. The World Health Organization (WHO) classification is the most commonly used, with four types of morphologic lesions being recognized: polyclonal early lesions, polymorphic PTLD, malignant monoclonal monomorphic PTLD (B-cell or T/NK-cell lymphoma), and classical Hodgkin lymphoma-type PTLD. Histologic changes observed in PTLD are similar to those in lymphomas occurring in nontransplant patients, with the vast majority being B-cell lymphomas, due to decreased T-cell immune surveillance, although T-cell and Hodgkin lymphomas, or even plasma-cell disease-resembling myelomas, may sporadically occur.

EBV-negative and/or T-lineage PTLD

A growing number of cases of EBV-negative PTLD have been reported, mainly in SOT recipients [4]. These cases tend to present later (>5 years after transplant), and an increased risk is observed as long as 10 years after transplantation [17]. In our opinion, these cases should be regarded as malignant lymphoma, not PTLD. T-lineage PTLD (T-PTLD) is usually EBV-negative and the relatively long latency between transplantation and T-PTLD onset may be explained by molecular events. The frequency of T-PTLDs ranges from 4 to 15% of all PTLD cases. EBV is present in approximately one-third of T-PTLDs [18,19]. For the majority of B-lineage PTLDs (B-PTLD), the role of EBV has been proposed and accepted [20], whereas no direct role for EBV has been confirmed in T-PTLD. The pathogenesis of B-PTLD is mostly based on B lymphocytes infected by EBV. In general, T lymphocytes do not express the EBV receptor CD21; however, some T-PTLDs might show aberrant T cells that are positive for CD21 and EBV [21].

Composite B-cell and T-cell lineage PTLD harboring both B- and T-cell clones either concurrently or successively in the same patient are extremely rare and only a few cases have been reported in the literature, exclusively after SOT, with poor outcome.

Clinical symptoms of PTLD

The median time to diagnosis of PTLD after HSCT is 2 months, with about 6% occurring within the first month and almost 90% within the first 6 months after HSCT [5]. Fever and lymphadenopathy are the most common symptoms and signs of EBV-PTLD and are commonly associated with rapidly progressive multiorgan failure and death if not promptly treated [22]. Other EBV-associated post-transplant diseases, also referred to as end-organ EBV diseases, include encephalitis/myelitis, pneumonia, and hepatitis. In recipients of an allo-HSCT, the 3-year cumulative incidence of the total of EBV-associated diseases, PTLDs, EBV fever, and EBV end-organ diseases was reported to be 15.6%, 9.9%, 3.3%, and 3.3%, respectively [22]. In the recipients of unrelated cord blood, the incidence of EBV-related complications was 3.3% for myeloablative and 7% for nonmyeloablative transplantations [14]. Fever was the most common symptom of EBV-associated diseases.

Diagnosis of PTLD

The diagnosis of PTLD is based on symptoms and signs, imaging, histologic confirmation, and the presence of EBV. A diagnostic work-up for suspected PTLD should therefore include physical examination (including examination for tonsillitis, adenopathy, and organomegaly), a complete blood count, serum electrolytes, calcium, blood urea nitrogen and creatinine, liver function tests, uric acid, lactate dehydrogenase, quantitative immunoglobulins, stools for occult bleeding, flow cytometry of lymphocytes (when possible), imaging (including ultrasound, PET, CT of neck/chest/abdomen/pelvis), a needle or excisional biopsy of the suspected lesion, or endoscopy in cases of gastrointestinal symptoms. EBV studies should also be performed, including serology (anti-EBNA, i.e., Epstein–Barr nuclear antigens, viral capsid antigen, and early antigen), EBV viral load from peripheral blood, and EBER (EBV-encoded RNA) and CD20 histochemistry studies on biopsy material.

EBV-related PTLD can be classified as either proven or probable disease [11]. PTLD is proven when EBV is detected in a specimen obtained from an organ by biopsy or other invasive procedure, using a test with appropriate sensitivity and specificity, together with symptoms and signs from the affected organ. Probable PTLD is defined as significant lymphadenopathy or other end-organ disease without a biopsy, accompanied by a high EBV DNA blood load, in the absence of other etiologic factors or established diseases. According to the definition of EBMT Infectious Diseases Working Party, histopathologic diagnosis of EBV-PTLD should have at least two and ideally three of the following features: (i) disruption of underlying cellular architecture by a lymphoproliferative process; (ii) presence of monoclonal or oligoclonal cell populations as revealed by cellular and/or viral markers; and (iii) evidence of EBV infection in many of the cells (i.e., DNA, RNA or protein). Detection of EBV nucleic acid in blood is not sufficient for the diagnosis of EBV-PTLD.

EBV DNAemia and PTLD

There is a high correlation between EBV DNAemia in peripheral blood and the development of PTLD and other EBV-associated disorders [4,6]. Prospective monitoring of EBV DNAemia can be performed in whole blood, plasma, or serum [5,11,23]. Usually, EBV DNAemia precedes the onset of clinical symptoms but this has not been a consistent finding [24].

Screening for EBV DNA should start on the day of HSCT and should continue for 3 months with a frequency of at least once weekly in high-risk patients; longer monitoring is recommended in patients on treatment for GVHD, after haploidentical HSCT, and in those having experienced an early EBV reactivation [11]. In EBV DNA-positive patients with rising EBV DNA load, a more frequent sampling might be considered since the viral load can rise very rapidly [25]. Current data do not allow the establishment of an EBV viral load threshold value for the diagnosis of PTLD (or other end-organ EBV disease) in HSCT patients [26]. It is also not possible to correlate the peak EBV viral loads with clinical disease manifestations [11].

EBV management strategies

Different approaches have been used for the prevention and treatment of EBV-PTLD. These include the administration of rituximab, reduction of immunosuppression, or use of EBV-specific CTL. These have been published as recommendations by the European Conference on Infections in Leukemia (ECIL) [11]. Despite a relatively wide range of antiviral drugs, none of them can be recommended for prevention or therapy of EBV-PTLD. This is due to the lack of activity of a viral thymidine kinase in latent EBV. PTLD lesions typically consist of EBV-immortalized B cells and only a minority of cells expressing lytic antigens of EBV. A novel approach has been recently used in which viral replication is promoted with the use of arginine butyrate upregulating the expression of the EBV thymidine kinase [27]. A new antiviral agent, brincidofovir, has excellent antiviral activity against EBV *in vitro* but whether prophylaxis with this drug will be able to reduce the risk for EBV replication and possibly PTLD will require further study.

Possible strategies for using these approaches include prophylaxis, preemptive therapy, and treatment of established PTLD. The following definitions are used.

1 Prophylaxis against EBV DNAemia is defined as treatment given with the aim of preventing EBV reactivation in a seropositive patient (or a primary infection when the donor is seropositive and the patient seronegative).

2 Preemptive therapy is defined as anti-EBV treatment given to an asymptomatic patient with EBV detected by a screening assay.

3 Treatment of EBV disease is defined as therapy given to a patient with EBV (proven or probable) disease.

Prevention of EBV-PTLD

The ECIL recommends that high-risk HSCT patients should be tested for EBV antibodies before allo-HSCT. If a patient is found to be seronegative, the risk for PTLD is higher if an EBV seropositive donor is used. Thus, HSCT donors should also be tested for EBV antibodies. When there is a choice, selection of a seronegative donor for an EBV-seronegative patient should be contemplated since EBV might be transmitted with the graft. CD34-positive selection does not prevent EBV-PTLD. Antiviral prophylaxis with currently available agents is not recommended for prevention of EBV-PTLD. Prophylactic use of rituximab before or early after allo-HSCT might reduce the risk of PTLD [28].

The selected monitoring and intervention strategy should depend on individual assessment of a patient [12]. Monitoring for EBV DNA is recommended after unrelated or HLA-mismatched, T-cell depleted, EBV-mismatched, or cord blood transplants [11]. The risk in HLA-identical sibling transplant recipients not receiving T-cell depletion is low, and no routine screening for EBV is recommended. The same is the case after autologous stem cell transplantation. For patients with hematologic malignancies receiving standard chemotherapy and in autologous HSCT recipients, EBV infection is of small importance. No routine diagnostics for EBV are recommended in these groups of patients, both before and after therapy.

Despite the lack of controlled studies and the cost of rituximab, many centers use rituximab-based preemptive therapy based on the presence of high or increasing EBV DNA levels [12,29]. An EBV viral load of 10^3 or 10^4 copies/mL in whole blood, serum, or plasma is commonly used to begin rituximab-based preemptive therapy. Rituximab is usually given for 2–3 weekly doses while monitoring EBV viral load. Additional doses might result in downregulation of CD20 expression and thereby possibly decreased efficacy. It is also possible to give EBV CTL preemptively in patients with high viral loads but not yet having developed PTLD.

Therapy of probable or proven EBV-PTLD

A summary of reported outcomes of EBV-related PTLD in HSCT recipients is shown in Table 26.1 [5,30].

Rituximab

Rituximab is the treatment of choice for EBV-related PTLD, with positive outcome reported in almost 70% of patients. Rituximab has been shown to be effective also when administered intrathecally in central nervous system (CNS) involvement [31].

Table 26.1 Estimated efficacy of specific therapies of EBV-PTLD.

	Preemptive therapy	Targeted therapy	Comments
Rituximab	89.7%	63–69%	Recommended first-line therapy, available in all centers
Reduction of immunosuppression*	56%	—	Recommended in combination with rituximab, if possible
EBV CTL	94.1%	88.2%	Very good and promising method, but not available to most centers
DLI*	—	41%	Rarely used
Chemotherapy*	—	26%	Rarely used
Antiviral agents*	—	34%	Should not be used

*In most cases, used in combination with other therapies.

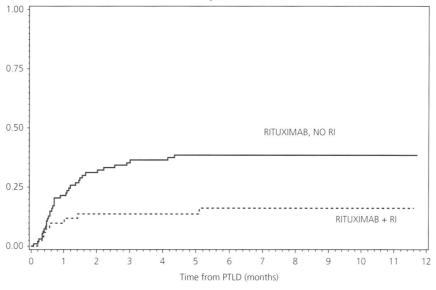

	Patients	Events	%PTLD mortality (95%CI)	P
No reduction of IS therapy	93	36	38.71 (29.98, 49.99)	0.006
Reduction of IS therapy	51	8	16.19 (8.55, 30.65)	

(a)

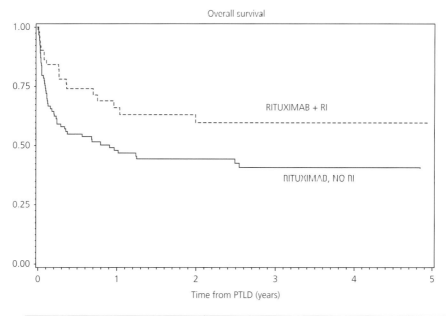

	Patients	Events	%OS from PTLD date (95%CI)	P
No reduction of IS therapy	93	53	40.89 (30.38, 51.12)	0.024
Reduction of IS therapy	51	18	59.86 (43.38, 72.96)	

(b)

Figure 26.1 Post-transplantation lymphoproliferative disease (PTLD)-related mortality (PRM), and overall survival (OS). a) Cumulative incidence of PRM of the 51 patients who could reduce immunosuppression therapy on PTLD diagnosis (RI) compared with the 93 patients who could not reduce immunosuppression (no RI). b) Probability of OS in patients with RI compared with patients with no RI. Combined approach with rituximab and RI was associated with significantly reduced PRM (P = 0.006) and improved OS (P = 0.024). From Styczynski *et al.* [5]. Reproduced with permission of Oxford University Press.

Reduction of immunosuppression

Reduction/withdrawal of immunosuppression (RI) remains the gold standard for first-line PTLD therapy after SOT [34]. However, RI is rarely successful as the sole intervention in PTLD following HSCT [32,33]. The obvious risk with RI is an increased risk of graft rejection or GVHD [6]. However, recent data show that RI when applied in combination with rituximab significantly improves the outcome (Figure 26.1) [5]. In this study, RI was defined as a sustained decrease of at least 20% of the daily dose of immunosuppressive drugs with the exception of low-dose corticosteroid therapy. RI was associated with a lower PTLD mortality (16% vs. 39%). Furthermore, a decrease in EBV DNAemia in peripheral blood during therapy was predictive of better survival. In contrast, older age, extranodal disease, and acute GVHD predicted poor outcome [5].

Cellular therapy

Donor leukocyte infusion (DLI) has been successful as treatment of PTLD post HSCT, but to achieve efficacy the donor must be EBV-positive. However, unselected DLI can be associated with severe GVHD [35,36]. Data on efficacy are very limited as DLI has usually been used in combination with other treatment modalities. In one study, overall survival was reported to be 41.0% (16/39) in DLI-treated patients [30].

Ex vivo-generated EBV CTL have been proven to be effective as prophylaxis, preemptive therapy, and treatment for PTLD post HSCT [37]. Such cells are associated with a low risk for severe GVHD in contrast to unselected DLI. EBV CTL can be isolated and expanded *in vitro* from EBV-seropositive stem cell donors or third-party donors. Recent advances have shown efficacy of multispecific viral CTLs (EBV, CMV, and adenovirus) obtained from third party donors [38]. EBV-specific T cells can also be selected directly from EBV-positive donors and infused to patients without expansion [39,40].

Chemotherapy in PTLD

Chemotherapy has traditionally been reserved for refractory and/or relapsing PTLD [6]. It can be considered for initial use in monomorphic PTLD occurring late in the post-transplant course. Overall response rates in the SOT setting have been determined as 65–75% including late mortality [41,42]. The newer approach is to limit the use of chemotherapy to only those patients who fail rituximab or to combine chemotherapy with the application of rituximab [43].

PTLD of the CNS is a rare complication of SOT and there is currently no consensus on an optimal therapy. Recurrent PTLD following rituximab and front-line chemotherapy represents a particularly difficult therapeutic challenge.

Chemotherapy for PTLD after HSCT is usually not recommended due to poor toleration in HSCT patients who have usually been heavily pretreated with chemotherapy and/or conditioning before HSCT [5,30].

Other therapies

Active immunization against EBV is not available. There are no data to support the use of intravenous immune globulin or interferon in therapy of EBV DNAemia or PTLD. Surgical therapy is of little benefit in PTLD after SOT and is not used in HSCT patients.

Conclusions

PTLD is a heterogeneous disease; it may occur early, within the first year post transplant, with the highest occurrence during the first 6 months after HSCT; or late, up to 10 years after SOT. Early-onset PTLDs are usually EBV-positive, histologically heterogeneous, including most polyclonal mononucleosis-like forms, and are associated with higher levels of EBV DNA copies in the peripheral blood. Nearly 30% of late-onset cases exhibit the biological pattern of EBV-negative malignant lymphoma.

The use of rituximab for EBV-related PTLD is a therapy of choice after HSCT. Recent data show that reduction of immunosuppression when applied in combination with rituximab significantly improves the outcome of HSCT patients. Reduction or withdrawal of immunosuppression remains the gold standard for first-line PTLD therapy after SOT, while rituximab is regarded as second-line therapy in this setting. Although attractive, adoptive cellular therapy is still not available for most HSCT centers.

References

1 Patriarca F, Medeot M, Isola M *et al*. Prognostic factors and outcome of Epstein–Barr virus DNAemia in high-risk recipients of allogeneic stem cell transplantation treated with preemptive rituximab. *Transpl Infect Dis* 2013;**15**:259–67.
2 Curtis RE, Travis LB, Rowlings PA *et al*. Risk of lymphoproliferative disorders after bone marrow transplantation: a multi-institutional study. *Blood* 1999;**94**:2208–16.

3 Cohen JI. Epstein–Barr virus infection. *N Engl J Med* 2000;**343**:481–92.

4 Green M, Michaels MG. Epstein–Barr virus infection and posttransplant lymphoproliferative disorder. *Am J Transplant* 2013;**13**(Suppl 3):41–54.

5 Styczynski J, Gil L, Tridello G *et al.* Response to rituximab-based therapy and risk factor analysis in Epstein Barr virus-related lymphoproliferative disorder after hematopoietic stem cell transplant in children and adults: a study from the Infectious Diseases Working Party of the European Group for Blood and Marrow Transplantation. *Clin Infect Dis* 2013; **57**:794–802.

6 Gross TG. Treatment for Epstein–Barr virus-associated PTLD. *Herpes* 2009;**15**:64–7.

7 Marshall NA, Howe JG, Formica R *et al.* Rapid reconstitution of Epstein–Barr virus-specific T lymphocytes following allogeneic stem cell transplantation. *Blood* 2000;**96**: 2814–21.

8 Landgren O, Gilbert ES, Rizzo JD *et al.* Risk factors for lymphoproliferative disorders after allogeneic hematopoietic cell transplantation. *Blood* 2009;**113**:4992–5001.

9 Sundin M, Le Blanc K, Ringden O *et al.* The role of HLA mismatch, splenectomy and recipient Epstein–Barr virus seronegativity as risk factors in post-transplant lymphoproliferative disorder following allogeneic hematopoietic stem cell transplantation. *Haematologica* 2006;**91**:1059 67.

10 Uhlin M, Wikell H, Sundin M *et al.* Risk factors for Epstein–Barr virus-related post-transplant lymphoproliferative disease after allogeneic hematopoietic stem cell transplantation. *Haematologica* 2014;**99**:346–52.

11 Styczynski J, Reusser P, Einsele H *et al.* Management of HSV, VZV and EBV infections in patients with hematological malignancies and after SCT: guidelines from the Second European Conference on Infections in Leukemia. *Bone Marrow Transplant* 2009;**43**:757–70.

12 Omar H, Hagglund H, Gustafsson-Jernberg A *et al.* Targeted monitoring of patients at high risk of post-transplant lymphoproliferative disease by quantitative Epstein–Barr virus polymerase chain reaction. *Transpl Infect Dis* 2009;**11**:393–9.

13 Cohen JM, Sebire NJ, Harvey J *et al.* Successful treatment of lymphoproliferative disease complicating primary immunodeficiency/immunodysregulatory disorders with reduced-intensity allogeneic stem-cell transplantation. *Blood* 2007;**110**:2209–14.

14 Brunstein CG, Weisdorf DJ, DeFor T *et al.* Marked increased risk of Epstein–Barr virus-related complications with the addition of antithymocyte globulin to a nonmyeloablative conditioning prior to unrelated umbilical cord blood transplantation. *Blood* 2006;**108**:2874–80.

15 Mautner J, Bornkamm GW. The role of virus-specific CD4+ T cells in the control of Epstein–Barr virus infection. *Eur J Cell Biol* 2012;**91**:31–5.

16 Omar H, Ahmed R, Rane L *et al.* Decreased IL-7 signaling in T cells from patients with PTLD after allogeneic HSCT. *J Immunother* 2011;**34**:390–6.

17 Caillard S, Lamy FX, Quelen C *et al.* Epidemiology of post-transplant lymphoproliferative disorders in adult kidney and kidney pancreas recipients: report of the French registry and analysis of subgroups of lymphomas. *Am J Transplant* 2012;**12**:682–93.

18 Herreman A, Dierickx D, Morscio J *et al.* Clinicopathological characteristics of posttransplant lymphoproliferative disorders of T-cell origin: single-center series of nine cases and meta-analysis of 147 reported cases. *Leukemia Lymphoma* 2013;**54**:2190–9.

19 Tiede C, Maecker-Kolhoff B, Klein C *et al.* Risk factors and prognosis in T-cell posttransplantation lymphoproliferative diseases: reevaluation of 163 cases. *Transplantation* 2013;**95**:479–88.

20 Pasquale MA, Weppler D, Smith J *et al.* Burkitt's lymphoma variant of post-transplant lymphoproliferative disease (PTLD). *Pathol Oncol Res* 2002;**8**:105–8.

21 Roncella S, Cutrona G, Truini M *et al.* Late Epstein–Barr virus infection of a hepatosplenic gamma delta T-cell lymphoma arising in a kidney transplant recipient. *Haematologica* 2000;**85**:256–62.

22 Xuan L, Jiang X, Sun J *et al.* Spectrum of Epstein–Barr virus-associated diseases in recipients of allogeneic hematopoietic stem cell transplantation. *Transplantation* 2013;**96**:560–6.

23 Kinch A, Oberg G, Arvidson J *et al.* Post-transplant lymphoproliferative disease and other Epstein–Barr virus diseases in allogeneic haematopoietic stem cell transplantation after introduction of monitoring of viral load by polymerase chain reaction. *Scand J Infect Dis* 2007;**39**:235–44.

24 Gartner BC, Schafer H, Marggraff K *et al.* Evaluation of use of Epstein–Barr viral load in patients after allogeneic stem cell transplantation to diagnose and monitor posttransplant lymphoproliferative disease. *J Clin Microbiol* 2002;**40**:351–8.

25 Stevens SJ, Verschuuren EA, Pronk I *et al.* Frequent monitoring of Epstein–Barr virus DNA load in unfractionated whole blood is essential for early detection of posttransplant lymphoproliferative disease in high-risk patients. *Blood* 2001;**97**:1165–71.

26 Weinstock DM, Ambrossi GG, Brennan C *et al.* Preemptive diagnosis and treatment of Epstein–Barr virus-associated post transplant lymphoproliferative disorder after hematopoietic stem cell transplant: an approach in development. *Bone Marrow Transplant* 2006;**37**:539–46.

27 Perrine SP, Hermine O, Small T *et al.* A phase 1/2 trial of arginine butyrate and ganciclovir in patients with Epstein–Barr virus-associated lymphoid malignancies. *Blood* 2007;**109**:2571–8.

28 Dominietto A, Tedone E, Soracco M *et al.* In vivo B-cell depletion with rituximab for alternative donor hemopoietic SCT. *Bone Marrow Transplant* 2012;**47**:101–6.

29 Gil L, Styczynski J, Komarnicki M. Strategy of pre-emptive management of Epstein–Barr virus post-transplant lymphoproliferative disorder after stem cell transplantation: results of European transplant centers survey. *Contemp Oncol (Pozn)* 2012;**16**:338–40.

30 Styczynski J, Einsele H, Gil L, Ljungman P. Outcome of treatment of Epstein–Barr virus-related post-transplant lymphoproliferative disorder in hematopoietic stem cell recipients: a comprehensive review of reported cases. *Transpl Infect Dis* 2009;**11**:383–92.

31 Czyzewski K, Styczynski J, Krenska A *et al*. Intrathecal therapy with rituximab in central nervous system involvement of post-transplant lymphoproliferative disorder. *Leukemia Lymphoma* 2013;**54**:503–6.

32 Cesaro S, Murrone A, Mengoli C *et al*. The real-time polymerase chain reaction-guided modulation of immunosuppression enables the pre-emptive management of Epstein–Barr virus reactivation after allogeneic haematopoietic stem cell transplantation. *Br J Haematol* 2005;**128**:224–33.

33 Cesaro S, Pegoraro A, Tridello G *et al*. A prospective study on modulation of immunosuppression for Epstein–Barr virus reactivation in pediatric patients who underwent unrelated hematopoietic stem-cell transplantation. *Transplantation* 2010;**89**:1533–40.

34 Paya CV, Fung JJ, Nalesnik MA *et al*. Epstein–Barr virus-induced posttransplant lymphoproliferative disorders. ASTS/ASTP EBV-PTLD Task Force and The Mayo Clinic Organized International Consensus Development Meeting. *Transplantation* 1999;**68**:1517–25.

35 Lucas KG, Burton RL, Zimmerman SE *et al*. Semiquantitative Epstein–Barr virus (EBV) polymerase chain reaction for the determination of patients at risk for EBV-induced lymphoproliferative disease after stem cell transplantation. *Blood* 1998;**91**:3654–61.

36 Papadopoulos EB, Ladanyi M, Emanuel D *et al*. Infusions of donor leukocytes to treat Epstein–Barr virus-associated lymphoproliferative disorders after allogeneic bone marrow transplantation. *N Engl J Med* 1994;**330**:1185–91.

37 Rooney CM, Smith CA, Ng CY *et al*. Infusion of cytotoxic T cells for the prevention and treatment of Epstein–Barr virus-induced lymphoma in allogeneic transplant recipients. *Blood* 1998;**92**:1549–55.

38 Leen AM, Bollard CM, Mendizabal AM *et al*. Multicenter study of banked third-party virus-specific T cells to treat severe viral infections after hematopoietic stem cell transplantation. *Blood* 2013;**121**:5113–23.

39 Uhlin M, Okas M, Gertow J *et al*. A novel haplo-identical adoptive CTL therapy as a treatment for EBV-associated lymphoma after stem cell transplantation. *Cancer Immunol Immunother* 2010;**59**:473–7.

40 Uhlin M, Mattsson J, Maeurer M. Update on viral infections in lung transplantation. *Curr Opin Pulm Med* 2012;**18**:264–70.

41 Lee JJ, Lam MS, Rosenberg A. Role of chemotherapy and rituximab for treatment of posttransplant lymphoproliferative disorder in solid organ transplantation. *Ann Pharmacother* 2007;**41**:1648–59.

42 Choquet S, Trappe R, Leblond V *et al*. CHOP-21 for the treatment of post-transplant lymphoproliferative disorders (PTLD) following solid organ transplantation. *Haematologica* 2007;**92**:273–4.

43 Knight JS, Tsodikov A, Cibrik DM *et al*. Lymphoma after solid organ transplantation: risk, response to therapy, and survival at a transplantation center. *J Clin Oncol* 2009;**27**:3354–62.

APPENDIX I

Follow-up calendar after autologous stem cell transplantation in lymphoma

Angela Moreschi Woods

Screening/testing	Day 100	6 months	1 year	Annually
T-cell and B-cell subsets	✓		✓	✓
Immunizations per transplant center or international guidelines		✓	✓	✓
Dental assessment		+	✓	✓
Tobacco avoidance/cessation	✓	✓	✓	✓
Liver function testing	✓	✓	✓	✓
BUN/creatinine testing		✓	✓	✓
Urine protein screening	✓	✓	✓	✓
Thyroid function testing			✓	✓
Gonadal function assessment				
Prepubertal male and female		✓	✓	✓
Postpubertal women			✓	+
Postpubertal men			+	+
Vitamin D (25-hydroxyvitamin D)	✓		✓	✓
Screening for secondary cancers			✓	✓
Pulmonary function testing		+	+	+
Chest radiograph		+	+	+
Cardiac testing: echocardiogram/MUGA		+	+	+

✓ Recommended for all transplant recipients.
+ Recommended for new symptoms or previous abnormality.
BUN, blood urea nitrogen; MUGA, multi-gated acquisition scan.
Source: Majhail *et al.* [1]. Reproduced with permission of Elsevier.

Reference

1 Majhail NS, Rizzo JD, Lee SJ *et al.* Recommended screening and preventive practices for long-term survivors after hematopoietic cell transplantation. *Biol Blood Marrow Transplant* 2012;**18**:348–71.

Clinical Guide to Transplantation in Lymphoma, First Edition. Edited by Bipin N. Savani and Mohamad Mohty.
© 2015 John Wiley & Sons, Ltd. Published 2015 by John Wiley & Sons, Ltd.

Follow-up calendar after allogeneic stem cell transplantation in lymphoma

Angela Moreschi Woods

Screening/testing	6 months	1 year	Annually
Encapsulated organism prophylaxis	*	*	*
PCP prophylaxis	✓	*	*
CMV and EBV PCR testing	*#	*#	*#
IgG	✓	✓	✓
T-cell and B-cell subsets		✓	✓
Immunizations per transplant center or international guidelines	✓	✓	✓
Fundus examination	+	✓	+
Schirmer's test	+	+	+
Dental assessment	+	✓	✓
Tobacco avoidance/cessation	✓	✓	✓
Liver function testing	✓	✓	✓
Serum ferritin testing		✓	+
BUN/creatinine testing	✓	✓	✓
Urine protein screening	✓	✓	✓
Bone density testing		✓	+
Thyroid function testing		✓	✓
Gonadal function assessment			
Prepubertal male and female		✓	✓
Postpubertal women	✓	✓	+
Postpubertal men		+	+
Vitamin D (25-hydroxyvitamin D)	+	✓	✓
Recommend frequent skin self-examinations	✓	✓	✓
Sun exposure counseling	✓	✓	✓
Gynecologic examination for women	+	✓	✓
Screening for secondary cancers		✓	✓
Pulmonary function testing	+	+#	+#
Chest radiograph	+	+#	+#
Cardiac testing: echocardiogram/MUGA	+	+#	+#

✓ Recommended for all transplant recipients.
* Recommended for patients with ongoing GVHD or immunosuppression.
+ Recommended for new symptoms or previous abnormality.
# According to your transplant center recommendation.
BUN, blood urea nitrogen; CMV, cytomegalovirus; EBV, Epstein–Barr virus; GVHD, graft-versus-host disease; MUGA, multi-gated acquisition scan; PCP, *Pneumocystis carinii* pneumonia; PCR, polymerase chain reaction.
Source: Majhail *et al.* [1]. Reproduced with permission of Elsevier.

Reference

1 Majhail NS, Rizzo JD, Lee SJ *et al.* Recommended screening and preventive practices for long-term survivors after hematopoietic cell transplantation. *Biol Blood Marrow Transplant* 2012;**18**:348–71.

Index

Page numbers in *italics* refer to illustrations; those in **bold** refer to tables

acquired immunodeficiency syndrome (AIDS) 223
  cancer risk 224
  see also HIV-related lymphomas; human immunodeficiency
    virus (HIV)
acute kidney injury (AKI) 97–98
adolescents 33
  see also pediatric lymphomas
adult T-cell leukemia/lymphoma (ATL) 215–220
  allogeneic HSCT 217
    conditioning regimen 217
    donor choice 217–218
  autologous HSCT 217
  case study 220
  clinical presentation 215
  diagnostic criteria 215–216
  graft-versus-ATL effect 218
  minimal residual disease follow-up 218
  subtypes 215, 218
  treatment 216
    algorithm *219*
    recommendations 218–219
    supportive therapy 219
AGNIS software 18, *18*
alemtuzumab 63, 137, 241
  chronic lymphocytic leukemia/small lymphocytic lymphoma
    management 140
    post-transplant chemotherapy 143
  diffuse large B-cell lymphoma management 156
  follicular lymphoma management 128–129
  Hodgkin lymphoma management 182, 186
  peripheral T-cell lymphoma management 197, 200
allogeneic HSCT 25, 59, 105
  adult T-cell leukemia/lymphoma 217
  anaplastic large-cell lymphoma 39
  Burkitt lymphoma 27, 207–208
  care delivery for survivors 107
  children, adolescents, and young adults 35–42
  chronic lymphocytic leukemia/small lymphocytic
    lymphoma 137–140

complications 106–107
  anemia 117
  infections 117, 118–119
  risk factors 106–107, **106**
  screening and prevention guidelines 107, **108–109**
  thrombocytopenia 117
  see also graft-versus-host disease (GVHD)
conditioning *see* conditioning regimens
cutaneous T-cell lymphoma 241–244, **241**
  relapse management 244
day zero 115
diffuse large B-cell lymphoma 26, 149–154
  after autograft failure 153–154
  refractory disease 154
donor/stem cell sources 63–65, 88–89, **90**
  bone marrow 88–89
  haploidentical transplantation 64–65, 91–92, 129–130,
    185, 242
  matched related donor 90
  matched unrelated donor 90–91, 129–130, 184–185, 242
  mismatched unrelated donor 91
  mobilized peripheral blood 88–89
  umbilical cord blood cells 64, 88, 92, 129, 185
first 100 days 115–119, **116**
  conditioning regimen impact 116
  mortality 119
  return home 118–119
  time to engraftment 117
follicular lymphoma 26–27, 127–130
  chemorefractory follicular lymphoma 131
  transformed follicular lymphoma 130
  versus autologous transplant 130
follow-up schedule 106, 269
historical background 7–10, 87
HIV-related lymphomas 231–233
Hodgkin lymphoma 26, 36–37, 179–185, *180*
  earlier phase disease 184
  patients failing after autologous HSCT 181–182
  relapse management 186

Clinical Guide to Transplantation in Lymphoma, First Edition. Edited by Bipin N. Savani and Mohamad Mohty.
© 2015 John Wiley & Sons, Ltd. Published 2015 by John Wiley & Sons, Ltd.

allogeneic HSCT(*cont'd*)
  long-term survival 105–106
  lymphoblastic lymphoma 38, 208–210
  lymphoplasmacytic lymphoma 249, 251, **251**
  mantle cell lymphoma 27, 165, 166, 168–170, **169**
    relapse management 172
  non-Hodgkin lymphoma 26–27, 40–41
  peripheral T-cell lymphoma 27, 192–193, 196–199
    relapse management 200
  preparation 59–66
    see also conditioning regimens
  primary CNS lymphoma 27
  primary mediastinal large B-cell lymphoma 255
  prognostic tools 27
  rationale 87–88
  vaccine strategies 65
  Waldenström macroglobulinemia 249, 251, **251**
anaplastic large-cell lymphoma (ALCL) 38–39, 191
  ALK-negative 191, 196
  ALK-positive 191, 193–195
anemia 112–113, 117
angioimmunoblastic T-cell lymphoma (AITL) 196
antithymocyte globulin (ATG) 242
antiviral therapy
  adult T-cell leukemia/lymphoma 216
  highly active antiretroviral therapy (HAART) 223–224,
    227, 231
apheresis 79–80
  complications 82
arsenic trioxide 216
Asia-Pacific BMT Registry (APBMT) 15
aspergillosis 10
  prophylaxis 96
atrial fibrillation 96–97
autologous HSCT 25
  adult T-cell leukemia/lymphoma 217
  anaplastic large-cell lymphoma 38–39
  Burkitt lymphoma 27, 207
  children, adolescents, and young adults 34–36, **34**,
    38–42
  chronic lymphocytic leukemia/small lymphocytic
    lymphoma 138–139
  complications 95–100, **99**
    anemia 112–113
    cardiovascular side effects 96–97, 99
    endocrine side effects 99–100
    engraftment syndrome 97
    infections 95–96, **96**, 113
    liver toxicity 98
    mucositis 96
    neurologic toxicity 98
    pulmonary complications 97, 99
    renal toxicity 97–98
    secondary malignancies 98–99

thrombocytopenia 112–113
  conditioning *see* conditioning regimens
  day zero 111
  diffuse large B-cell lymphoma 26, 149–153
    refractory disease 153
    relapsed disease 152
  first 100 days 111–114, **112**
    conditioning regimen impact 112
    mortality 114
    returning home 114
    time to engraftment 112–113
  follicular lymphoma 26–27, 123–127
    graft purging 126–127
    relapsed disease 124–126, **126**
    transformed follicular lymphoma 130
    versus allogeneic transplant 130
  follow-up calendar 267
  historical background 8–9
  HIV-related lymphomas 226–229, **230**
    immunological recovery after transplant 229–230
  Hodgkin lymphoma 9, 25–26, 36, 178–179
    prognostic factors 178
    relapse management 185–186
  lymphoblastic lymphoma 38, 208
  lymphoplasmacytic lymphoma 249–251, **250**
  mantle cell lymphoma 27, 165–168
    first-line treatment results 166–168, **167**, **168**
    prognosis 170, *171*
    relapse management 170–172
    salvage treatment results 168
    second transplantation after failure 171–172
  non-Hodgkin lymphoma 8–9, **34**, 40–41
  peripheral T-cell lymphoma 27, 191–196
    front-line therapy 193–195, **194**
    post-transplant relapse management 199–200
    relapsed/refractory disease 195–196
  preparation 47–53
    see also conditioning regimens
  primary CNS lymphoma 27
  primary mediastinal large B-cell lymphoma
    254–255
  prognostic tools 27
  Waldenström macroglobulinemia 249–251, **250**
  see also stem cell mobilization

B-cell receptor (BCR) 143
BCNU regimen 48–52
  follicular lymphoma 125
  see also chemotherapy
BEAM regimen 48–52
  chronic lymphocytic leukemia/small lymphocytic
    lymphoma 139
  diffuse large B-cell lymphoma 150–151
  follicular lymphoma 125, 126

HIV-related lymphomas 227, 228
    Hodgkin lymphoma 178, 182
    see also chemotherapy
bendamustine 142, 156, 186, 200, 248–249
"Berlin" patient 232–233
bexarotene 240
bleeding risk 113, 117
Blood and Marrow Transplant Clinical Trials Network
        (BMT CTN) 16, 52, 65, 92
bone marrow transplantation 88
    versus mobilized peripheral blood 88–89
bortezomib 59, 158, 172, 248–249
brentuximab 41, 63, 185–187, 200, 241
British National Lymphoma Investigation 9
Bruton's tyrosine kinase 143
Bu/Mel regimen 52
    see also chemotherapy
Burkitt lymphoma 27, 205–208, **206**
    allogeneic HSCT 27, 207–208
        reduced-intensity conditioning 208
    autologous HSCT 27, 207
    children, adolescents and young adults 39
    HIV-related 207, 225–227
busulfan 48–49, 52, 64

Candida prophylaxis 96
cardiovascular side effects 96–97, 99
carfilzomib 158
CBV regimen 48, 49
    diffuse large B-cell lymphoma 150
    HIV-related lymphomas 226–227, 231
    Hodgkin lymphoma 178–179
    see also chemotherapy
Center for International Blood and Marrow Transplant
        Research (CIBMTR) 15, 21–23, 105
    case example 21–22
    data flow 18, *18*
    data quality 18
    data reporting 16–18
        challenges 17–18
    registry structure 16
    value for public 22
    value for young investigators 22
    working committees 16, **16**
chemotherapy 112
    adult T-cell leukemia/lymphoma 216
    Burkitt lymphoma 207
    chronic lymphocytic leukemia/small lymphocytic
        lymphoma 139, 140, 142
        post-transplant chemotherapy 142–143
    complications 95
        early toxicities 95–98, 112
        late toxicities 98–100
    diffuse large B-cell lymphoma 150–152, 158

relapse after transplantation 156
        salvage chemotherapy response 150
    follicular lymphoma 123–126, 128–129
        chemorefractory patients 131
    HIV-related lymphomas 225–228
    Hodgkin lymphoma 178–179, 182
    lymphoblastic lymphoma 37, 208
    lymphoplasmacytic lymphoma 249
    mantle cell lymphoma relapse management 170–171
    mycosis fungoides 240–241
    non-Hodgkin lymphoma 8–9, 26–27, 39
    pediatric lymphomas 34, 37, 39, 42
    peripheral T-cell lymphoma 193–197
        relapse management after transplantation 199–200
    post-transplant lymphoproliferative disorders 264
    primary mediastinal large B-cell lymphoma 253–254
        relapsed/refractory disease 255
    rejection prevention 118
    Sézary syndrome 240–241
    traditional conditioning regimens 47–49
children 33
    stem cell mobilization 82
    see also pediatric lymphomas
chimeric antigen receptor (CAR) T-cell therapy 2, 41
    chronic lymphocytic leukemia/small lymphocytic
        lymphoma 144
CHOP regimen
    adult T-cell leukemia/lymphoma 216
    chronic lymphocytic leukemia/small lymphocytic
        lymphoma 139
    diffuse large B-cell lymphoma 158
    follicular lymphoma 123, 124
    HIV-related lymphomas 225, 226
    lymphoplasmacytic lymphoma 249
    peripheral T-cell lymphoma 191, 195, 197
    primary mediastinal large B-cell lymphoma 253–254
    see also chemotherapy
chronic lymphocytic leukemia/small lymphocytic lymphoma
        (CLL/SLL) 137–145
    allogeneic HSCT 137, 138
        outcome 139–140
        reduced-intensity conditioning regimens 137, 138, 140
    autologous HSCT outcome 138–139
    case study 145
    donor-derived CLL 142
    novel therapies 143–145
    relapse management after transplantation 140–143
        early versus late relapses 141
        recommended treatment approaches 141–142
    timing and preparation for transplantation 138
    transplantation indications 137–138
Collaborative Trial in Relapsed Aggressive Lymphoma
        (CORAL) 27, 52, 150
competing risk data 19

conditioning regimens 47, 112, 115
  allogeneic HSCT 59–66, 115
    complications 116
  autologous HSCT 47–53, 112
    complications 95, 112
  cutaneous T-cell lymphoma 242–243
  dose intensity role 182–184
  future directions 52–53
  monoclonal antibody incorporation 49–52, 63
    radioimmunotherapy 49–52, **51–52**
  novel agents 52
  traditional regimens 47–49
  see also myeloablative conditioning (MAC) regimens;
    reduced-intensity conditioning (RIC) regimens; *specific*
    lymphomas
Cox model 21
crizotinib 201
cutaneous T-cell lymphoma (CTCL) 239
  allogeneic HSCT 241–244, **241**
    conditioning regimen 242–243
    donor selection and stem cell source 242
    GVHD prophylaxis 243
    indications for 242
    monitoring for recurrence 243–244
    post-transplant infectious prophylaxis 243
    relapse management 244
  autologous HSCT 241
  see also mycosis fungoides (MF); Sézary syndrome (SS)
C.W. Bill Young Cell Transplantation Program 16, *17*
cyclophosphamide 8–9, 52, 60, 64
  chronic lymphocytic leukemia/small lymphocytic lymphoma
    management 139, 140
    post-transplant chemotherapy 142
  cutaneous T-cell lymphoma management 242
  follicular lymphoma management 123–125, 128
  HIV-related lymphoma management 227, 231
  Hodgkin lymphoma management 178–179
  stem cell mobilization regimens 79
  T-cell depletion 91
  see also CBV regimen; chemotherapy; CHOP regimen
cyclosporine 128, 182, 243
cytarabine 27
cytomegalovirus (CMV) reactivation 10, 96

diabetes mellitus 81
diffuse alveolar hemorrhage (DAH) 97
diffuse large B-cell lymphoma (DLBCL) 21–22, 26,
    149–159
  allogeneic HSCT 26, 149–150, 153–154
    after autograft failure 153–154
    conditioning regimen role 154
    outcomes **155**
    reduced-intensity conditioning (RIC) regimens 26,
      60, 154

    refractory disease 154
  autologous HSCT 26, 149–153
    consolidation in first remission 152
    refractory disease 153
    relapsed disease 152
  case study 158–159
  children, adolescents and young adults 39
  histologic transformation to DLBCL 27
  HIV-related 225, 227
  myeloablative conditioning 26, 154
  novel therapies 157–158
  post-transplantation disease monitoring 154–156
  relapse management after transplantation 156–157
    treatment algorithm *157*
  salvage chemotherapy response 150
  timing and preparation for transplantation 150–151
  transplantation indications 149–150
  treatment algorithm *151*
  see also primary mediastinal large B-cell lymphoma
    (PMBL)
dimethyl sulfoxide (DMSO) side effects 111
disease testing 73
donor sources 63–65, 72, **90**
  adult T-cell leukemia/lymphoma 217–218
  chronic lymphocytic leukemia/small lymphocytic
    lymphoma 138
  follicular lymphoma 129–130
  haploidentical transplantation 64–65, 91–92, 129–130,
    185, 242
  matched related donors 217, 242
  matched unrelated donors 129, 184–185, 217, 242
  mismatched unrelated donors 91
  umbilical cord blood cells 64, 88, 92, 129, 185
donor–recipient matching *see* donor sources; HLA
    matching
doxorubicin 241
drug fever 113, 117

endocrine side effects 99–100
engraftment 117–118
engraftment syndrome 97
enteropathy-associated T-cell lymphoma (EATL) 196
EPOCH regimen 39
  diffuse large B-cell lymphoma 158
  HIV-related lymphomas 225–226
  see also chemotherapy
epratuzumab 158
Epstein–Barr virus (EBV) 41, 224
  Burkitt lymphoma association 205–207
  management strategies 261–264, **262**
  post-transplant lymphoproliferative disorders 259,
    260, 261
    EBV DNAemia and 261
    prevention 262

etoposide 52, 60
  follicular lymphoma management 123–124
  stem cell mobilization regimens 79
  see also BEAM regimen; CBV regimen; chemotherapy
European Inter-Group for Childhood NHL (EICNHL) 39
European Society for Blood and Marrow Transplantation
    (EBMT) 9, 15, 53
  adult T-cell leukemia/lymphoma report 218
  data flow 18, *18*
  data reporting 17–18
evaluation *see* patient evaluation

febrile neutropenia 95
  management 96
filgrastim 77, 82
flavopiridol 144–145
fludarabine 8, 36–37, 64
  chronic lymphocytic leukemia/small lymphocytic lymphoma
    management 139, 140
    post-transplant chemotherapy 142
  cutaneous T-cell lymphoma management 242
  follicular lymphoma management 128, 129
  HIV-related lymphoma management 231
  peripheral T-cell lymphoma management 197
follicular lymphoma (FL) 26–27, 123–132
  allogeneic transplant 26–27, 127–130
    chemorefractory follicular lymphoma 131
    nonsibling donor 129–130
    reduced-intensity conditioning regimens 60–62
    versus autologous transplant 130
  autologous transplant 26–27, 123–127, 130
    consolidation for first remission 123–124
    graft purging 126–127
    relapsed follicular lymphoma 124–126, **126**
  minimal residual disease detection 131
  post-transplant relapse 131
  transformed follicular lymphoma 130
  transplant recommendations **132**
FormsNet™ reporting system 17
Foundation for the Accreditation of Cellular Therapy
    (FACT) 15

gemcitabine 52, 199, 241
gene therapy 233–234
graft purging 126–127
graft-versus-host disease (GVHD) 7, 87–92, 118
  adult T-cell leukemia/lymphoma 217
  chronic GVHD 11, 89, 105
    Hodgkin lymphoma 181
  chronic lymphocytic leukemia/small lymphocytic
    lymphoma 138, 142
  cutaneous T-cell lymphoma 242–243
    prophylaxis 243
  follicular lymphoma 128–129

hepatic acute GVHD 11
  HIV-infected patients 231–232
  mantle cell lymphoma 168
  patient education 73
  prevention 11, 118, 243
  relapse relationship 37
graft-versus-lymphoma (GVL) effect 8, 9, 37, 87, 118
  adult T-cell leukemia/lymphoma 218
  children, adolescents, and young adults 35, 37, 40–41
  chronic lymphocytic leukemia/small lymphocytic
    lymphoma 140, 141
  cutaneous T-cell lymphoma 241
  diffuse large B-cell lymphoma 149, 153, 156
  Hodgkin lymphoma 177, 179
    evidence for 184, **184**
  lymphoplasmacytic lymphoma 249
  mantle cell lymphoma 168, 172
    evidence for 169
  peripheral T-cell lymphoma 193, 197
granulocyte colony-stimulating factor (G-CSF) 77
  adverse effects 82
  neutropenia reduction 95
  stem cell mobilization 77–79, 82–83, 229
  see also filgrastim

hair loss 112, 113, 116
haploidentical transplantation 64–65, 91–92, 129–130,
    185, 242
hematopoietic stem cell transplantation (HSCT) 1–2
  as a platform for gene therapy 233–234
  children, adolescents, and young adults 33
  historical background 7–11
  indications **26**
  see also allogeneic HSCT; autologous HSCT; *specific*
    lymphomas
hepatic venoocclusive disease (VOD) 98
herpes simplex prophylaxis 96
high-dose therapy/autologous stem cell transplant (HDT/
    ASCT) *see* autologous HSCT; conditioning regimens
highly active antiretroviral therapy (HAART) 223–224,
    227, 231
histologic transformation to DLBCL 27
histone deacetylase inhibitors 201
HIV-related lymphomas 223–235, *229*
  allogeneic HSCT 231–233
  autologous HSCT 226–229, **230**
    immunological recovery after transplant 229–230
  "Berlin" patient 232–233
  Burkitt lymphoma 207
  chemotherapy 225–226
  clinical presentation 225
  prognosis 225
  stem cell mobilization 229
  see also human immunodeficiency virus (HIV)

HLA matching 89–91, **90**
  chronic lymphocytic leukemia/small lymphocytic
      lymphoma 138
  haploidentical transplantation 64–65, 91–92, 129–130,
      185, 242
  historical background 8
  Hodgkin lymphoma 184–185
  outcome relationships 90–92
Hodgkin lymphoma (HL) 25–26, 177–187
  allogenic HSCT 26, 36–37, 179–185, *180*
    earlier phase disease 184
    increasing the pool of donors 184–185
    patients failing after autologous HSCT 181–182
    reduced-intensity conditioning regimens 36, 37, 63,
        179–184, *181*
    relapse management 186
  autologous HSCT 25–26, 36, 178–179
    historical background 9
    preparative regimen 178–179
    prognostic factors 178
    relapse management 185–186
  children, adolescents and young adults **34**, 35–37
  debulking therapy 178
  HIV-related 224–227
  novel therapies 186–187
  post-transplantation disease monitoring 185
  relapsed disease 9, 35–37
  transplantation indications 177
human immunodeficiency virus (HIV) 223, *224*
  cancer risk 224
  gene therapy potential 233–234
  highly active antiretroviral therapy (HAART) 223–224, 227,
      231
  see also HIV-related lymphomas
human lymphotropic virus I (HTLV-I) 215, 218
hyperviscosity syndrome 247–248
  see also Waldenström macroglobulinemia (WM)

ibritumomab 50, 63
ibrutinib 22, 53, 59
  chronic lymphocytic leukemia/small lymphocytic lymphoma
      management 143
  lymphoplasmacytic lymphoma management 248–249, 250
  mantle cell lymphoma management 172
idelalisib 143–144, 249, 250
idiopathic pneumonia syndrome (IPA) 97
immune escape 141
infections 95, **96**, 113
  opportunistic 10
  prophylaxis 95–96, 113, 117
  risk avoidance 114, 118–119
infertility 100
inotuzumab ozogamicin 53
insurance approval 74

interferon alpha (IFN) 216, 241
International Bone Marrow Transplant Registry
    (IMBTR) 15
International Prognostic Index (IPI) 191, 225, 254
International Prognostic Scoring System for Waldenström
    Macroglobulinemia (IPSSWM) 248
invasive fungal diseases 10

Joint Accreditation Committee of ISCT and EBMT
    (JACIE) 15

Kaplan–Meier survival curves 19
Kaposi sarcoma (KS) 224

lenalidomide 158, 172, 201
lenograstim 78
liver toxicity 98
lymphoblastic lymphoma (LBL) 37–38, 205, 208–210, **209**
  allogeneic HSCT 38, 208–210
  autologous HSCT 38, 208
Lymphoma Working Committee 19
lymphoplasmacytic lymphoma (LPL) 247
  clinical manifestations 247–248
  epidemiology 247
  HSCT role 249–251, **250**
    allogeneic HSCT 249, 251, **251**
    management at relapse 249–251
  novel agents 248–249, **250**
  prognostic factors 248

maintenance therapy 27
mantle cell lymphoma (MCL) 27, 165–172
  allogeneic HSCT 27, 165, 166, 168–170
    outcome 169–170, **169**
    reduced-intensity conditioning regimens 63, 169–170
    relapse management 172
  autologous HSCT 27, 165, 166–168
    first-line treatment results 166–168, **167**, **168**
    prognosis 170, *171*
    relapse management 170–172
    salvage treatment results 168
    second transplantation after failure 171–172
  novel therapies 172
  post-transplantation disease monitoring 170
  timing and preparation for transplantation 166
  transplantation indications 165, **166**
melphalan 52, 231, 242
methotrexate
  GVHD prevention 7, 11, 118, 243
  Hodgkin lymphoma management 179, 182
  lymphoplastic lymphoma management 37
  mycosis fungoides management 241
  peripheral T-cell lymphoma management 196, 197
  see also chemotherapy

mogamulizumab 201
monoclonal antibodies 49, 63
   radioimmunotherapy 49–52, **51–52**
   see also specific antibodies
monoclonal B-cell lymphocytosis (MBCL) 141
mucositis 96
mycophenolate mofetil 243
mycosis fungoides (MF) 239
   allogeneic HSCT *see* cutaneous T-cell lymphoma (CTCL)
   nontransplant therapies 240–241
   pathology 239
   staging 239–240, **240**
myeloablative conditioning (MAC) regimens 60, **61**,
      115, 210
   adult T-cell leukemia/lymphoma 217
   children, adolescents and young adults 37, 38, 41–42
   chronic lymphocytic leukemia/small lymphocytic
      lymphoma 138
   cutaneous T-cell lymphoma 242
   diffuse large B-cell lymphoma 26, 154
   follicular lymphoma 127–128
   historical background 9–10
   Hodgkin lymphoma 26, 37
   lymphoblastic lymphoma 38, 210, 211
   peripheral T-cell lymphoma 195
   transplant-related mortality and 127–128
myelodysplastic syndrome/acute myelogenous leukemia (t-
      MDS/AML) 98

National Marrow Donor Program (NMDP) 15, 25, 90
neurologic toxicity 98
neutropenia 95–96
   management 96
non-Hodgkin lymphoma (NHL) 26–27
   allogeneic HSCT 26–27
   autologous HSCT 26–27
      historical background 8–9
   children, adolescents and young adults **34**
   HIV-related 224–225
   see also specific types
nonmyeloablative (NMA) conditioning regimens 59, 91
   see also reduced-intensity conditioning (RIC) regimens
nonrelapse mortality (NRM) 35, 37, 60
   diffuse large B-cell lymphoma 154
   see also transplant-related mortality (TRM)
novel therapies 27–28
   see also specific lymphomas

obese patients 81
obinutuzumab 41, 59, 144, 158
ofatumumab 59, 143, 158
older patients 2, 25
   reduced-intensity regimens 115
opportunistic infections 10

oral mucositis assessment scale (OMAS) 96
organ function testing 73

patient education 73–74
patient evaluation 72–74
   data review **72**
   disease testing 73
   organ function testing 73
   post-evaluation review 74
   preparation for 72–73
PD-1/PD-L1 pathway 53
pediatric lymphomas
   anaplastic large-cell lymphoma 38–39
   future directions 41–42
   Hodgkin lymphoma 35–37
   HSCT principles 34–35
   lymphoblastic lymphoma 37–38
   mature B-cell lymphomas 39–41
   proposed treatment paradigm **42**
pegfilgrastim 78, 82
pentostatin 142
peripheral blood stem cells (PBSCs) 77
   guideline recommendations **192**
   mobilized peripheral blood transplantation 88
      versus bone marrow 88–89
   transplantation indication 191–193
   see also stem cell mobilization
peripheral T-cell lymphoma (PTCL) 27, 191–201
   allogeneic HSCT 27, 192–193, 196–199
      relapse management 200
   angioimmunoblastic T-cell lymphoma (AITL) 196
   autologous HSCT 27, 191–192, 193–196
      front-line therapy 193–195, **194**
      relapse management 199–200
   enteropathy-associated T-cell lymphoma (EATL) 196
   novel therapies 200–201
   post-transplant disease monitoring 199
   prognostic indices 191–192
   reduced-intensity regimens 193, 196–197, **198**
   relapsed/refractory disease 193, 195–196
   skin involvement 239
   timing and preparation for transplantation 193
   see also adult T-cell leukemia/lymphoma (ATL)
phosphatidylinositol 3-kinase (PI3K) 143
phototherapy, mycosis fungoides/Sézary syndrome 240
pidilizumab 53
platelet transfusions 112, 117
plerixafor
   adverse effects 82
   stem cell mobilization 77, 79, 82–83
      poor mobilizers 80–82, *81*
pneumonia 95, 113
   idiopathic pneumonia syndrome (IPA) 97
   Pneumocystis jirovecii pneumonia 96

post-transplant lymphoproliferative disorders (PTLD)
259–264
  clinical symptoms 260
  diagnosis 261
  EBV association 259–264
  EBV-negative PTLD 260
  epidemiology 259
  pathogenesis 260
  prevention 262
  risk factors 260
  therapy 262–264
  T-lineage PTLD 260
pralatrexate 200–201, 241
preparative regimens *see* conditioning regimens
primary CNS lymphoma 27
  HIV-related 224
primary mediastinal large B-cell lymphoma (PMBL) 253–256
  allogeneic HSCT 255
  autologous HSCT 254–255
  case study 256
  first-line therapy 253–254
  prognostic factors 254
  relapsed/refractory disease treatment 255
Prognostic Index for PTCL (PIT score) 191–192
prognostic tools 27
pruritus 239
pulmonary complications 97, 99
  diffuse alveolar hemorrhage (DAH) 97
  pulmonary edema 97
  see also pneumonia

radiation therapy 48–49
  chronic lymphocytic leukemia/small lymphocytic
    lymphoma 142
  cutaneous T-cell lymphoma 242
    total body skin electron beam radiation (TBSEB) 243
  diffuse large B-cell lymphoma 156
  lymphoblastic lymphoma 37
  radioimmunotherapy 49–52, **51–52**
  see also total body irradiation (TBI)
red blood cell transfusions 112, 117
reduced-intensity conditioning (RIC) regimens 2, 59,
    60–63, **62**, 91
  adult T-cell leukemia/lymphoma 217
  Burkitt lymphoma 208
  children, adolescents, and young adults 36, 37, 42
  chronic lymphocytic leukemia/small lymphocytic
    lymphoma 137, 138, 140
  cutaneous T-cell lymphoma 242
  diffuse large B-cell lymphoma 26, 60, 154
  follicular lymphoma 60–62, 128, **129**
  historical background 10
  Hodgkin lymphoma 36, 37, 63, 179–184, *181*
  mantle cell lymphoma 63, 169–170

older patients 115
  peripheral T-cell lymphoma 193, 196–197, **198**
reduction of immunosuppression *see* withdrawal of
    immunosuppression (WIS)
referral 71–72
rejection *see* graft-versus-host disease (GVHD)
renal toxicity 97–98, 100
respiratory complications *see* pulmonary complications
rituximab 49, 63
  adverse effects 63
  Burkitt lymphoma management 207
  chronic lymphocytic leukemia/small lymphocytic lymphoma
    management 139
    post-transplant therapy 143
    relapse management 140, 142
  combination chemotherapy 8–9, 26, 27
  diffuse large B-cell lymphoma management 150–152,
    157–158
    relapse after transplantation 156
  follicular lymphoma management 124, 125, 127,
    128, 130
    graft purging 127
  HIV-related lymphomas 225–226
  Hodgkin lymphoma relapse management 186
  lymphoplasmacytic lymphoma management 248, 249
  maintenance therapy 26, 27, 52–53
  mantle cell lymphoma management 167, 170
  post-transplant lymphoproliferative disorder
    management 261, 262
  primary mediastinal large B-cell lymphoma
    management 253–254
  radioimmunotherapy 49, 52
  targeted immunotherapy 27–28, 35, 39, 41
romidepsin 201, 241

secondary malignancies 98–99
Sézary syndrome (SS) 239–244
  nontransplant therapies 240–241
  pathology 239
  staging 239–240, **240**
  see also cutaneous T-cell lymphoma (CTCL)
statistical methods 19–21
  adjusted comparison 21
  at-risk population definition 19
  competing risk data 19
  survival data 19
  time to event 19
  unadjusted comparison 19–21
stem cell collection 79–80
stem cell mobilization 77
  adverse effects 82
  children 82
  HIV-infected patients 229
  methods 77–79, *78*

obese patients 81
poor mobilizers and mobilization failure 80–81
    remobilization 81
    risk factors **80**
supermobilizers 79
Stem Cell Therapeutic Outcomes Database (SCTOD) 16
    data reporting 16–17
Streptococcus viridans infections 96
stromal-derived factor (SDF)-1 77
supportive care 10–11
survival data 19

tacrolimus, GVHD prevention 11, 243
targeted immunotherapy 27–28, 35, 41–42
T-cell based therapies 41
T-cell depletion 91
    follicular lymphoma management 128–129
T-cell lymphoma *see* adult T-cell leukemia/lymphoma (ATL);
        cutaneous T-cell lymphoma (CTCL); peripheral T-cell
        lymphoma (PTCL)
temsirolimus 172
thrombocytopenia 82, 112–113, 117
    bleeding risk 113, 117
thyroid side effects 99–100
tositumomab 50–52
    diffuse large B-cell lymphoma management 151
total body irradiation (TBI) 47, 48–49, 60
    chronic lymphocytic leukemia/small lymphocytic
        lymphoma 139
    cutaneous T-cell lymphoma 242
    diffuse large B-cell lymphoma 150
    follicular lymphoma 123–127
    HIV-related lymphomas 227, 231
    Hodgkin lymphoma 178
    mantle cell lymphoma 167

peripheral T-cell lymphoma 195
    see also radiation therapy
total body skin electron beam radiation (TBSEB) 243
transplant-related mortality (TRM) 19, 35, 95, 138
    diffuse large B-cell lymphoma 26
    follicular lymphoma 127–128
    see also nonrelapse mortality (NRM)

umbilical cord blood cell transplantation 64, 88, 92
    adult T-cell leukemia/lymphoma 217–218
    follicular lymphoma 129
    Hodgkin lymphoma 185
UV radiation therapy, mycosis fungoides/Sézary
        syndrome 240

vaccine strategies 65
Varicella zoster prophylaxis 96
vinorelbine 52
vorinostat 241

Waldenström macroglobulinemia (WM) 247
    clinical manifestations 247–248
    epidemiology 247
    HSCT role 249–251, **250**
        allogeneic HSCT 249, 251, **251**
        prognostic factors 248, **248**
withdrawal of immunosuppression (WIS)
    chronic lymphocytic leukemia/small lymphocytic
        lymphoma 141
    diffuse large B-cell lymphoma 156–157
    mantle cell lymphoma 172
    post-transplant lymphoproliferative disorders 262–264, *263*

zeta-chain-associated protein (ZAP) 140
zidovudine 216, 223, 231